S0-ASG-631

# Dr. Mary's Monkey

*Dr. Mary's Monkey*

# Dr. Mary's Monkey

How the unsolved murder of a doctor,
a secret laboratory in New Orleans and
cancer-causing monkey viruses are linked to
Lee Harvey Oswald, the JFK assassination and
emerging global epidemics

## Edward T. Haslam

Foreword by
## Jim Marrs

DR. MARY'S MONKEY: HOW THE UNSOLVED MURDER OF A DOCTOR, A SECRET LABORATORY IN NEW ORLEANS AND CANCER-CAUSING MONKEY VIRUSES ARE LINKED TO LEE HARVEY OSWALD, THE JFK ASSASSINATION AND EMERGING GLOBAL EPIDEMICS

Copyright © 2007 Edward T. Haslam. All rights reserved.

Book layout and cover by Ed Bishop

TrineDay
PO Box 577
Walterville, OR 97489
1-800-556-2012
www.TrineDay.com
support@TrineDay.com

Library of Congress Control Number:  2006911309

---

Haslam, Edward T.
    Dr. Mary's Monkey: How the Unsolved Murder of a Doctor, a Secret Laboratory in New Orleans and Cancer-Causing Monkey Viruses are Linked to Lee Harvey Oswald, the JFK Assassination and Emerging Global Epidemics / Edward T. Haslam ; with forward by Jim Marrs — 1st ed.
        p. cm.
    ISBN 978-0-9777953-0-6   (acid-free paper)
    1. Kennedy, John F. (John Fitzgerald), 1917-1963—Assassination. 2. Oswald, Lee Harvey. 3. Poliomyelitis vaccine—Contamination—History—Popular works. 4. Political Corruption—United States. 1. Title
    364.1'524—dc20

---

FIRST EDITION
10 9 8 7 6 5


Printed in the USA

Distribution to the Trade by:
    Independent Publishers Group (IPG)
    814 North Franklin Street
    Chicago, Illinois 60610
    312.337.0747
    www.ipgbook.com

Dedicated to my father:

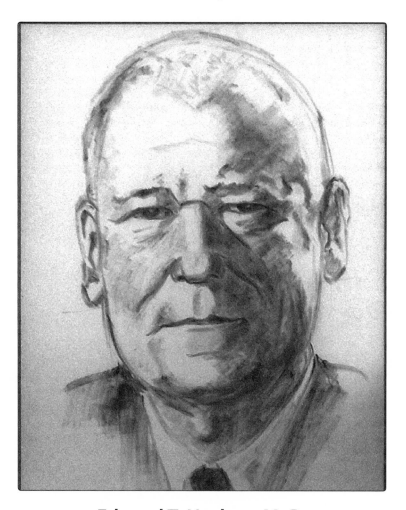

# Edward T. Haslam, M. D.
## 1915-1971

Commander, United States Navy
Professor of Orthopedic Surgery
Tulane University, New Orleans

A doctor committed to upholding medical ethics.

# *Dr. Mary's Monkey*

# CONTENTS

*How the Unsolved Murder of a Doctor, a Secret Laboratory in New Orleans and Cancer-Causing Monkey Viruses are Linked to Lee Harvey Oswald, the JFK Assassination and Emerging Global Epidemics*

# FOREWORD

## By Jim Marrs

*There is nothing new to learn about the assassination of JFK.*

WORDS LIKE THESE HAVE BECOME ALMOST a mantra among sanctimonious media pundits and complacent publishers. The problem is that they're not true.

In this book, Ed Haslam takes our knowledge of the dark underpinnings of the 1960s to a new level by offering a whole new look at events surrounding the assassination of President John F. Kennedy. He focuses on activities in New Orleans during 1963, reaching far beyond Lee Harvey Oswald's leafleting or his contacts with anti-Castro Cubans, government agents and mobsters.

Anyone who has seen the Oliver Stone film *JFK* or has read one of the many books on the assassination knows of New Orleans District Attorney Jim Garrison's ill-fated prosecution of International Trade Mart Director Clay Shaw.

We know of Guy Banister, the ex-FBI agent who was connected to the CIA, anti-Castro Cubans and the accused assassin Oswald. We know of David Ferrie, a defrocked priest who was connected to the Mafia, the CIA and Oswald.

Shaw was able to successfully argue that he had never met Ferrie or Oswald. Today, we know that claim is simply untrue.

It is now well-accepted that officials within the federal government of the United States of America took steps to effectively block and derail Garrison's probe. It seemed the New Orleans investigation was at an end.

But what if all that activity in New Orleans had nothing to do with the assassination? What if there was some other reason for sabotaging Garrison's investigation?

After all, there is not one hard piece of evidence linking the Shaw-Ferrie axis to the events in Dealey Plaza. Ferrie, the man connected to Oswald, the Mob and the CIA, never got closer to Dallas than a Houston phone booth, and there was never any serious accusation that Clay Shaw went to Dallas.

Could there have been a deeper secret reason why the Garrison investigation had to be shut off? And could that reason have had more to do with contaminated polio vaccines and the secrecy of a deadly biological weapon experiment than any plotting against President Kennedy?

In his 1995 book *Mary, Ferrie & the Monkey Virus*, Haslam opened a whole new can of worms when he revealed the medical experiments that had taken place in David Ferrie's apartment in 1963.

He was one of the first to bring to the public the now well-documented story of how the polio vaccines of the 1950s was adulterated with a cancer-causing virus derived from monkey glands. Federal certification officers were aware of the possibility of the polio vaccine being defective but were pressured into approving the vaccine by powerful medical interests, including Dr. Alton Ochsner of New Orleans.

Once the magnitude of the cancer-causing viruses in the polio vaccines became known, a massive covert effort was undertaken in an attempt to find a cure or preventative. All this was clandestine work, very hush-hush. No one wanted the American public to know that the polio vaccines inoculated into millions of our citizens were contaminated with dangerous monkey viruses, perhaps causing the cancer epidemic of recent years.

But then the story took an even darker turn: the CIA began to take an interest in the work. After all, this was a time when documented efforts were under way to find a subtle way of assassinating Fidel Castro. Military and intelligence eyes sparkled at the prospect of somehow injecting Castro with cancer. His death would appear natural, and there would be no accusations from the Soviet Union.

But what was Oswald's role in all this activity? The evidence of Oswald's intelligence work for the U.S. Government is overwhelming. Did he become involved in a biological weapons experiment so monstrous that its secret had to be maintained at all costs?

Diligent researchers know that Oswald was playing intelligence games in New Orleans in the summer of 1963. One day he was handing out pro-Castro literature on street corners, some of it stamped with the same address as Banister's anti-Castro office at 544 Camp Street. Another day, Oswald was offering his services to anti-Castro militant Carlos Bringuier. Oswald's duplicity resulted in what appeared to authorities as a staged fight between Oswald and Bringuier on a New Orleans street.

Oswald was arrested for disturbing the peace. While in jail, he did not ask to see a lawyer but instead someone from the FBI. Despite being outside normal business hours, FBI Agent John Quigley arrived and spent more than an hour with Oswald, who commenced to detail his activities since arriving in New Orleans, almost as though he was making a report to superiors. Yet Oswald made no public mention of David Ferrie or his work at Ferrie's cancer lab.

According to information gathered by Haslam, Oswald also was much more closely connected to his uncle, Charles "Dutz" Murret, and New Orleans crime lord Carlos Marcello than previously suspected.

But Haslam's primary focus is on the strange and horrible death of Dr. Mary Sherman, whose charred body was found in her home in July 1964. She had been stabbed multiple times. Her body exhibited the effects of extreme scorching and heat, yet there was only superficial fire damage to her bed and home. He also delves into Oswald's work with Ferrie in the covert cancer lab and its fatal results. His research provides a plausible explanation for the caged white mice reported in Ferrie's apartment, Oswald's missing time at the Reily Coffee Company, and for the never fully understood trip to Clinton, LA, by Oswald, Ferrie and Shaw.

Readers of Haslam's previous book, *Mary, Ferrie & the Monkey Virus*, will recall the author's suspicion that Dr. Sherman's death may have been the result of an accident involving a linear particle accelerator used in the cancer research. In this updated account, Haslam lays out strong evidence that just such a device was in use on the U.S. Public Health Service Hospital grounds near Tulane in the 1960s.

His previous work was embraced by the late Mary Ferrell, that indefatigable Dallas JFK assassination researcher. When asked her opinion of Haslam's research, Mary replied, "Based on what we know today, I think it's totally accurate."

In this new volume, Haslam brings the one thing missing from his earlier work — a living witness.

The importance of this new testimony was summed up by consummate conspiracy debunker John McAdams, who stated, "If Judyth Vary Baker is telling the truth, it will change the way we think about the Kennedy assassination."

Ed Haslam's research may indeed change the way we think about the assassination, about Lee Harvey Oswald and about the greatest health scandal in history.

The tragic assassination of President John F. Kennedy may come to be seen as a mere bump in the road of a series of national scandals and conspiracies which have plagued the United States right up to today.

JIM MARRS, SPRING 2007

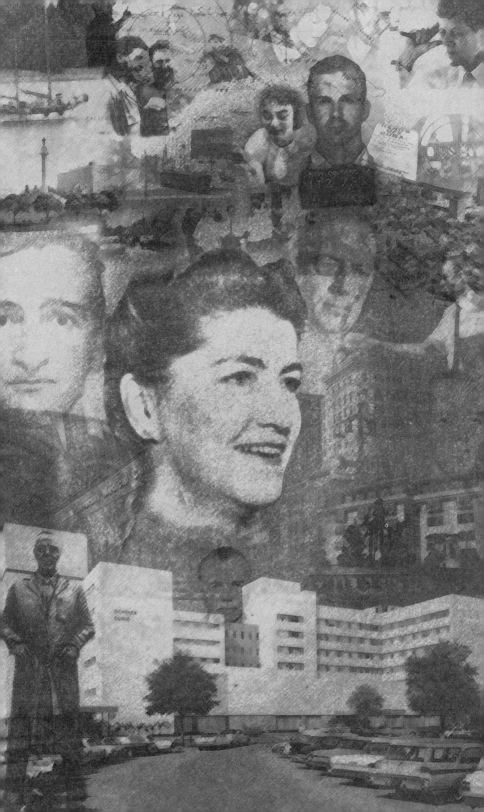

# PROLOGUE

# The Warning

O N ONE LEVEL THIS BOOK is a cold-case investigation into the 1964 murder of Dr. Mary Sherman in New Orleans — a murder which remains unsolved and is remembered as one of the most mysterious ever committed in a city that has known so much mystery and so many murders. But there is more to this story than murder and mystery.

Understanding the death of this one woman unravels much of our nation's secret history. It illuminates the darkness. It connects great medical disasters of our time to important political events of the day. It unveils the contamination of hundreds of millions of doses of the polio vaccine with dozens of monkey viruses. It spotlights the epidemic of soft tissue cancers that swept our country. And it exposes dangerous secret experiments which used radiation to mutate cancer-causing monkey viruses. It connects leaders of American medicine to the accused assassin of the President of the United States. This one murder helps us understand why we have been lied to with such conviction for so many years — and why those lies are likely to continue.

But this is not a murder mystery: fascinating perhaps, but hardly entertainment. For me, writing this book was difficult, stressful and dangerous. What began as an investigation into this single murder morphed into consideration of epidemics which killed millions of people and which cost billions of dollars. It became an investigation into an underground medical laboratory that was accidentally discovered during an investigation into the JFK assassination — a laboratory which secretly irradiated cancer-causing monkey viruses to develop a biological weapon.

This story seems to have followed me throughout my life, and its recurring pattern is eerie indeed. Had I realized its importance, I would have paid closer attention. What I do remember are fragments that I pieced together later in life: a name here, an incident there, pieces of a puzzle often separated by years of unrelated distractions. I even remember sitting on Mary Sherman's lap once as a child. She and my father worked together at Tulane Medical School in New Orleans. They had taken a British doctor out to dinner and then to our family's home for an after-dinner drink.

When she died in the summer of 1964, I saw my father cry for the first time. As a Navy doctor during World War II, my father had seen more than his share of burned and broken bodies. Someone (I don't know who) had asked him to go to the morgue to look at Mary Sherman's body to get a second opinion on her unusual death. He came home from the morgue that day, fixed himself a drink, sat down in his chair, and cried silently. I wondered what was wrong. My mother told me that a woman he knew from the office had died. It was only later that I learned it was Mary Sherman.

Seeing my father cry was memorable for me — a once in a lifetime experience. Having spent his career amputating limbs and standing in an Emergency Room making life-or-death decisions about people pulled from mangled vehicles, he was not prone to show much emotion. I mention this incident here because it is important to our story. It is how

I learned about the evidence that unraveled the mystery of Mary Sherman's murder. My father told my mother, and my mother later told me: Mary Sherman's right arm was missing.

This key fact in the case was never told to the press. Why not? Can you imagine the O.J. Simpson trial without "the glove"? Why was the press not told the most obvious fact in this case? Who was trying to protect whom? Were there powerful forces controlling the story from the beginning? If so, what did they not want us to know? And why did they not want us to know it?

That same summer, I overheard my father complain bitterly when he learned about certain activities going on at the U.S. Public Health Service Hospital. His anger and frustration seemed out of character for this deep-keeled man. I remember his words: "We fought wars to keep people from doing things like this."

IN THE SUMMER OF 1964 my father learned something about what had been going on at the USPHS hospital. I do not recall if this was before or after Mary Sherman's death, but it was around that time. He was particularly insulted by the idea that it was taking place on the grounds of the U.S. Public Health Service Hospital, a facility that was supposed to protect the American public from deadly diseases.

When he vented his frustration to my mother, she reminded him that there was probably nothing he could do about it "at this point." His response: "It just that I gave up so much to keep stuff like this from happening." I have always understood this comment to be about leaving the Navy and ending his admiral-track career. Despite this high price, he remained dedicated to the idea of medical ethics, a commitment he acquired from his father — a bio-chemist, veterinarian, and medical doctor who helped develop the first anthrax vaccine. Thus he was not only not a part of these secret radiation experiments, but was also disturbed to learn about them.

In the late 1960s, I heard about Mary Sherman's connection to an underground medical laboratory run by a suspect in the murder of President Kennedy. I was told they were using monkey viruses to create cancer. The possibility of this being used as a biological weapon was clear. The dark specter of unleashing a designer virus on the world haunted me. I even offered a sarcastic comment at the time: "The good news is if there's a bizarre global epidemic involving cancer and a monkey virus thirty years from now, *at least we'll know where it came from.*"

IN 1971, during what might be described as a deathbed conversation, I confronted my father about Mary Sherman. He was getting ready to go to the hospital. For the first time in his life, he was going as a patient. His cancerous lung was scheduled to be surgically removed in the morning. We both knew that, due to his fragile health, he would probably not survive the surgery. We discussed it. We both realized that this would probably be the last conversation we would ever have with each other. He stoically gave me instructions about caring for my mother. I listened and pondered the strength of this quiet man who had seen so much death in his professional life. I studied the courage with which he faced his own.

When he finished, I acknowledged his requests and confirmed my willingness to carry out his instructions. Then I said that I had a few questions of my own. Questions that I would never be able to ask him again. Questions that I thought were important for him to answer, so that the truth would not die with him. I asked him to tell me about Mary Sherman and about all that spooky stuff that was going on at the U.S. Public Health Service Hospital. "Wasn't she some kind of cancer expert?" I ventured.

He shook his head slowly from side to side, to let me know that he would not tell me.

I persisted. I wanted to know why he would not tell me. Solemnly he said, "There might be repercussions. I have to think about the family first. I have to protect them."

"What if I figure it out myself?" I challenged.

"I'm hardly in a position to stop you," he said with the casual resignation of a man who never expected to see another football game. Then he collected his thoughts and, in a grave voice, he gave me this warning: "Ed, I need you to listen to me carefully. I will not be able to say this to you again. If you do figure out what happened down there and decide to tell the world what you found, I need you to realize that you will be crossing swords with the most powerful people in our country. And you should think twice before crossing them."

THE 1980S USHERED IN THE EPIDEMICS that I had feared in the 1960s. The mainstream scientific community stated that AIDS was caused by the unexplained mutation of a monkey virus. They estimated the date of the mutation to be around 1960. The logical question (who had been mutating monkey viruses around 1960) was not even asked in the press. And, yes, I was concerned about what I had heard in New Orleans. It all sounded so similar. Could there be a connection? And if there was, was there any point in speaking up about it? Trade places with me for a moment: If you were in my shoes, would you have?

I went to medical libraries and read scientific articles hoping to find facts that would make my fears unfounded. I was anxious to find a flaw in my own argument, which would enable me to walk away from a project that was starting to consume all of my free time. I did not find the flaw, but I did find something else.

As I poured over the official cancer statistics from the National Cancer Institute, I saw the dimensions of the massive epidemic of soft-tissue cancers that had swept our country. An epidemic that had been all but ignored by our watchdog press. An epidemic that could reasonably be explained by the cancer-causing monkey viruses that had contaminated the polio vaccine of my youth. Whatever I felt my options were prior to that moment, they suddenly narrowed.

I also noticed that names connected to the polio vaccine were names connected to Mary Sherman and to the investigation of the JFK assassination. I began to suspect that these secrets were somehow intertwined. A web of secrecy surrounding our national health. Interlocking secrets that protected each other. Secrets which presented serious accountability problems for the people in power. I remembered the warning my father had given me. I could see how unwelcome this news would be in many circles.

IN THE 1990S I FOUND DOCUMENTATION and witnesses to support much of what I had heard as a child. My fears were now based in facts. I met highly-credentialed scientists who understood both the history and the science behind these events clearly, and they took my concerns seriously. Some quietly helped me find people who knew things that I needed to know. They helped me connect the dots.

Finally, I found evidence of the radioactive machine used to mutate the monkey viruses. I now had motive, opportunity and what detectives call propinquity (right people, right place, right time). I decided it was time to speak out — even if I did not have all the information in hand at the moment.

In July 1995 I self-published my story as *Mary, Ferrie & the Monkey Virus: The Story of an Underground Medical Laboratory*. I could only afford to print 1,000 copies, but I hoped that getting the story out might attract a publisher. After the first thousand books were gone, I could not afford a reprint. Still without a publisher, I switched tactics and started photocopying comb-bound manuscripts in batches of ten. This new technique enabled me to update the book with new information as I found it and kept me in print for years. A handful of orders trickled in each week. By the end of 1999, a second thousand books had been shipped. With copies in all fifty states and five foreign countries, I felt that "the cat" was now "out of the bag," and I could finally go back to my advertising career and try to make a living — which I did in 2000.

It was at this exquisitely inconvenient moment that *60 Minutes*, the CBS News TV show, contacted me. They were investigating a woman who said that she had been in the underground medical laboratory that I had written about in my book. That she knew Mary Sherman. That she had been trained to handle cancer-causing viruses. That she had been part of the effort to develop a biological weapon. That she knew Lee Harvey Oswald. Would I meet with them for an off-camera interview? I accepted.

By the time *60 Minutes* interviewed me in November 2000, they had already interviewed their witness for hours. They got additional input from other researchers and journalists. Finally, they decided not to air her story.

Three years later, in November 2003, the History Channel aired a story about this same underground medical laboratory. It mentioned Dr. Mary Sherman, David Ferrie, and Lee Oswald, but not my book. The episode, featuring a young woman who had handled the cancer-causing monkey viruses for the secret project, was part of their series *The Men Who Killed Kennedy*. A week later the History Channel reversed course. The episode was withdrawn from circulation, and has not been aired again.

OUR STORY COMES FROM A FERMENTING MASH of science, secrecy, patriotism, power, paranoia and extremism. It is not a pretty picture. It involves death, disease, covert wars, and the quiet hand of power. In our path sit innocent people whom I am sure would prefer not to be involved. I apologize to them in advance. Then there are others who claim to have forgotten everything they know about this matter or who know but refuse to talk. To them I offer no apology.

This story casts a shadow that is so dark and so long that I have chosen to tell it simply. Some have said that it has the nightmarish quality of an anxiety dream. I prefer to see it in a different light. It is, as songwriter Jackson Browne once said, "the fitful dream of some greater awakening." We are just beginning to wake up to the responsibilities of being a free society. It is much more complicated than dropping bombs on an obvious enemy. It is time we began to question what the people of power did with the trust and money we gave them.

I doubt we will ever hear the Surgeon General stand up at a press conference and acknowledge this operation. This one still possesses serious accountability problems for those who hold positions of power. Further, it comes from the land of unvouchered expenditures, where the trails of accountability were obscured by professionals decades ago.

There are reasons for such secrecy. Powerful reasons. Reasons capable of destroying careers and toppling governments. A full exposure here would threaten the treasure of our nation's wealthiest corporations, the reputations of some of the powerful political figures of the day, and the precious confidence we give our national institutions. While we can understand why they kept these matters secret, we have a different goal.

Our task is to unmask these secrets because they were hidden from us for reasons. Powerful reasons. Reasons that affect decisions being made today. Reasons that involve politics and medicine. Reasons that affect our health and ultimately our freedom.

To investigate such secrecy is a formidable task. We tread lightly for we walk upon tender ground, over the bones of children, through sour rooms of tumor-bearing mice, and into the blood-stained bedroom of one of our nation's most respected cancer researchers. It is here we search for knowledge that was not meant to be known. We will use published sources and official records as best we can. At times we examine these more closely and in greater detail than anyone before us. But we must be prepared to look beyond the official paper trail and to use less certain methods to find our way. Methods like oral history, personal testimony, feeble press accounts, censored government documents, and our own capable and curious intellects.

Complicating our task further is the catastrophic flood of 2005 that followed Hurricane Katrina. Irreplaceable documents (like the crime-scene photos) and precious physical evidence (like the blood-soaked gloves found in Mary Sherman's apartment, which could still yield DNA or other clues) may have been lost forever when the waters of Lake Pontchartrain engulfed the city of New Orleans. Yet we can proceed with what we *do* know. As you will see, plenty of evidence had been collected previously.

You will find this book as much of a personal odyssey as a journalistic work. But that's what happens when you investigate a murder only to discover an epidemic. Either way the destination is the same. I will tell you why I am deeply suspicious of certain activities that occurred in New Orleans in the 1960s, and why you should be too. We will begin with what I personally saw and heard over the years. To that we add years of research. Then we get questions. Fair and honorable questions. Questions which deserve answers. Questions which have their own purpose, their own energy, even their own dignity. Questions which will eventually help us coax this Orwellian monster out of its swamp of secrecy.

EDWARD T. HASLAM, SPRING 2007

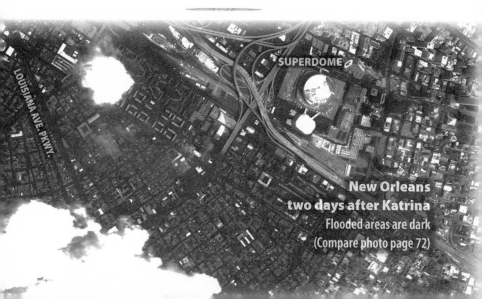

LOUISIANA AVE. PKWY.

SUPERDOME

New Orleans
two days after Katrina
Flooded areas are dark
(Compare photo page 72)

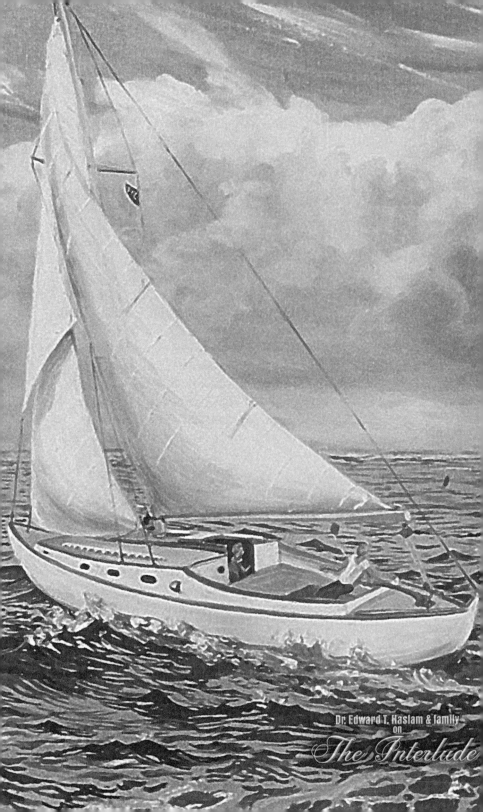

Dr. Edward T. Haslam & family
on
*The Interlude*

# CHAPTER 1

# The Pirate

I N THE SPRING OF 1962 I WAS A CHILD OF TEN YEARS. Those innocent, sun-filled days were spent swimming and sailing on Lake Pontchartrain in New Orleans.

This particular day, my father and I had been sailing on his boat, the *Interlude*, a modest double-ended wooden sloop whose leaky hull showed its age. The *Interlude* was a noticeable step down the status ladder from the larger, newer, more glamorous boats which flanked it on the pier. Boats tend to be metaphors of their owners, and this was no exception. It was an unpretentious boat for an unpretentious man.

My father was dressed in his habitual sailing clothes, baggy khaki pants, a blue cotton shirt, and a dark blue baseball cap that covered his short-cropped head of completely grey hair. This attire was as close as he could get to his old Navy uniform, and he wore it whenever he sailed. With his omnipresent cigarette in hand, he shuffled down the concrete pier in a casual gait with me at his side. This quiet man honored simplicity and enjoyed the peace that followed a long, terrible war.

This rumpled façade concealed a complex and accomplished man who had witnessed more than his share of human suffering. The son of a country doctor, he graduated from Harvard Medical School in the late 1930s and then served as an officer in the U.S. Navy, in both the Atlantic and the Pacific, during World War II. By the end of the war, he was planning medical support for an invasion of Japan, where they anticipated *one million* American casualties. In 1946-47, he was stationed (with his wife and infant daughter) in the smoldering Philippines. Upon returning to the states, he left the Navy and specialized in orthopedic surgery. After several moves, he settled in New Orleans in 1952. Now he made his living teaching at Tulane Medical School, performing surgery, and working with crippled children. He sailed to relax.[1]

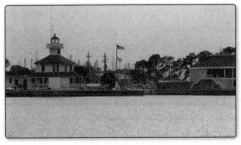

As we walked, we approached a section of the pier referred to as the Visitor's Dock, where sailors from around the world occasionally stopped on their travels. Since New Orleans was the northern port of the Gulf of Mexico, salty boats and weathered crews frequently came straight from the Caribbean and Central America. Some of these boats were remarkably picturesque, more reminiscent of ships from "the great age of sail" than the sleek modern designs which populated yacht club harbors. This day, an exceptionally nautical-looking boat had slipped into the Visitor's Dock while we were out sailing.

"Look, Dad! It's a pirate ship," I said with great excitement. The boat was a gaff-rigged schooner about fifty feet long with a carved wooden figurehead on the bow. A live parrot was perched on a cross beam in the rigging. Freshly-washed clothes were hung out to dry.

"And there's the pirate," I whispered, letting my wide eyes announce the importance of the news. Coming down the pier towards us was the boat's skipper, a bare-chested barefoot gypsy, looking every bit like the Ancient Mariner himself. Never before had I seen such a character in person. His leathery skin held a deep brown tan set off sharply by his tattered sun-bleached pants cut below the knee. Long curls of grey hair haphazardly fell from under the bandanna tied around his head. On his shoulder sat a small, mischievous monkey about twelve inches tall, tethered on a leash. As we passed, the pirate smiled at us; his 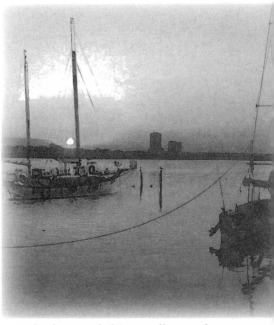 eyes sparkled. The monkey studied us with his small round head and big brown eyes. Despite my intrigue, I gave them a wide berth and tried not to stare, but it was difficult. My thoughts were now focused on the monkey.

I had seen plenty of monkeys before, mostly in the zoo, but I had never thought about having a monkey as a pet. We had a dog. Why not a monkey? It would be much more interesting. So I asked my father, "Dad, can I get a monkey for a pet?"

"No," was his immediate answer. After a pause, he anticipated my next question by adding, "They carry diseases."

I had heard my mother mention that monkeys occasionally carried rabies. I reasoned to myself for a moment: Dogs could carry rabies, but we had a dog. A vet could tell you if your dog carried rabies, so a vet should be able to tell you if your monkey carried rabies. And nothing (to my ten-year-old mind) could possibly be worse than rabies! I decided to give the monkey pet idea a second try. "Like rabies?" I countered.

"Yes," he answered in a flat tone. "They can carry rabies, but they carry a lot of other diseases, too. Some are weird viruses that we don't understand yet. Some of them can kill you."

I was puzzled by his comment. I wondered how my father, an orthopedic surgeon whom the children in my family jokingly referred to as "old sawbones," knew about weird monkey viruses which were still being researched at the leading edge of medical science. So I asked him, "Where did you learn about that?" He paused to take a long drag off his cigarette and seemed to be thinking about the question. In the interim I decided to speculate: "Did you learn about that in the Philippines?"

"No," he said, blowing out his cigarette smoke in a short breath. "I don't suppose there's *any harm in telling my ten-year-old son*," as if talking to a cloud. Then he turned to me and said, "They're researching monkey viruses down at the med school. Some of the more deadly ones are coming in from Africa."

*Africa?!!!* I may have been ten years old, but I did not need Joseph Conrad to tell me that Africa was mysterious. From what I had seen in school and on television, Africa was a wild, poverty-stricken continent riddled with starvation and horrifying diseases. It was also full of bizarre forms of life which defied your imagination, like ants the size of your foot and snakes as long as your car. I was not interested in catching any weird fatal virus from Africa, no matter how cute the monkey. I wondered if the pirate knew the danger he was in.

The fact that these diseases obviously concerned my father more than rabies made a huge impression upon me. His comments ended my desire for a pet monkey, but they were the beginning of my curiosity about the monkey virus research being conducted in New Orleans. My first real question arose from my dad's cautiousness: Why were Tulane's doctors not supposed to talk about the monkey virus research program?

SEVERAL DAYS AFTER THE PIRATE INCIDENT we had a substitute teacher at school. In the middle of the day she turned her attention to science and started talking about germs and diseases. She reviewed the basics about how germs caused diseases and how our bodies fought back. She went on to explain the differences among bacteria, fungi, and viruses. As her lecture continued, she confidently explained how modern medicine had triumphed over bacteria and fungi with medicines and antibiotics. Then she moved the discussion to the frontier of medicine, where researchers were battling the mysterious world of viruses.

I raised my hand to make a contribution to the discussion: They were researching viruses down at Tulane Medical School. (I knew the monkey subject was taboo, so I did not mention it.) "No," she said immediately, and turning toward the entire class, she said, "That's wrong," in a definitive voice. "Tulane is just a college and its purpose is to teach students, not to do research. Virus research," she continued, "is a very complex subject and is only done by very intelligent specialists at faraway places like Harvard and Johns Hopkins universities and at special government research centers which have special equipment."

I was embarrassed by her response, but there was nothing I could do about it. I knew she was both right and wrong. Tulane's faculty was full of people from Harvard and Hopkins. My father was one of them. Many of them were doing research. For over 100 years the reputation of Tulane had been based on battling tropical diseases like yellow fever and malaria.

It was true that the names Harvard and Johns Hopkins were in the news more often than Tulane, each time announcing some medical breakthrough or at least updating the public on their progress in fighting some dreaded disease. Other than announcing its pathetic football scores, Tulane's name hardly ever appeared in the local press. Public news about Tulane Medical School was basically non-existent in the 1960s.[2] The teacher had stated the public's perception accurately enough. More importantly, I knew that nothing I could say would change her mind. More than likely she just could not grasp that idea that something "local" might be important. Beaten for the moment, I held my tongue.

THE NEXT TIME I HAD A CHANCE to talk to my father I asked him why it was that we always heard on the news about the medical research being done at faraway places like Harvard and Johns Hopkins, but we never heard about the research being conducted at Tulane.

"Not everybody wants publicity," he patiently explained. "Yes, some people do research because they want to be famous and tell the world how great they are; but other people are not interested in publicity, and they do research to get information and knowledge. It's just part of being involved in academic medicine."

While I understood that he was trying to communicate the nobility of quiet scholarship, his answer did not make sense to me. Such an explanation might explain the bragging of an upstart school, but it did not explain why we heard about research from first-class schools like Harvard and Hopkins, but not Tulane. I thought about his comment for a minute and asked, "What sort of people wouldn't want the public to know about their research?"

He hid his exasperation with my relentless questioning in his quiet bedside manner, and said that much of the research at Tulane was financed by money from drug companies and from the U.S. government. These grants were frequently for experiments with drugs that were not yet ready for the public. Therefore, there was no reason to tell the public about them.

That still did not answer the question to my satisfaction. Sooner or later those drugs would be ready, but somehow I knew we still would not hear about them. The not-ready-yet argument was as true for Harvard and Hopkins as for Tulane. But I did understand his main points clearly. First, Tulane did not have enough money to fund its own research and was dependent upon others, like drug companies and the U.S. government, who consequently dictated what was to be researched and what was to be talked about. And secondly, Tulane Medical School did not get publicity because it did not want publicity. While this was not much of a victory for me, at least I understood why the teacher and the public did not know about Tulane's virus research programs.

Actually there were some very good reasons to keep subjects like researching monkey viruses quiet. The main ones were (1) potential public panic over an accidental epidemic, (2) growing public pressure from the animal rights movement, and (3) the secrecy demanded by covert operations.

The possibility of public panic over an accidental epidemic was a real and present danger to both researchers and their financial backers. One bad incident might trigger a public outcry that would effectively shut down all such research for years. The possibility of such an accidental epidemic was very real, and the scientists knew it.[3]

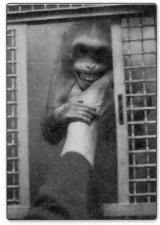

During the early 1960s there were numerous outbreaks of infectious diseases among the animal handlers in monkey labs around the country.[4] Waterborne diseases were transferred through saliva, moisture in the breath, and urine. They could be caught just by being around the primates. Cleaning out animal cages was dangerous. Feeding a monkey was dangerous. Taking a monkey out of a cage was dangerous. Holding a monkey was dangerous. Primates are intelligent mammals, and they quickly figured out that a trip with a handler often meant getting stuck with needles, or having the top of the skull chopped off with a power saw, or being injected with psychoactive drugs. The monkeys fought back. They bit their handlers. They urinated on them. They tried to escape.

Monkey handlers who drew blood from one cancerous monkey to inject it into another occasionally stabbed themselves with needles full of blood laced with carcinogenic monkey viruses.[5] The dangers were enormous, and the controls were feeble by today's standards. The generality of all this is well documented in medical libraries around the country. One book published during the 1960s made the point clearly in its title, *The Hazards of Handling Simians*, and listed the numerous outbreaks of diseases in the primate research facilities during the previous two decades.[6]

Then, the monkey handlers would go home and resume their normal lives, including sexual activities. The potential for zoonoses (diseases jumping from animal to man) was very real, and the medical community knew it.

Consider these comments written in the 1960s by Richard Fiennes, Britain's leading primate researcher, about the dangers of primate research:

> There is ... a serious danger that viruses from such closely related groups as the simian primates could show an altered pathogenesis in man, of which malignancy could be a feature. The dangers of such happening are enhanced by man's exposure in crowded cities to oncogenic agents and increased radiation hazards ...
>
> The danger of transmitting simian viruses in vaccines is a real and alarming one ...
>
> The further danger is that simian viruses might become adapted to human populations, and spread with appalling rapidity, and under circumstances in which there were no possible immediate means of control ...
>
> Knowledge of prophylaxis against viral diseases is in its infancy, and time must elapse before any effective vaccine could be prepared, tested, and manufactured in bulk to protect populations against a pandemic caused by a new virus ...
>
> Plainly, it is in the realms of virology that primate zoonoses present the greatest danger ...
>
> Far too little is known of the virology of simians ...[7]

Does this sound familiar? Does it not predict the current AIDS epidemic? Speaking further of this danger, Fiennes discussed O'nyong-nyong, a mildly lethal virus that swept Africa:

> Had O'nyong-nyong been attended by a high death-rate... the human population of a large part of East and Central Africa would have virtually ceased to exist. To such an extent, in spite of twentieth-century medicine, is man still vulnerable to attack from new viruses.[8]

The danger was real. The fear of public panic was real. With experimental animals, unpredictable viruses and exposed animal handlers intermingled in a sweltering tropical city of nearly a million people (like New Orleans), the opportunity for a biological disaster was ripe.

The idea of an epidemic suddenly sweeping the streets of an American city was not foreign to the public. In fact, a movie called *Panic in the Streets* won the Academy Award for best screenplay in 1952. *Panic in the Streets* depicted a U.S. Public Health Service officer battling a modern day outbreak of bubonic plague on the streets of New Orleans. But the press of the 1950s and 1960s either did not consider the public's interest in medical matters substantial enough to warrant coverage, or they felt they had a higher duty to prevent public panic. Either way, the press did a poor job of covering the issue then. But, they do a better job of covering it today.

For example, an accident occurred at a Yale laboratory in the 1990s. The headline in *Time* shouted, "A Deadly Virus Escapes." The sub-headline continued, "Concerns about lab security arise as a mysterious disease from Brazil strikes a Yale researcher."[9] The researcher worked at a Biohazard-3 lab and was studying a rare, potentially lethal virus when he broke a test tube. He failed to report the incident, which sprayed this virus into his nostrils. Instead, he went to visit friends in Boston. When the incident was discovered, the researcher was quarantined, and his friends were put under medical surveillance. The article concluded, "If researchers do not tighten some of their procedures, the next outbreak might not be so benign." All of which makes one wonder: What safety procedures were enforced in the monkey labs of the 1960s? And what procedures would have been followed in an underground medical laboratory with no visible sponsor?

To understand the type and extent of monkey virus research being done in medical schools in the 1950s and 1960s, I went to medical libraries and started reading the history of virology. While even an overview of these activities is beyond our scope at the moment, there are a few points worth mentioning. First is that it was well established in these medical research circles around the world *prior to 1960* that certain monkey viruses caused various types of cancer, including cancers of the skin, lungs, and bones.[10]

Secondly, experimentation with carcinogenic viruses was widespread throughout the network of primate research centers, from the U.S., to Europe, to the U.S.S.R. Blood, tumor cells, and viral extracts were routinely taken from a variety of animals and injected into monkeys like a game of viral roulette. One lab created tumors in as little as eight days.[11] Another lab injected human volunteers with the known cancer-causing monkey viruses to observe the effects.[12]

New diseases started to appear — diseases which were unknown in the wild. One such disease that first appeared in the lab is now called SAIDS or Simian AIDS.[13] It occurred when *African* monkey viruses were given to *Asian* monkeys. SIV, the retrovirus that collapsed the immune systems of Asian monkeys, did not cause disease in its natural host, the African Green monkey.[14]

In addition to viral roulette, researchers experimented with radiation therapy, beaming x-rays and gamma rays directly into tumors to encourage remission. The medical researchers of the 1960s irradiated tumors in laboratory animals, including primates, and shot radiation directly into the tumors of human patients.[15] Think this one through before we proceed. When you shoot a radioactive beam at a tumor, you not only hit the tumor, but you also hit the blood and viruses in and around the tumor. Was the type of radiation used to dissolve cancer tumors strong enough and focused enough to damage the DNA and RNA of the viruses floating in the patient's blood?

At this point, the medically sophisticated reader might say, "Wait a minute! The radiation exposure of a clinical x-ray machine does minimal damage to DNA or RNA, and very many people receive very many x-rays without getting cancer." And this is true where we are talking about the exposure and energy levels associated with common clinical use, which have been clinically established as relatively safe for humans.

However, in the late 1950s a powerful new device emerged from the physics lab and quietly began to be distributed to selected medical research facilities. It was called a *linear particle accelerator*.[16] Never before had a machine of this magnitude been put into the commercial workplace. You might think of it as a poor-man's atom-smasher. These high-voltage scientific machines were capable of doing things never done before, and they spawned new ultra-hi-tech applications that stretched the imagination. Their basic capabilities included producing high-energy radiation and hurling sub-atomic particles near the speed of light into whatever object one desired.[17] To illustrate their ability to change things generally considered to be unchangeable, let's look at a commercial application of a linear accelerator in South Africa. Shooting sub-atomic particles through imperfect yellow diamonds stripped the impurities out of the yellow diamonds and turned them into clear marketable white diamonds. These linear accelerators were capable of destroying anything in their path. There is *nothing* they could not cut, if directed to do so.

This particular point was dramatically demonstrated by a man named Jack Nygard, an engineer at a company in Boston which manufactured linear accelerators.[18] Nygard developed ingenious new commercial applications for linear accelerators, from preserving bananas to cross-bonding wood. By shooting particles laterally through plastic-laminated wood, Nygard created a new structural matrix inside the wood. The result was an ultra-hard super-wood that would never warp. It was the perfect low-maintenance solution for the bowling industry. Nygard turned entrepreneur and set up shop in the heart of the lumber industry near Seattle, Washington, where he began producing his super-wood on a commercial scale. His success continued until the day the technician running his accelerator did not notice that Jack had stepped into the wood-processing area. When the technician flipped the switch on the 5,000,000 volt machine, it was the last anyone ever saw of Jack Nygard.[19] The beam of electro-magnetic radiation burned him to the point of disintegration. They swept up his ashes. (Or so the story goes.)

The medical applications of linear particle accelerators included destroying cancer tissue and conducting various types of viral and genetic research. These machines were quite capable of either killing viruses or simply mangling the molecules in the genome necessary for reproduction.

In the field of virus research, radioactive medical experiments greatly increased the danger of an already dangerous scenario. They introduced the capability of mutating viruses already known to be deadly, and raised the possibility of creating both *new vaccines* and *new super-diseases*.

Some of the scientists involved in the field of monkey virus experiments got *extremely* nervous about the dangers of such experiments, and warned their colleagues in the mid-1960s that if one of these monkey viruses mutated into a more lethal form and got into the human blood supply, there could be a *global epidemic* which would be *unstoppable*, given the current level of medical knowledge![20]

In 1959, the U.S. Congress finally took the danger of an accidental monkey virus epidemic seriously, and financed seven regional primate centers in order to get the experiments out of the cities.[21]

In Louisiana, the Delta Regional Primate Center opened its doors in November 1964 with Tulane University serving as the host institution.[22] This took the monkey virus research out of downtown New Orleans and put it in 500 wooded acres near Covington, Louisiana, across Lake Pontchartrain. Today that laboratory has over 4,000 primates, thirty scientists, and 130 support workers, plus a public relations director whose job it is to boast of the center's virus research, especially on AIDS, and to point to the improvements in lab security, such as the high-security zone, where researchers and staff shower and change clothes before approaching or leaving the 500 monkeys infected with simian AIDS. Despite these security measures, Delta was back in the headlines in 1994, when eighty-three monkeys escaped. The public

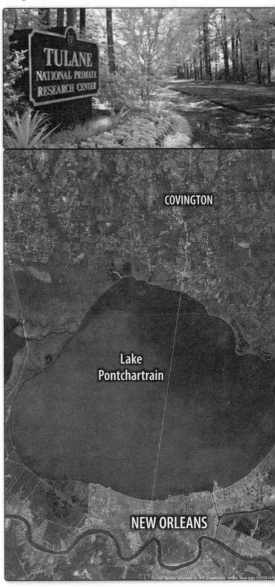

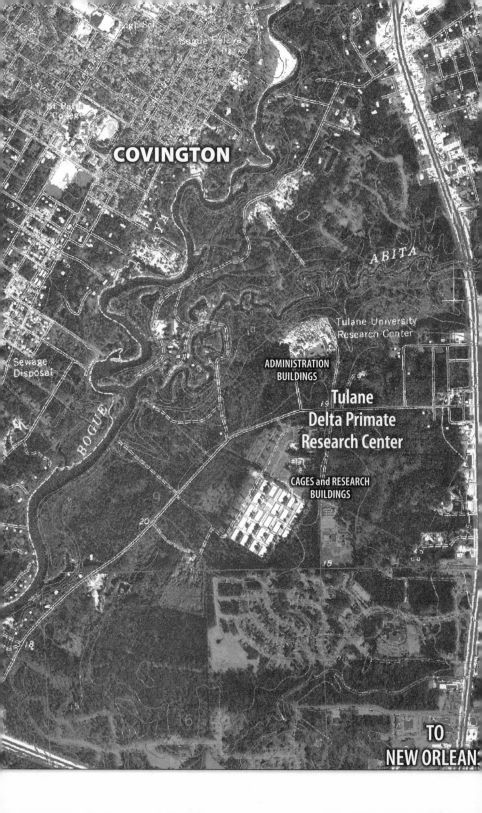

was told to call Delta to report any monkeys seen swinging through the trees,[23] the center having claimed the week before that *nearly* all of them had been captured.[24]

The Delta primate lab's $4,000,000 per year operating budget comes directly from the U.S. government's National Institutes of Health, as it has for the past forty years. One critic of animal research, Dr. Peggy Carlson of the Physicians' Committee for Responsible Medicine, claimed that animal research is big business, and said, "They are taking money away from other areas and dumping it into a sinkhole."[25] Other critics opposed animal research on humanitarian grounds, many believing that animal research actually contributes more to advancing professional careers than to advancing human medicine.

A case in point involved ten monkeys, which were transferred to the Delta Regional Primate Center from Silver Springs laboratory after their infamous experiments triggered a national animal-rights debate in the 1980s. Delta terminated eight of the monkeys following heavy-handed experiments. The other two monkeys which had their spinal cords deliberately severed at Silver Springs in the mid-1980s were kept alive at the Delta Regional Primate Center until the early-1990s.[26]

Dana Dorson, an activist from a group called Legislation in Support of Animals, saw little improvement in the new experimental oversight procedures: "Those committees just rubber stamp whatever is presented to them."[27] Attempting to counter the animal rights critics, Delta Regional Primate Center's director Peter Gerone said, "Sometimes the public perception is that we do anything we want to monkeys, but that's a myth. Maybe it was like that thirty years ago, but it's not like that now."[28]

OK, so just what was it like then? Gerone surely knew. A virologist, Gerone had been director of the Delta Primate Center for *twenty-three years* before making that statement in 1994. Appointed in 1971, he had left the U.S. Army's

Biological Warfare Center at Fort Detrick, where he had been one of their experts on airborne transmission of diseases.[29] In 1975 he collaborated with representatives of the Defense Nuclear Agency, the Armed Forces Institute of Pathology, and the U.S. Army Medical Research Institute of Infectious Diseases to attend an NCI-sponsored symposium on "Biohazards and Zoonotic Problems of Primate Procurement, Quarantine, and Research." There he presented his paper on "Biohazards of Experimentally Infected Primates."[30]

I CAN SAY FROM PERSONAL EXPERIENCE THAT, despite the establishment of the Delta Regional Primate Center in 1964, other primate research continued at Tulane Medical School in downtown New Orleans for years to come.

One day in the spring of 1970 I had gone down to the Tulane Medical School to help my father with a clerical project. After

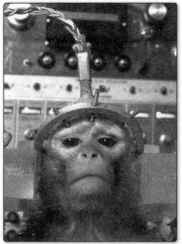

several hours I took a break and, as a distraction, set out to explore the mysteries of the medical school. Near the elevator on one floor, I found an incredible display of mutated human fetuses stored in glass jars. This mind-boggling collection of genetic malfunctions featured two-headed babies, Mongoloid fetuses, and Siamese twins. I decided to explore the other floors to see what else they had.

At the end of one hall I found an open door and a room full of cages. Inside there were monkeys. Each appeared to be wearing a flat-topped organ grinder's hat. But a closer look revealed these were not hats.

A voice came from inside the room. "Come in. Come in. Who are you? And what can I do for you?" A professor sat in his chair looking at me, his head cocked to one side. He was dressed

*Dr. Mary's Monkey*

casually, a plaid shirt, no coat, no tie, no medical jacket. I introduced myself saying that I was visiting my father who was a professor in orthopedics. He invited me to come in and see the monkeys. He explained that the tops of their skulls had been removed with a bone saw and electrodes had been placed deep inside their brains. He held a sample electrode up for me to see.

It was a copper wire with a silver ball on the end which acted like a microphone inside the monkey's brain, sensing and amplifying electrical signals. Once fifteen or so of these electrodes were implanted in the monkey's brain, they were soldered to a data plug which was then glued to the monkey's skull. Once everything was in place, the monkeys would be plugged into a electronic data-collection machine, similar to an EEG, and then injected with experimental psychoactive drugs. The machine measured the reaction of the various parts of their brains to the drugs. The professor held up a haphazardly folded scroll of paper full of squiggly lines to show me how the raw data was collected. "It's amazing work," I commented gesturing to the monkeys.

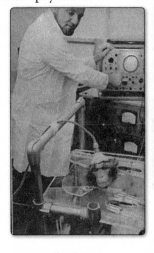

"Putting in the plugs is nothing," he said in a tone that could only be described as arrogant. "The technicians do that. The hard part is figuring out what's happening inside their brains." I thanked him and left. I had to get back to my task.

FROM WHAT I CAN FIND IN THE MEDICAL LIBRARIES, the history of primate research in America started with psychology experiments. An American psychologist named Robert Yerkes originally became famous for developing and administering the first large-scale intelligence test to American soldiers during World War I. Later, as a professor at Yale, Yerkes started exploring the biological basis for intelligence by comparing the brain functions of a wide variety of animals. He called this niche "psycho-biology." In the 1920s Yerkes went further still, getting as close to the human brain as he could, by dissecting and analyzing the brains of gorillas and other high primates. His 1924 book *The Mind of the Gorilla* catapulted him to become the world's leading authority on brain function. In 1928 he established the first large-scale scientific primate laboratory for Yale University, not in Connecticut,

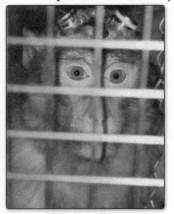

but in the warmer suburbs of Jacksonville, Florida.[31] There they used lobotomies and other techniques to isolate brain function further. In 1942 the laboratory was renamed in his honor. The Yerkes lab was eventually moved to Emory University in Atlanta, nearer the Center for Disease Control. Today it is one of the seven federally funded primate research centers. Only seven, if you do not count the U.S. military's primate laboratories.

For some reason, before the Delta Regional Primate Center was established, the Tulane/LSU monkey lab was unofficially referred to as the "Yerkes lab." I say this mostly from personal experience. Growing up I repeatedly heard the New Orleans lab referred to as "Yerkes." As my seventh grade teacher put it, "It's not the famous Yerkes lab, but it's *like* the Yerkes lab." During the course of researching and writing this book, I heard three separate people refer to the Delta primate lab as "Yerkes." Further, I found a reference in a 1967 medical book to "an outbreak of hepatitis

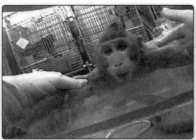

at Yerkes in New Orleans,"[32] reported by Dr. Arthur Riopelle in 1963, a year before the Delta Regional Primate Center opened.

Dr. Riopelle was a psychologist specializing in brain function at the LSU Medical School in New Orleans, and he soon became the first director of the Delta Regional Primate Center. I wrote him a letter asking for clarification on the Yerkes name. He did not write back. The use of the Yerkes name for a lab in New Orleans remains somewhat of a mystery to me. But it certainly would have helped deflect any reports of misconduct in a lab if one circulated the name of another lab hundreds of miles away. When confronted with an accusation, one could say, "What are you talking about? The Yerkes lab is in Florida. You must be confused."

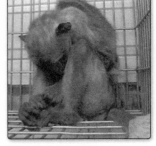

Monkey research in the 1930s and 1940s was by no means confined to psychology. Monkeys were the primary means of studying many viruses, including polio. Then in the late 1940s John F. Enders, a microbiologist from Harvard, and several students figured out how to grow viruses in a test tube full of human cells. At the time, the breakthrough was hailed as the end of the monkey era.[33] Today, however, there are approximately 20,000 monkeys sitting in cages in scientific laboratories across the country who might disagree with that prediction.

The second reason for maintaining a low profile was that the animal rights movement was just starting to grow. Antivivisectionists groups were protesting the treatment of experimental animals, and were distributing literature which showed the horrors of life and death in the animal labs. Keeping a low profile prevented such publicity from creating negative pressures on researchers and their employers.

The third reason for keeping a low profile was the secrecy demanded by covert Cold War operations. Simply said, Tulane was conducting sensitive research for the U.S. government, some of which was for the CIA. This was as much a matter of political pork as national security. Louisiana had one of the most powerful delegations in Washington, and much of that power was concentrated in the hands of legislators who controlled the military budgets. Congress works on the seniority system, and very few people had been in Washington longer than Louisiana's most powerful members:

> ⮞ **F. EDWARD HEBERT,** Chairman of Armed Services Committee of the U.S. House of Representatives. Taxes start in the House, and budgets start in Committee. As Chairman of the House Armed Services Committee, the entire U.S. military budget and the vast majority of the CIA budget started on Hebert's desk. One of his jobs was to hide most of the CIA budget in the U.S. military budget. He was known as "the military's best friend."[34]

> ⮞ **ALLEN ELLENDER** had been in the U.S. Senate for over 40 years. He was the senior senator when Huey Long was the junior senator in 1930s. Ellender sat on the Armed Services Committee of the U.S. Senate and got Hebert's budget through the Senate. Between the two, they made sure that Louisiana received its fair share of military and space contracts.[35]

> ⮞ **RUSSELL LONG,** the son of Huey Long, was Majority Whip of the U.S. Senate, Chairman of the Senate's powerful Ways and Means Committee, and a member of the Senate Banking Committee.

> ⮞ **HALE BOGGS,** Majority Whip of the U.S. House of Representatives, was the 3rd most powerful man in that body, and was considered by many to be LBJ's "man-in-the-House."

TULANE WAS A MAJOR WATERING HOLE for the Louisiana delegation, and it got "pork" whenever they could dish it out. Hebert and Ellender were in terrific position to assure that Tulane received pork in the form of CIA research contracts. CIA projects were hidden from both Soviet and American scrutiny by placing them in other agencies' budgets, such as the National Institutes of Health, in the various military branches, or in private foundations.[36] From what I heard through Tulane's student grapevine over the years, I must conclude that Tulane was definitely involved in both NIH-

and CIA-sponsored projects, especially research with psychoactive drugs.

Why would the CIA be interested in doing medical research? There were three main reasons: (1) mind control, (2) to get rid of Castro or other foreign leaders, and (3) to keep up with the Soviets.

First, mind control. The CIA's much-publicized LSD experiments were just the beginning of their efforts to get people to talk when they wanted, to sleep when they wanted, and to kill when they wanted. Their general mind-control project was called OPERATION ARTICHOKE.[38]

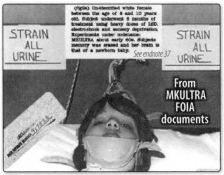

(fig2a) Un-identified white female between the age of 8 and 10 years old. Subject underwent 6 months of treatment using heavy doses of LSD, electroshock and sensory deprivation. Experiments under codename: MKULTRA about early 60s. Subjects memory was erased and her brain is that of a newborn baby. *See endnote 37*

STRAIN ALL URINE

STRAIN ALL URINE

From MKULTRA FOIA documents

Secondly, the CIA was trying to get rid of Fidel Castro and Communism in the Western Hemisphere. They tried to use their mind-altering resources and other medical tactics to discredit Castro. The project was called MKULTRA.[39] One specific plan was to spray a hallucinogenic drug in Castro's personal radio studio, so that he would make a fool out of himself during a national radio broadcast. Then they decided to kill him. Their new team was called ZR-RIFLE, and its job was to explore exotic ways of advancing the date of his death.[40] The CIA's medical director for these projects was brain-function expert Dr. Sidney Gottlieb.[41]

(The name "Gottlieb" shows up frequently in AIDS literature. Dr. Michael S. Gottlieb is an immunologist at UCLA Medical School who "discovered AIDS" in 1981. Dr. A. Arthur Gottlieb is also an immunologist and is a professor at Tulane Medical School, as is his wife. In 1972 A. Arthur Gottlieb was chosen by the U.S. Army's Biological Warfare Laboratory at Fort Detrick, Maryland to edit its book on

Dr. Sidney Gottlieb

infectious diseases.[42] Please note that I have no information to suggest whether or not there is any relationship between Dr. Sidney Gottlieb, Dr. Michael S. Gottlieb, or Dr. A. Arthur Gottlieb, so the reader should be cautious about any such conclusions.)

One of the best sources of information on "The Secret War Against Cuba" is a book called *Deadly Secrets: The CIA-Mafia War Against Castro and the Assassination of J.F.K.*, written by Warren Hinckle and William Turner. Turner is an ex-FBI agent who specialized in the political right. He worked with Jim Garrison on his JFK probe and was inside David Ferrie's apartment. His writing partner Warren Hinckle was editor of *Ramparts* magazine. In *Deadly Secrets* they made numerous references to the fact that the CIA was getting the best minds in America, and particularly from the universities, involved in figuring out exotic ways to eliminate Castro and his government from Cuba.[43]

Hinckle and Turner explained the frustration of the Kennedy White House. After spending hundreds of millions of dollars and recruiting thousands of Cuban exiles for OPERATION MONGOOSE (a free Cuba paramilitary operation based on the campus of the University of Miami), the Kennedy brothers wanted to see some action. They pressured the CIA for more tangible and immediate results and encouraged the use of alternative means to remove Castro and Communism from Cuba. Consider this passage:

> ... The pressure for more spectacular results was on Lansdale (CIA), who was in almost daily contact with the attorney general (Bobby Kennedy). He passed the pressure on to an interagency group formulating plans for approval by the SGA (Special Group Augmented — a CIA/White House task force focused on Cuba), saying that "it is our job to put the American genius to work on this project, quickly and effectively. This demands a change from the business as usual and a hard facing of the fact that we are in a combat situation — where we have been given full

command." Lansdale hinted that "we might uncork the touchdown play independently of the institutional program we are spurring."[44]

Other than naming the University of Miami, *Deadly Secrets* does not say which universities were involved. Was Tulane one of the universities asked "to put the American genius to work"? It certainly would have fit into the economic interests and anti-Communist sentiment of the New Orleans business community. It would have fit into the tradition of close cooperation between CIA officials and certain members of the Tulane Board, most notably Sam Zemurray (who was chairman of both the United Fruit Company and the Tulane University Board of Directors in 1954, when the CIA produced a coup d'etat in Guatemala to reclaim 250,000 acres of United Fruit land which had been nationalized by Guatemala's democratically elect-ed government).[45] And the proj-ect would have been considered "pork" by the elected political officials who were in a position to ap-prove the budget.

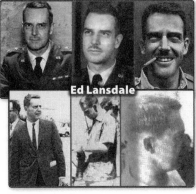

And what of Lansdale's proposal to "*uncork the touchdown play* independently of the institutional program"? Does this not suggest that there were some back channels open which were not officially or overtly connected to institutions? Was he referring to the CIA's much-publicized use of the Mafia to try to kill Castro? Or might he have been referring to an underground medical laboratory run by politically sympathetic scientists who might develop a biological means of eliminating the entire Cuban leadership?

Thirdly, the CIA would have been interested in medical research for political reasons. In the 1950s and 1960s, Soviet scientists were ahead of U.S. scientists in certain areas of medical research, one of which was the investigation

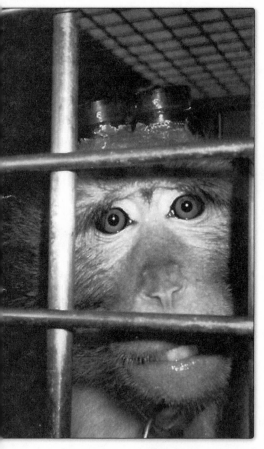

of cancer-causing monkey viruses. The Soviets were explicit, as early as 1951, about their demonstration that certain simian viruses caused a variety of cancers.[46] This was six to eight years before American government researchers produced the same results. This Soviet edge was a concern for American Cold War planners, who monitored Soviet scientific journals. From their perspective, this was just another Soviet threat. Either the Soviets might use this information to develop a sexually-transmitted biological weapon to undermine freedom in the promiscuous West, or they might develop a cure for cancer before the U.S. did and thereby cause a major American political embarrassment. Either could provide sufficient reason for the CIA not to want the U.S. to fall behind the Soviets in this important area.[47]

Whatever the motive, the U.S. government wanted the work done. The money was provided for researching monkey viruses through convenient channels, but the doctors were not supposed to talk about it. In the process, New Orleans became one of the leading centers of knowledge about immunology and retroviruses. The doctors at Tulane who specialized in cancer and pathology had access to this knowledge, to these monkeys, and to their viruses.

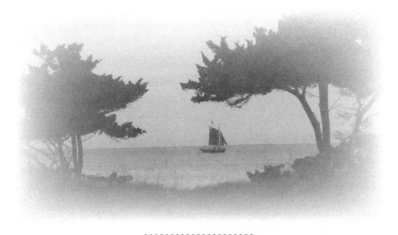

1  My father was a limb surgeon whose specialties were reconstructive surgery and the rehabilitation of amputees. He was President of the Crippled Children's Hospital and Medical Director of the Physical Rehabilitation Center at Delgado College. He knew Mary Sherman because they both taught orthopedic surgery at Tulane Medical School in the 1950s and early '60s. He never worked at Ochsner's clinic or hospital. He was not a virus researcher and was not involved in the underground medical laboratory in any way.

2  Tulane did publish the *Bulletin of the Tulane Medical School*, but it was an industry relations piece sent to other medical schools.

3  An outbreak of infectious hepatitis was reported in New Orleans in 1962 by A. Riopelle and J.F. Molloy: "Infectious Hepatitis at Yerkes Laboratories of Primate Biology," *Laboratory Primate Newsletter*, 1962, Vol. 1 (4), p. 12. See also Fiennes, *Zoonoses of Primates as related to Human Disease* (Cornell, 1965), p. 146.

4  Fiennes, *Zoonoses of Primates*, p. 142, plus *Hazards of Handling Simians* (International Association of Microbiological Associations, 1969).

5  Allison, A.C., "Simian Oncogenic Viruses," *Hazards of Handling Simians*, p. 172.

6  *Hazards of Handling Simians* (International Association of Microbiological Associations, 1969), table.

7  Fiennes, *Zoonoses of Primates*, pp. 144-150.

8  Ibid., p. 149

9  Lemonick, Michael D., "A Deadly Virus Escapes," *Time* magazine, September 5, 1994, p. 63.

10  Petrov, a Soviet scientist, used viruses to produce bone cancer in monkeys in 1951: Lapin, B.A., et al., "Use of Non-Human Primates in Medical Research, Especially in the Study of Cardiovascular Pathology and Oncology," Institute of Experimental Pathology and Therapy, U.S.S.R., in *Some Recent Developments in Comparative Medicine* (London: 1966), ed. Richard Fiennes, p. 204. In the U.S., in 1957, Stewart and Eddy discovered "polyoma," a virus that caused a variety of cancers in various animals; reported in Edward Shorter, *The Health Century* (New York, 1987), p. 198. By 1959, polyoma was considered to be essentially the same as SV-40, a monkey virus that caused various cancers in a variety of animals: Ibid., p. 201.

11  Lapin, "The Use of Non-Human Primates...," *Some Recent Developments in Comparative*

*Medicine*, ed. Fiennes, p. 206; also Spencer Munroe, "Viral Oncogenesis in the Rhesus Monkey," Ibid., p. 229; also J.S. Munroe & W.F. Windle, "Tumors induced in Primates by a Chicken Sarcoma Virus," *Science* (1963), vol. 140, p. 1415.

12  Grace, J. T. Jr. & E. A. Mirand, "Human Susceptibility to a Simian Tumor Virus," *Annals of the N.Y. Academy of Science* (1963), vol. 108, p. 1123.

13  Essex, Max  & Phyllis J. Kanki, "The Origins of the AIDS Virus," *Science of AIDS: A Scientific American Reader* (New York, 1989), p. 30.

14  Ibid., p. 32.

15  Three references to the use of radiation on tumors can be found in *Tumors of Bone and Soft Tissue* (Chicago: 1964). In "Histogenesis of Bone Tumors," p. 16, Mary Sherman discusses genetic damage inflicted on cells by irradiation. In "Giant Cell Tumor of Bone," p. 166, Sherman questions the claim that x-ray therapy turns benign tumors into deadly sarcomas. On p. 10 R. Lee Clark says, "X-ray therapy in the management of soft tissue of tumors is almost limited to Kaposi's sarcoma."

16  "The New War on Cancer via Virus Research and Chemotherapy," *Time*, July 27, 1959, p. 54.

17  Dr. John Roberts, surgeon and president of the Medical Legal Foundation, interviewed by author, October 3, 1994. Roberts was one of the doctors who used linear particle accelerators to destroy cancer tissue, preferring it to Cobalt-60 because it could be controlled more precisely, minimizing destruction of healthy tissue.

18  Roberts interview.

19  Roberts interview.

20  Fiennes, *Zoonoses of Primates*, p. 149.

21  Eyestone, Willard H.,  "Scientific and Administrative Concepts Behind the Establishment of the U.S. Primate Centers," *Some Recent Developments in Comparative Medicine*, ed. Fiennes, p. 2.

22  Ibid., p. 6.

23  Willits, Stacy, "Escapees Swinging Through Trees," *Times-Picayune/States-Item* (New Orleans), September 1, 1994, Metro News

24  Willits, Stacy, "Primate Center Back in Spotlight," *Times-Picayune* (New Orleans), September 8, 1994, p. B-1.

25  Ibid.," p. B-2.

26  Guillermo, Kathy Snow, *Monkey Business* (Washington, 1993). This book chronicles the decade-long battle between two tenacious whistle-blowers and the federal government over extreme animal cruelty in the name of science. The level of animal cruelty described in this book can only be described with words like "mutilation" and "torture." Criminal charges resulted. In the process, the whistleblowers founded PETA (People for the Ethical Treatment of Animals) and took their battle to both the U.S. Congress and the U.S. Supreme Court. The high court ruled in their favor, but not soon enough to save 60% of the monkeys from further experimentation and death. Scientific experimentation on monkeys continues today and is financed annually by $20,000,000 of U.S. taxpayer dollars.

27  Willits, "Escapees Swinging Through Trees." *Times-Picayune* (New Orleans) September 1, 1994, Metro News

28  Willits, "Primate Center Back in Spotlight." *Times-Picayune* (New Orleans) September 8, 1994, p. B-1

29  Guillermo, *Monkey Business*, p. 173.

**30** Richard Hatch, "Cancer Warfare," *Covert Action*, Winter 1991-92, p. 18.

**31** Eyestone, Willard H., "Scientific and Administrative Concepts Behind the Establishment of the U.S. Primate Centers," *Some Recent Developments in Comparative Medicine*, ed. Fiennes., p. 6.

**32** Fiennes, *Zoonoses of Primates*, p. 142; A. Riopelle and J.F. Molloy, "Infectious Hepatitis at Yerkes Laboratories of Primate Biology," *Laboratory Primate Newsletter*, 1962, vol. 1-4, p. 12.

**33** Shorter, *Health Century*, p. 65.

**34** Word-of-mouth description of Congressman Hebert which this author personally heard in his district in the 1960s.

**35** Not the least of which was the NASA facility that builds the huge fuel tank for the space shuttle. Vice-President Lyndon Johnson was head of NASA when this facility was announced, and President when it was built.

**36** Marks, John, *Search for the Manchurian Candidate* (New York, 1980).

**37** (fig2a) "Un-identified white female between the age of 8 and 10 years old. Subject underwent 6 months of treatment using heavy doses of LSD, electroshock and sensory deprivation. Experiments under codename: MKULTRA about early 60s. Subjects memory was erased and her brain is that of a newborn baby."

**38** Russell, Dick, *The Man Who Knew Too Much* (New York, 1992), p. 380-381.

**39** Ibid., p. 380., and *Project MKULTRA, the CIA's Program of Research in Behavioral Modification*, U.S. Senate Select Committee on Intelligence, August 3, 1977

**40** Russell, *The Man Who Knew Too Much*, p. 381.

**41** Ibid., p. 380.

**42** Gottlieb, A. Arthur, et al., *Transfer Factor* (New York, 1976).

**43** Hinckle, Warren and Turner, William, *Deadly Secrets* (New York, 1992), p. 122.

**44** Ibid., p. 135. Caution: James DiEugenio told me that the source of these statements is ultimately CIA officer Howard Hunt, and that he may have fabricated them to make his anti-Castro activities to appear to have been authorized by the White House. If so, we should remember that fabricating the authorization does not equal fabricating the activity. In fact, there is little reason to fabricate the authorization unless one was trying to legitimize an otherwise illegal activity. Or to put it bluntly, it is unlikely that someone would try to legitimize an activity that did not exist.

**45** Ibid., p. 40.

**46** B.A. Lapin et al, "Use of Non-Human Primates in Medical Research, Especially in the Study of Cardiovascular Pathology and Oncology," Institute of Experimental Pathology and Therapy, U.S.S.R., *Some Recent Developments in Comparative Medicine*, ed. Fiennes, p. 204.

**47** Who would synthesize a disease for which there is no cure? Consider the Defense Appropriations Hearing in the U.S. House of Representatives in 1970: "Within the next 5 to 10 years, it would probably be possible to make a new infective microorganism which would differ in certain important aspects from any known disease-causing organisms. Most important of these is that it might be refractory to the immunological and therapeutic processes upon which we depend to maintain our relative freedom from infectious disease." While I personally do not think that this conversation led to HIV-1, it does show the thinking of a biological weapons developer. Of course, the rationale was defensive: we'd better do it before some bad guy does.

～～～～～～

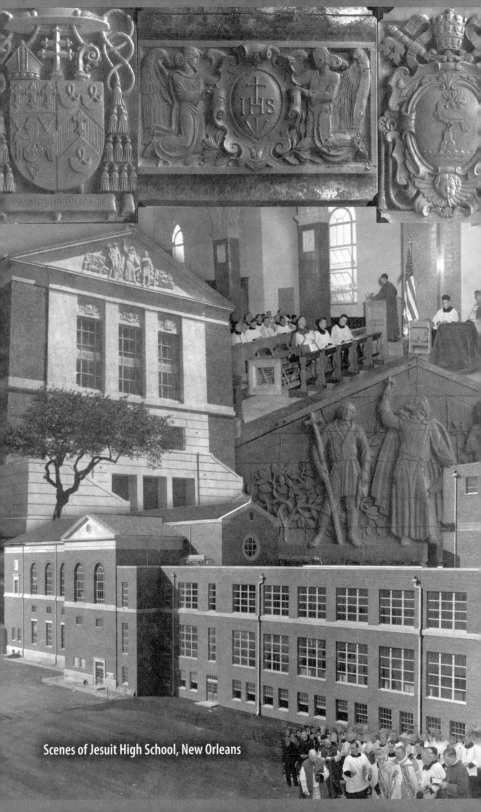

Scenes of Jesuit High School, New Orleans

# CHAPTER 2

# The Classroom

CARROLLTON AVENUE is a wide, tree-lined boulevard which runs north and south, bisecting New Orleans and connecting the Mississippi River to Lake Pontchartrain. At its mid-point, in a residential neighborhood near the corner of Canal Street, stands a huge four-story brick building resembling a fortress. It covers an entire city block. This is Jesuit High School, where the Jesuit priests have been educating the future leaders of New Orleans for over 100 years. The Jesuits are famous, even notorious, for demanding academic excellence. Therefore, the economic and power elite of this predominantly Catholic city send their male children to the Jesuits to be educated. Admission is highly competitive. Discipline is strict. Military uniforms are worn. High performance is required. And nobility is expected. The students are trained for success and for leadership roles in tomorrow's society. Above all else, they are expected to carry the militant social conscience and uncompromising values of their Jesuit educators with them into their future roles.

I attended Jesuit High School from 1966 to 1969. During this time, New Orleans District Attorney Jim Garrison was investigating the assassination of President Kennedy. This investigation culminated in the trial of New Orleans businessman Clay Shaw in early 1969. The amount of press coverage this received in New Orleans was staggering. And much of this was a contrived media smog, aggressively negative toward Garrison. The national press had been particularly vicious, with anti-Garrison articles like "Jolly Green Giant in Wonderland."[1] They basically claimed that the New Orleans District Attorney had completely lost his marbles, was recklessly prosecuting homosexuals for spite, and suffered from paranoid delusions of grandeur.

Garrison, in turn, appeared on national television and stated in unambiguous language that a faction within the U.S. Central Intelligence Agency had murdered the President of the United States. Gesturing to the camera, he waved sworn statements from witnesses who claimed that their testimony to the Warren Commission had been altered to distort important information. If that was not enough, he went further, reminding the American people that the order to hide the hard evidence (Kennedy's x-rays and the autopsy photos) from the American people came directly from the Oval

Jim Garrison announcing the arrest of Clay Shaw

*Dr. Mary's Monkey*

Office in the White House. Garrison said bluntly that there had been a "coup d'etat" right here in the United States and that the press had ignored it.

This was a difficult time for people whose families were connected to the Garrison investigation. Several of my close friends had family members involved, and I saw their dilemma first hand. The basic situation was this: If Kennedy's murder had been planned in New Orleans, then something should be done about it. Many people supported Garrison's efforts. He was, after all, a legally-elected law enforcement official investigating a murder within his jurisdiction.

On the other hand, Garrison was investigating some sensitive issues and some very important people. On the national front, he had discovered the U.S. government's secret war against Cuba, uncovering in the process that elements of the CIA were involved with the Mafia and were trying to kill Castro. (Today we know that this is true, since it was established beyond any reasonable doubt in 1975 by the U.S. Senate Intelligence Committee, but back in the 1960s it was political heresy.) On the local front, Garrison was investigating, and in some cases arresting, some of New Orleans' most prominent citizens.

For example, Clay Shaw, whom Garrison arrested and charged with conspiring to murder John Kennedy, was former General Manager of the International Trade Mart, one of the city's most important business institutions. Garrison claimed that Shaw had personally been associated with Lee

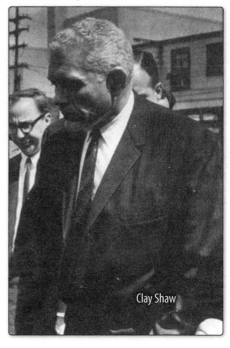

Clay Shaw

Harvey Oswald and had helped Kennedy's killers by setting up Oswald to take the fall for Kennedy's death. Shaw, of course, claimed he never knew Oswald and had never worked for the CIA. (Today, both Shaw's association with Oswald and his association with the CIA have been established.[2] But at the time both Shaw and the CIA denied it.)

Particularly baffling was Garrison's inability to get the press on his side, especially the local press. The whole situation was very confusing, even embarrassing at times. Garrison was under a gag order. We all waited for the trial. On Sunday, March 1, 1969, the jury acquitted Clay Shaw of all charges in less than one hour. Everyone was stunned. After two solid years of heavy publicity and waiting for the evidence to come out in the trial, it seemed like it should have taken more than one hour for the jury to decide the verdict. What was going on? Was Garrison really crazy as his critics claimed, or had he been successfully shut down by forces inside the federal government?

In the days following the announcement of the "not guilty" verdict, I went to school as usual. There was a remarkable silence. From Monday morning to Friday afternoon, I did not hear the names Kennedy, Garrison, or Shaw once from any student or teacher! Then on Friday afternoon all that changed.

In one of my classes there was a student named Nicky. His father was Dr. Nicolas Chetta, the Coroner of Orleans Parish (an officer known as the Medical Examiner in many locales) who was involved with Garrison's investigation. Dr. Chetta was somewhat of a local celebrity for us. Not only was he an elected politician whose name was frequently in the press, but he was the team physician for our football team. Once he even took our class on a memorable field trip to the city morgue.

Nicky, the son, was well liked. He was a friendly, modest, boy-next-door who was well-intentioned and sincere. He did not strive for any "star" position and certainly did not trade on his father's reputation. I never knew anybody that did not like him. He and I were friends, but we were not what you would call "close." We went to the same school, lived in the same neighborhood, and both had fathers who were doctors.

So, I was sitting in class at Jesuit High School in early March of 1969. The lesson finished early, and the teacher asked the class if anyone had any thoughts on the Clay Shaw verdict.

Nicky erupted, saying in a loud, tense voice that Garrison had gotten a "raw deal." We all knew Nicky to be quiet and even-keeled. This outburst seemed quite out of character. But we all respected his sincerity. We knew who his father was, and we all saw the same ridiculous news coverage night after night. We were all confused, and we wanted to hear what he had to say. No one counterattacked. The room was quiet. We waited to see what would happen next. The teacher said patiently, "What do you mean?"

Then Nicky started talking. He held the class spellbound for fifteen minutes with information about the investigation, much of which had either not been revealed to the press or which they had basically ignored. We all listened carefully. His points included:

- that someone, presumably the FBI or the CIA, had bugged Garrison's office and conference rooms, had stolen and/ or photocopied his files concerning Clay Shaw, and had turned them over to Shaw's attorneys;
- that *all* of Garrison's extradition requests for witnesses from other states had been turned down, as had *all* of his requests to subpoena former federal officials, preventing him from assembling the pieces of his puzzle in a court of law;
- that an ex-airline pilot named David Ferrie and a former high-ranking FBI official named Guy Banister had been training anti-Castro Cubans for paramilitary as-

saults against Cuba at a secret training camp across Lake Pontchartrain; and

⚐ that Ferrie and Banister had stolen weapons for this operation from a company in Houma, Louisiana which was operating as a CIA front. Nicky said he couldn't pronounce the name of the company, but said that the name "looked German, but sounded French." (It turns out that he was referring to the Schlumberger Tool Company, pronounced locally "Slum-ber-jay.")

Someone asked Nicky why we had not heard all this in the press.[3] It was a fair question. We had all been taught that the press was the "Watchdog of Government." How could they have overlooked these obvious and important points. Nicky paused and repeated Garrison's favorite saying: "Treason never prospers, for if it prospers, none dare call it treason." This was just the sort of riddle that made it hard for the public to understand what Garrison was up to.

Then Nicky turned his attention to David Ferrie and started talking about him in more detail. (Today Ferrie is considered a central character in several assassination theories, but back then he had been little more than a blip on the television screen during the first year of Garrison's investigation.) His sudden death on the eve of his arrest for conspiracy to murder the President was considered by many to be a very suspicious coincidence, even though his death had officially been ruled to be from "natural causes."

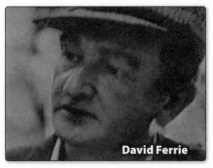
David Ferrie

Ferrie was an unusual man in many respects. Professionally, he was a pilot. Politically, he was a notorious right-wing extremist.[4] Personally, he was completely bald from head to toe, and was a homosexual who favored teenage boys. Ferrie's bizarre appearance and personal history was one of the things that earned six-foot six-inch

Jim Garrison the nickname "Jolly Green Giant," because "he put fruits and nuts in the can." Ferrie died several days after Garrison's investigation was made public. Garrison, who was about to arrest Ferrie for conspiring to murder President Kennedy, thought that either Ferrie had been murdered to silence him or that Ferrie had silenced himself. But it was the Coroner's job, not the District Attorney's, to rule on the cause of death. Dr. Chetta, Nicky's father, was the Coroner, and said that he found *no evidence* of foul play. Therefore, he ruled that Ferrie died of natural causes (a ruptured blood vessel in the brain), and noted that Ferrie had been under enormous stress.

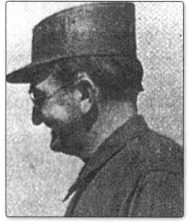

Nicky continued: Ferrie had known Lee Harvey Oswald when he was a cadet at the Civil Air Patrol and had been seen with him that summer. Ferrie's role in the assassination was as a get-away pilot. He reportedly spent the two weeks before the assassination at Mafia boss Carlos Marcello's hunting camp across the Mississippi River. He may have been flying people and supplies around to position them for the assassination.

Now all this seemed pretty wild, but it got even wilder. Nicky said that the day they announced Ferrie's death, Bobby Kennedy had called his house to discuss the cause of death with his father.[5] A murmur shot through the room. Nicky countered by saying he had answered the phone himself. Thinking it was a prank, he hung up on the then-Senator. But Kennedy called back. This time Nicky's father answered the phone himself.

Then Nicky started talking about Ferrie's apartment, which his father had seen the day Ferrie died. Ferrie lived alone. But in his closets they had found both women's clothing and priest's robes. They also found a small medical laboratory with a dozen mice in cages which he used for medical experiments. His medical equipment included microscopes, syringes, surgical tools, and a medical library. When they talked to Ferrie's other landlords, they were told of a full-scale laboratory in his apartment with thousands of mice in cages. It seemed clear that he was *inducing cancer* in the mice! Ferrie claimed that he was looking for a cure for cancer, but Garrison's investigators thought that he was trying to figure out a way to use cancer as an assassination weapon, presumably against Castro and his followers. Nicky added, almost as an aside, that Garrison's investigative team thought that this may have been how Jack Ruby died, murdered by induced cancer to silence him.

By this point, you could have heard a pin drop in the room. Back in 1969, we (and presumably the public) were taught that cancer was "a spontaneous disease," meaning it *could not* be created, transferred, caught or induced. Words like "carcinogenic" and "cancer-causing chemicals" were not yet part of the popular American vocabulary. Viral cancers were not discussed. The idea of "inducing cancer" was very strange indeed, and, scientifically, we (the students) considered it somewhere between "questionable" and "impossible."

A student asked, "How could they induce cancer?" The question was sincere, but doubting. I remember hoping, for both Nicky's sake and Garrison's, that the answer made some kind of common sense. Garrison's case already looked like Mardi Gras to the rest of the country. It did not need another bald, right-wing, counter-revolutionary, contraband pilot wearing a wig and a dress and saying the Catholic mass in Latin. And this particular claim, about inducing cancer, was not only out of John Q. Public's experience, it was also over the edge of what we understood to be scientific reality. Nicky sensed the doubt. You could see he felt it. He remained calm. Slowly and cautiously, he said that they had been "injecting mice with monkey viruses."

*Dr. Mary's Monkey*

*Monkey viruses!* The room groaned. I rolled my eyes and dropped my forehead into my hand. Why did it have to be monkey viruses? Garrison was already misunderstood because his plot was stranger than jazz — too complex, too subtle, and too bizarre for the American TV audience. Why couldn't it have been something simpler, like injecting rats with radiation. Cancer from plutonium! The public might follow that. But cancer from monkey viruses? The rest of the country would never buy it. The very words conjured up a dark collage of alienating images — diseases imported from tropical jungles in the bellies of insects and mixed with monkey heads boiled in voodoo rituals on the edge of the Louisiana swamp at midnight. It was all "so New Orleans."

You could feel that everyone in the room wanted to believe Nicky, but it was hard to know what to say. Then somebody said, "I don't get it. How could a monkey virus cause cancer?" Nicky said he didn't understand that part either. My brain was about to bust, but I wasn't about to bring Tulane into the conversation.

Then another student blurted out that there was a "kid" down at Tulane Medical School who was dying from the total collapse of his immune system. They couldn't figure out what was causing it. They gave him every antibiotic they had and nothing worked. He would get better for a while, and then he would get worse. While this comment was interesting, it sounded "off the wall." Two thoughts raced through my head. First, what did the uncontrollable collapse of an immune system have to do with our discussion about monkey viruses? And I also said to myself, I'm obviously not the only student at Jesuit that has a family member working at Tulane Medical School. I was certain that this was "insider information." It was the first time I had ever heard it. (But not the last!)

Then another student jumped into the exchange: "That means they were developing a *biological weapon!* What happens if it escapes into the human population?"

The room fell to a new level of silence. Let's call it fear. No one breathed. The Jesuits drilled social responsibility into us until it came out of our ears. Everybody knew that developing a biological weapon was high taboo. Twenty teenagers sat in dead silence pondering this mind-boggling question for a moment that hung like an hour. Then the bell rang.

In a routine voice, the teacher thanked Nicky for sharing his thoughts and dismissed the class. As I gathered my books together, I turned to the student next to me and made that nervous remark:, "Well, the good news is if there's a bizarre global epidemic involving cancer and a monkey virus thirty years from now, *at least we'll know where it came from.*"

I left the class and went back to my homeroom. I didn't talk to anyone else for the rest of the day. All I could think about were the monkey viruses, and I wasn't about to try to explain that to anyone.

When I got home that afternoon, I put my books away and called to my mother who was in the other end of the house. I said, "Do you have time for some *useless information?*" These were code words we frequently used for discussing things of interest. "Useless information" was one step above gossip. It could be anything from a new scientific theory about how the dinosaurs died, to speculation on who was going to get indicted next in the growing grain scandal. Her voice rang back down the hall. She would be right there.

When she came into the room, I told her that Dr. Chetta's son was in one of my classes and that he told us an amazing story about Garrison's investigation. "Oh, yes," she said. "I know who he is." I recapped Nicky's comments and ploughed through the stories of Ferrie's wigs, his dresses, and his religious vestments. She listened attentively, acknowledging each point as I went, but exhibiting no surprise whatsoever. Frankly, I was expecting a little bit more of a reaction, but New Orleans is a very tolerant place. If the transvestite stuff didn't get a reaction out of her, I was sure the medical stuff would. So I told her about the medical experiments and the laboratory with the thousands of white mice and waited for a response. Nothing. She was unfazed. I was getting frustrated. So I told her about the monkey viruses, expecting it to fall on her like a bombshell, like it had on me. Still nothing.

"But Mom," I said in an exasperated and serious tone, "weren't they researching monkey viruses down at Tulane Medical School? Do you think there could be a connection?"

"Well," she said, "one of the doctors from Tulane was involved in that lab."

Now, I was stunned. "Wait a second," I countered and tried to get my bearings. "Are you telling me that a *professor* from Tulane Medical School was involved in David Ferrie's underground medical laboratory? The one with the thousands of mice?"

"Oh, yes," she said matter-of-factly. "Everybody down at the medical school was talking about it. It was in that *Playboy* interview with Garrison that you had around here a couple of years ago. I took it to Boston with me that Christmas to see your sister."

"Who was the doctor?" I muttered. I could barely get the question out.

"Her name was Mary Sherman. Daddy knew her. He had a lot of respect for her. I think she was a pathologist. You know, she was more of a researcher than a physician. A cancer researcher, I think."

"What happened to her?" I asked, resigning myself to the fact that some terrible fate must have befallen her.

"She was killed. Murdered. A terrible thing. Slashed with a knife, dismembered, and set on fire. It looked like a sexual killing, you know. But the grapevine said that whoever killed her knew what they were doing with a knife ... maybe they even had a high level of medical knowledge, just judging by the way the cuts were done. What a terrible way to go!"

"Did they figure out who did it?" I queried hopefully.

"No. The investigation was shut down all of a sudden. It was all very hush-hush, like it had been shut down from above. But they think she knew her murderer and probably let them into her apartment."

"You said Daddy knew her?"

"Oh, yes. They worked together for years. She was older and considerably higher up the ladder than he was, but Daddy always said that she was one of the top people in her field. He had a lot of respect for her. Professional respect, I mean."

"Did you ever meet her?"

"Yes, we had dinner at her apartment one night. A strange woman, but very sophisticated and very well travelled. And very into theatre and literature. I felt very out of place. All I could talk about was my children. I remember that her friends were very strange."

"What do you mean by *strange*?"

"Oh, they were not the type of people we were used to associating with. They lived in the French Quarter and were involved in the theatre and all that. Mary was somewhat of an outcast at the medical school. Most of the doctors we knew had wives and children. Everyone respected Mary professionally, but she ran in different social circles. I remember driving home after the dinner. The normal protocol, like we used to do in the Navy, said the next step would have been for us to invite her over to our house for dinner. So I asked your father if he wanted to do that. He thought about it for a while and said, 'No,' adding that Mary's social circle was a little weirder than he wanted to be associated with. That was the last time we discussed it."

Suddenly I felt exhausted. I shook my head in dismay and breathed deeply. This was stranger and more disturbing than even Nicky's story had been. It's one thing for a crackpot to be doing home-brewed cancer experiments in his apartment, but it's something else to have the involvement of a highly respected and professionally competent cancer researcher working in the crackpot's lab. What was going on here? And to have it all so close to my family! I didn't know what else to say. I thought again about my wise-crack: "If there's a bizarre

50                                          *Dr. Mary's Monkey*

global epidemic ... *at least we'll know where it came from.*" I was depressed. We were silent. My mother went back to her task down the hall. I changed clothes and walked over to a friend's house, trying to forget about it.

1   "Jolly Green Giant in Wonderland," *Time*, August 2, 1968, p. 56.

2   Davy, Bill "License & Registration Please," *Probe*, June 1994, p. 5 & July 1994, p. 1. The Clinton incident is discussed in detail later. *Probe* is the newsletter from the CTKA, Citizens for the Truth about the Kennedy Assassination.

3   Actually, much of the information which Nicky discussed had been disclosed by Garrison in *Playboy* in October 1967. It was startling to us, because most of it had been systematically ignored by the press.

4   How extreme is extreme? In the *Playboy* interview Garrison said Ferrie had belonged to the Minutemen, an ultra-right-wing paramilitary group. Ferrie claimed that he left the group because they were too moderate. On the other hand, the Minutemen may have simply objected to Ferrie's mental instability, or his personal life, and kicked him out.

5   Robert F. "Bobby" Kennedy was President John F. Kennedy's younger brother, and served as U.S. Attorney General during his presidency. After the JFK assassination, Bobby was elected U.S. Senator from New York, and was then himself assassinated in 1968 as he sought the Democratic nomination for President.

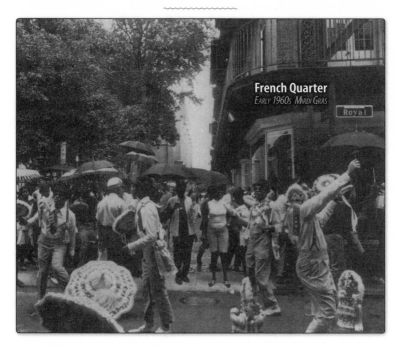

French Quarter
*Early 1960s Mardi Gras*
Royal

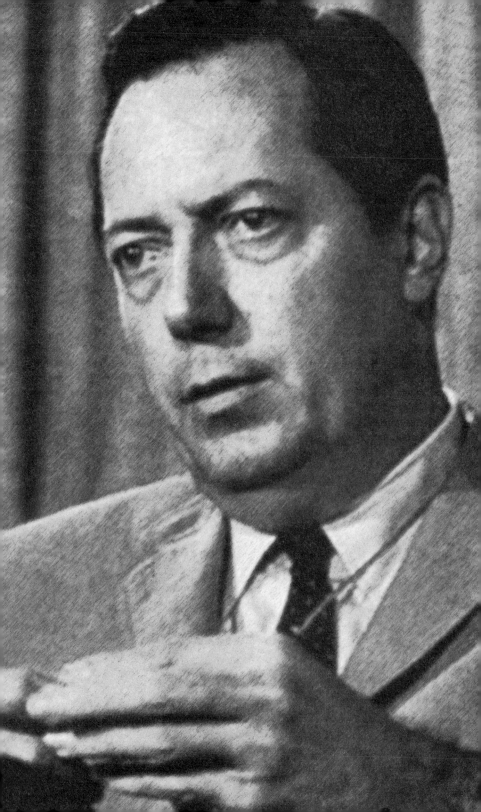

# CHAPTER 3

# Jimbo

JIM GARRISON WAS ONE OF THE MOST CONTROVERSIAL figures in modern American history. Attitudes about him tend to be polarized. To his supporters, he was a hero, the only public official to have the courage to dig for the truth about President Kennedy's assassination and to confront the American government and the American people with it. To his critics, he was a politically ambitious tyrant whose ruthless use of power was driven by his wild imagination. We do not need to judge Garrison, but we do need to understand him, because his statement recorded in an interview with a national magazine was for a long time the only documentary evidence we had in hand connecting Dr. Mary Sherman to David Ferrie's underground medical laboratory. So who was he?

Jim Garrison was born in Iowa in 1921.[1] His father abandoned his family when he was three. His mother moved him to Chicago and then to New Orleans. His original name was Earling Carothers Garrison. He changed it to "Jim" in 1946. His nickname "Jimbo" was a friendly corruption of the words "Jim" and "jumbo," based on his enormous size, six-feet six-inches.

His other nickname, "The Jolly Green Giant,"[2] was also based upon his size, but was intended to ridicule him in the press.

In 1940 Garrison joined the U.S. Army at the age of nineteen and became a pilot. During World War II he flew missions over France and Germany, acting as a forward observer for artillery units. At the end of the war, his unit liberated the infamous Dachau Concentration Camp, where he witnessed the horrors of Nazi incarceration first hand. It was there that he came to understand what one human being was capable of inflicting upon another in the name of a flag. It solidified his hatred of fascism, and his fear of autocratic governments.

After the war, he returned to New Orleans and earned a law degree from Tulane University. Soon he started working for the FBI, knocking on doors for background checks in the Northwest. Preferring combat to boredom, he re-enlisted in the army for the Korean War and, when that was over, returned to New Orleans. There he joined the National Guard and, like many young attorneys in New Orleans, became an assistant DA for a few years before starting a private practice.

In 1960, Garrison mounted his first political campaign: to become a judge in Criminal District Court; he lost. In 1961, he mounted a second political campaign, for the District Attorney of Orleans Parish, and surprised the political establishment by winning. Re-elected twice, he held that position for twelve years, until 1974 when he was defeated by Harry Connick, father of the popular singer/musician Harry Connick, Jr.

As District Attorney, Garrison positioned himself as "a tough-on-crime enforcer." He cracked down on prostitution and gambling in the French Quarter. Self-righteous and outspoken, he criticized police for being soft on crime and criminal court judges for refusing to finance his investigations into organized crime. His moralistic stance made him popular with some groups and unpopular with others. (The

*Dr. Mary's Monkey*

drummer in Jack Ruby's nightclub told me, "Garrison was a terrible man who ruined a lot of people.")

Perhaps his most important contribution to American law was a landmark victory in the U.S. Supreme Court in 1964. The New Orleans criminal court judges he criticized for being soft on crime had sued him for defamation. Garrison counter-sued on the grounds that he, as a citizen, had the right to criticize public officials. It was, as he called it, "the essence of self-government." The high court agreed.

A second indication of Garrison's penchant for rights of the individual against the state was his intervention in a racial-integration crisis on behalf of a New Orleans merchant who had been arrested for selling books by black author James Baldwin. The New Orleans Police Department felt the book, *Another Country,* violated the prevailing political and racial sensibilities, and should not be sold. To Garrison, it was just another book burning. Politically, this event solidified his support among the black population in New Orleans, since they had never seen anyone from the District Attorney's office intervene on their behalf before.

These actions gave Garrison strong political viability across all Louisiana. He was a potential candidate for any statewide office, such as State Attorney General, Governor, or U.S. Senator.

Garrison moved swiftly into the JFK probe. The day after Kennedy's death, the press announced that Lee Harvey Oswald had spent the summer before the assassination in New Orleans. Before Oswald was even buried, Garrison was tracking down New Orleanian David Ferrie on a tip that Ferrie was a getaway pilot in a larger assassination plot. Garrison's office raided David Ferrie's apartment, picked up Ferrie for questioning, and turned him over to the FBI. The FBI promptly released Ferrie, and Garrison dropped the matter.

Three years later, in November 1966, Garrison was persuaded to re-open his investigation into the JFK assassination by U.S. Senator Russell Long. Senator Long arranged to finance Garrison's inquiry secretly through an organization called Truth and Consequences, formed specifically for that purpose at Long's request by New Orleans oil man Joe Rault. In February 1967, a press leak concerning Garrison's secret investigation into the JFK assassination, followed immediately by the death of his prime suspect David Ferrie, catapulted Jim Garrison into the world media spotlight overnight. If it was fame he sought, he got it. And with it, the focus of assassination speculation shifted from Dallas to New Orleans.

In March 1967 Garrison arrested New Orleans businessman Clay Shaw for conspiring to assassinate President Kennedy. At first Garrison called the assassination a crime organized by extremist elements of the anti-Castro community, and to prevent any misinterpretation, he specifically pointed out that his team had not found any evidence of involvement by the CIA itself. But in May 1967, all that changed.

Garrison upped the stakes by announcing on national television that Kennedy's death was a coup d'etat organized by elements inside the CIA, particularly in its Plans Division.[3] What followed was two years of heavy character assault on Garrison.

The heart of Garrison's case was that he had associated Clay Shaw with Lee Harvey Oswald during the summer of 1963. Garrison believed Shaw's contact with Oswald was part of a deliberate attempt to set up Oswald to take the blame for Kennedy's impending assassination.[4] In particular, Garrison claimed that Shaw tried to help Oswald get a job at a mental hospital in Jackson, Louisiana, near the town of Clinton. According to Garrison, Shaw drove Oswald to Clinton so Oswald could register to vote in hopes of improving his chances of getting the job at the hospital.

As luck would have it, the Congress for Racial Equality was sponsoring a voter registration for black voters that day. When a black Cadillac drove into the center of the small Louisiana town, folks watched closely and curiously. Were these FBI agents? The press? Outside agitators? A young white man emerged from the back of the Cadillac and got in line to register. He made a memorable impression, since he was the only white person in the line and since he was not a resident of the area. Numerous eyewitnesses identified the person who got out of the Cadillac as Oswald, and, of course, the man had given his name to the registrar of voters as Lee Harvey Oswald.

The more difficult question: Who was driving the car? Witnesses said he looked like Clay Shaw, a white male in his fifties with wavy gray hair and a stern face. This described Shaw well enough, but it also described other people equally well. There was less difficulty identifying the other passenger in the car. His orange hair and painted-on eyebrows made seeing David Ferrie a truly unforgettable experience for anyone. Since it was already established that Ferrie knew Guy Banister and Oswald (all of whom were dead by '69), it was difficult for Garrison to prove that the man driving the car was actually Clay Shaw and not someone else, like Banister. Shaw, of course, claimed he never knew Oswald or Ferrie and had never been to Clinton. Garrison failed to prove the connection to the satisfaction of the jury. Shaw was acquitted.

Garrison counterattacked, claiming that Shaw had lied under oath and charged him with thirteen counts of perjury, confident that he would win the perjury conviction in the next trial. The federal government intervened, however, and dismissed the perjury charges; thus with the acquittal of Clay Shaw in 1969, Garrison was neutralized as a political force.

A decade later, the U.S. Congress's House Select Committee on Assassinations took a second look at the Clinton incident. On March 14, 1978, they took the testimony of Clinton town marshal John Manchester in Washington.[5] Manchester said that he approached the black Cadillac from which Oswald had emerged that summer day in 1963 and, acting as the town's law enforcement officer, instructed the driver to identify himself and to produce his driver's license.

The driver gave his name as "Clay Shaw from the International Trade Mart" and produced a driver's license which matched. For some reason, the HSCA took his testimony in "Executive Session" and kept this information *secret from the American public* for sixteen years.

We only know about it today because of documents released through the JFK Assassination Materials Act of 1992.[6] With information of this magnitude continuing to come to light, it will be tomorrow's historians, and not yesterday's press, who will have to judge Jim Garrison and his assassination theory. To call him "discredited" is extremely premature, despite the numerous attempts to make him appear so. We may owe Garrison an apology before it's all over.

In 1971, Garrison's life grew still more entangled. Based on information from a disgruntled former DA-office employee named Pershing Gervais, attorneys for the federal government charged Garrison with accepting kickbacks in exchange for not prosecuting illegal pinball operations. The trial lingered until August of 1973. Garrison defended himself, arguing that the charges against him were fabricated and that the evidence had been tampered with. The jury found him not guilty.[7]

The federal attorneys immediately struck back, charging Garrison with failing to pay income taxes on the same alleged kickbacks. Again, Garrison defended himself and was found not guilty. But the years of negative publicity had been too much for any publicly elected official to survive. He was now politically destroyed, and subsequently lost the 1974 election.

After four years of low visibility in private practice, he ran for a prestigious (yet lower profile) office, a judgeship on Louisiana's 4th Circuit Court of Appeal. He won the ten-year term and was re-elected in 1988.

During these post-investigation years, he wrote several books about the JFK assassination, the last of which was *On the Trail of the Assassins*, which Oliver Stone used as one basis for his movie *JFK*. Garrison even made a cameo appearance in *JFK*, ironically playing the role of U.S. Chief Justice Earl Warren.

Jim Garrison died in 1992 after a long illness, at the age of seventy-one.

At the height of his media visibility in 1967, *Playboy* magazine offered Garrison an interview.[8] Distrustful of the press and their motives, Garrison accepted the interview on the condition that Playboy present his whole story unedited. The 12 hour interview covered 25 pages, and presented his complex case to the American public for the first time. *Playboy* cannot be accused of being sympathetic. They began their interview with a series of questions, not about the assassination, but about the accusations that Garrison had bribed, drugged, and threatened witnesses. Even the title of the interview referred to him as *"the embattled district attorney"* [italics and lower case in original].

We find the first mention of the Ferrie-Sherman cancer experiments in this interview, in the midst of a barrage of questions about Jack Ruby.[9] Garrison was busy baffling his interviewer with answers like: "In Jack Ruby's case, his murder of Lee Harvey Oswald was the sanest act he ever committed." We pick up the interview there, right before the critical section:

GARRISON: ...and he (Ruby) became the prisoner of the Dallas police, forced over a year later to beg Earl Warren to take him back to Washington, because he wanted to tell the truth about "Why my act was committed, but it can't be said here ... my life is in danger here." But Ruby never got to Washington, and he's joined the long list of witnesses with vital information who have shuffled off this mortal coil.

PLAYBOY: Penn Jones, Norman Mailer and others have charged that Ruby was injected with live cancer cells in order to silence him. Do you agree?

GARRISON: I can't agree or disagree, since I have no evidence one way or the other. But we have discovered that David Ferrie had a rather curious hobby in addition to his study of cartridge trajectories: cancer research. He filled his apartment with white mice — at one point he had almost 2,000, and neighbors complained — wrote a medical treatise on the subject and worked with a number of New Orleans doctors on means of inducing cancer in mice. After the assassination, one of these physicians, Dr. Mary Sherman, was found hacked to death with a kitchen knife in her New Orleans apartment. Her murder is listed as unsolved. Ferrie's experiments may have been purely theoretical and Dr. Sherman's death completely unrelated to her association with Ferrie; but I do find it interesting that Jack Ruby died of cancer a few weeks after his conviction for murder had been overruled in appeals court and he was ordered to stand trial outside of Dallas — thus allowing him to speak freely if he so desired. I would also note that there was little hesitancy in killing Lee Harvey Oswald in order to prevent *him* from talking, so there is no reason to suspect that any more consideration would have been shown Jack Ruby if *he* had posed a threat to the architects of the conspiracy.

Let's go back through this passage carefully. First, who are Penn Jones and Norman Mailer?

William Penn Jones, Jr. was a retired U.S. Army officer who became an editor of a local newspaper in a small town outside of Dallas. He was famous for his "stir-the-shit" editorial style, particularly when it came to the JFK assassination. I asked two people who worked for him over the years if they knew anything about this claim. They said they did not, adding that Penn frequently said things that he could not back up. I tried to contact him, but was told that, due to his frail health, his wife no longer let people interview him. He died in 1998.

Norman Mailer is a New York-based writer whose strand of credibility traces back to a Pulitzer Prize he won for his World War II combat novel, *The Naked and the Dead*. He is a colorful character who is as famous for his personal behavior as for his stunning prose style.

I did contact Mailer and asked him what was behind his comment about Ruby's cancer. He emphatically, thoroughly, and completely denied ever having made any such comment about Jack Ruby or his cancer. So either *Playboy*'s interviewer was operating from bad information, or perhaps Mailer forgot what he had said. Either way, I was not able to gain any helpful information by tracking down Penn Jones and Norman Mailer.

Back to the interview:

> GARRISON: But we *have* discovered that David Ferrie had a rather curious hobby in addition to his study of cartridge trajectories: cancer research.

Cartridge trajectories? Isn't a cartridge the part of the bullet that stays in the gun after the slug flies out of the barrel? Yes, it is. And doesn't trajectory mean the flight path of the projectile? Yes, it does. And when you pull back the bolt to clear the chamber before inserting another bullet, the empty cartridge flies out of the rifle, to the right and to the rear. So what was Garrison talking about?

Earlier in the same interview, Garrison discussed some of the materials they found in Ferrie's apartment. His investigators found unusual notations in the margins of one of his books, a reference manual on high-powered rifles. It showed that Ferrie had measured exactly how many feet an empty cartridge flew when ejected from that rifle and at what angle.[10] Hence the apparent oxymoron "cartridge trajectory."

Why would someone want to measure cartridge trajectories? One reason is it would facilitate removing undesired evidence from a sniper's nest. On the other hand, if you wanted to construct a phony sniper's nest, you would know exactly where to place the cartridges.

But for this investigation the important words in that sentence are the last two: "cancer research." It is widely reported by people who knew Ferrie personally that he was actively involved in cancer research. For example, one of Ferrie's friends said, "Ferrie was going to fix everything. Find a cure for cancer. Get rid of Communism."[11] This activity stretched from his days as an airline pilot (late 1950s) until his death in 1967.

Continuing with the interview, Garrison states that Ferrie wrote a medical treatise. Ferrie wrote a medical treatise? What did it say about viral cancer experiments? Did it talk about using x-rays? Where is it today?

When I started this investigation, we did not know the answer to any of these questions. But today we do, and it is an important link in the chain of evidence, as we shall see.

It is also clear from his interview that Garrison thought that there was *more than one doctor* working with David Ferrie. Who were the other doctors? What was this claim based upon? If a group of doctors were working with Ferrie, it might be safe to assume that it was really their lab and not Ferrie's. This is an important point. If Ferrie was simply an executor, instead of the main instigator, the dimensions of the project change dramatically. It also means that the lab may have continued operating after Ferrie's death in 1967.

It should be noted that, in the summer of 1967, Garrison was talking about arresting one particular New Orleans doctor: Dr. Alton Ochsner.[12] (William Gurvich, one of Garrison's staff who resigned from the case, is said to have disclosed this fact to Ochsner.) Was Ochsner one of the other doctors Garrison was referring to in this interview when he said "a number of New Orleans doctors"? And if so, was Garrison saying this as a threat to get Ochsner, a political enemy, to stop his anti-Garrison activities? Or did he have information that he could not (or would not) disclose about Ochsner? I will say, speaking as a political observer, that if Garrison had attacked Ochsner openly in 1967, it would have been very bad for him. He needed all the support he could get from the people of New Orleans. Attacking the city's most famous doctor would have cost him significant political support. He did not need to open up another front in his war.

The most incredible thing about this interview from our current perspective is the reaction from the press. Or should we call it "the *non-reaction* from the press"? First, after being told that a District Attorney of a major American city who was investigating a murder in his jurisdiction had accidentally discovered an underground medical laboratory which was *inducing cancer*, and which was run by a known political extremist with a history of violent political activities and with no formal medical training, the interviewer did not even ask a follow-up question! Then, the members of our national press, the so-called Watchdogs of Democracy, simply continued to bash Garrison from coast to coast.

Had they bothered to read what Garrison had to say for himself? Had they read it and then somehow discredited it without bothering to tell anyone? Or did they think, "What's wrong with having a couple of thousand mice full of cancer viruses in your apartment?" Or perhaps, "This is too weird for my audience"? Whatever the reason, the press did nothing. Now Garrison is dead, and we cannot ask *him* any more questions.

But two important questions remain: Who was Dr. Mary Sherman? And what was she doing in David Ferrie's underground medical laboratory?

The few JFK researchers who remembered the cancer passage in Garrison's *Playboy* interview assumed that Dr. Mary Sherman was a local doctor and, therefore, that she was not significant. This was based on the assumption that no one of any measure would be associated with David Ferrie's cancer research, since Ferrie had no formal medical training. But this was not the case.

Dr. Mary Sherman was one of America's leading cancer experts and had all the credentials to prove it. The newspaper articles about her death refer to her as "an internationally-known bone specialist."[13] She was an Associate Professor at a prominent medical school engaged in monkey virus research, director of a cancer laboratory at an internationally famous medical clinic, and Chairman of the Pathology Committee of one of the most elite medical societies in America. The medical articles she wrote were quoted for half a century. So we ask the question again: What was a highly trained medical professional with impeccable credentials doing in an underground medical laboratory run by a political extremist with no formal medical training?

This question is so vexing that it puts enormous importance on the credibility of this one passage. What other evidence of the Ferrie-Sherman experiments do we have? Unfortunately, for many years, this interview was the single document connecting Sherman to Ferrie's cancer experiments. Perhaps even more unfortunately, however, this link has now been corroborated.

But back in the early stages of my investigation, I tried to find out what Garrison's claim was based upon. I succeeded in talking to a number of people who knew Garrison personally, but they did not know anything about the matter. In the process, I determined that the person most likely to know the answer was Lou Ivon, Garrison's Chief Investigator, who personally handled Ferrie. What did Lou Ivon know about the Ferrie-Sherman connection?

I wrote Lou Ivon letters, explaining the questions I wanted to ask, called his house, donated to his political campaign, even offered him royalties on this book, but I could not get Ivon to talk to me about the Ferrie-Sherman cancer experiments.[14] I finally gave up.

Therefore, I have never known what Lou Ivon knows (or does not know) about the Ferrie-Sherman cancer experiments, but my guess is that he probably knows more than anybody else about the basis for Garrison's claim that Dr. Mary Sherman worked with David Ferrie in his underground medical laboratory. I hope he will talk about it on the record one day. In the meantime, all I can say is that the investigator who probably knows the most about this important subject would not discuss it with me. He may also know who the other doctors were that Garrison had linked with Ferrie.

1   Most of Garrison's biography is from James DiEugenio, *Destiny Betrayed: JFK, Cuba, and the Garrison Case* (New York, 1992), p. 126 and Jim Garrison, *On the Trail of the Assassins: My Investigation and Prosecution of the Murder of President Kennedy* (New York, 1988).

2   "Jolly Green Giant in Wonderland," *Time*, August 2, 1968, p. 56. (*Time* was owned by Henry Luce, an active arch anti-Communist who personally financed raids by Cuban exiles against Cuba, in violation of the Neutrality Act, but with the tacit approval of the CIA: see Hinckle and Turner, *Deadly Secrets*, p. 186. Therefore, *Time's* reporting cannot be assumed to be objective on related issues.

3   The Federal Communications Commission found NBC's coverage of Garrison biased and ordered NBC to give Garrison 1/2 hour of national TV time to respond. Portions of this broadcast were included in a video called *The Garrison Tapes*, which aired on cable in the 1990s.

4   Garrison, *On the Trail of the Assassins*, p. 126. Garrison thought Shaw was an accessory to Guy Banister, and believed Banister to be primarily responsible for "sheep-dipping" Oswald, a deliberate attempt to associate the patsy with the evidence before the crime.

5   Davy, Bill, "License & Registration Please," *Probe*, June 1994, p. 5, and July 1994, p. 1.

6   Ibid., June 1994, p. 7,

7   Garrison, *On the Trail of the Assassins*, p. 298-306 & 318. Also see DiEugenio, *Destiny Betrayed*, p. 268-269.

8   Garrison, "Playboy Interview," *Playboy*, October 1967, p. 59.

9   Ibid., p. 175. Jack Ruby (Jacob Rubenstein) was the Dallas nightclub owner who murdered Lee Harvey Oswald "live" on national television. Ruby had a long history of Mafia contact dating back to Al Capone in Chicago.

10  Garrison, *Playboy*, p. 165.

11  Perry Russo, interview with author, January 1993.

12  Carpenter, Arthur, "Social Origins of Anti-Communism: The Information Council of the Americas," *Louisiana History*, Spring 1989, p. 117. His source: Letters, Ochsner to Butler, June 29 and July 12, 1967, *Ochsner Papers*, Historic New Orleans Collection.

13  "Police Check Ex-Patients of Slain Medic," *New Orleans States-Item*, July 22, 1964, p. 1.

14  Ivon did call me back once. He thanked me for the donation to his political campaign, and said he would take me "through Ferrie's cancer research" sometime, but it never happened.

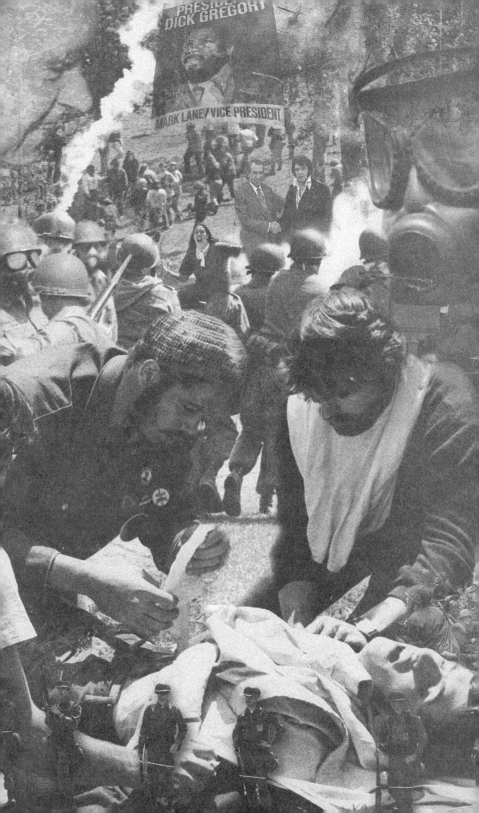

# CHAPTER 4

# College Daze

IN THE FALL OF 1969 I WENT AWAY TO COLLEGE. What a turbulent period! Each night the news brought fresh frustrations. Daily footage from Vietnam showed the bleeding and the dead. Body bags of mounting American casualties swept the screen. The smog of an incomprehensible and undeclared war settled over our land. Its endless drifting nature, its unbelievable cost, and its potential for expansion flared anger throughout the country. College campuses rioted. ROTC buildings burned. Congress revoked the student draft deferment, exposing all male college students to potential slaughter.

Each night the drama was played out on television. Police beat demonstrators with night sticks and dragged them through the streets by their hair. Some applauded the protestors, some the police. Angry words divided friends and families. The generation gap widened. Boomer disillusionment jelled into a sense of national betrayal and challenged the loyalty of the pre-Watergate generation. In return, the Boomer's parents pondered their questions: "What's wrong with this new generation? Where is their patriotism? Why don't they rush to support our war?" The Supreme Court sat and watched as 58,000 Americans died in an undeclared war.

Then Nixon ordered the bombing of Cambodia. The shock wave of this news rushed across the country. Campuses erupted. In Ohio, soldiers gunned down four college students at a demonstration on the Kent State campus. The second shock wave: "They've started killing us." Mass demonstrations broke out spontaneously, shutting down college campuses all across America. The protestors converged on Washington for a showdown demonstration. Tear gas flowed through the streets of our capitol.

Those were crazy and bitter days, which were made even more difficult for me personally by the death of my father. I dropped out of college and waited for them to pass. And when they were over, I was anxious to forget them. Completely free of any responsibilities, I hitchhiked around the country just to see what was out there. During the summer of 1971, I returned to my home in New Orleans to re-group and to plan my next steps.

On my travels I had developed an interest in writing, and started working on a book about my hitchhiking experiences. As the summer wore on, the publicity about the trial of the Manson murders in California took root, and the image of hitchhiking changed. Charles Manson and his companions had hitchhiked their way to one of the most grotesque multiple murders in American history. Everyone became aware of the real and present danger that lurked on the shoulders of our highways. Jack Kerouac's romantic vision of hitchhiking from *On the Road* was replaced by Jim Morrison's stark warning: "There's a killer on the road." My "hitchhiking for the fun of it" perspective suffocated, and my book project died. I started looking for something else to write about.

Mary Sherman's murder still intrigued me, and I thought it might have good potential for a screenplay. So I decided to track down the real facts. My first call was to the public library to see if there were any newspaper articles. I was informed that the indexing system stopped in 1963. If I wanted a newspaper, I would need to have the exact date. But I did not know the date, so I decided to try to get a copy of the police report. Based on what I knew about Sherman's murder and her connection to Ferrie, I figured this might be difficult. So instead of calling the police department myself, I decided to call someone "on the inside" who might be able to help me get a copy of the report quietly. I called Big Mike.[1]

He was known as "Big Mike" due to his enormous size. He stood six-feet five-inches and weighed close to 300 pounds. Big Mike worked in the Orleans Parish District Attorney's office and was an investigator for the Grand Jury. I knew him socially, but not well. We lived in the same neighborhood, and his daughter had been a friend of mine during high school. It had been several years since I had been to his house, and I wasn't sure if he would remember me. It was a Wednesday evening when I picked up the telephone to call him. His wife answered. Yes, she remembered me, and promptly called him to the phone.

When Big Mike came to the phone, I introduced myself and reminded him who I was. He was friendly, and greeted me with "Yeah, kid, I remember you." Then he proudly detailed his daughter's recent accomplishments at college. When he was finished, I told him the purpose of my call: I was doing research for a screenplay and wanted to know how I could get a copy of the police report on the Mary Sherman murder. He was accommodating and in a casual voice said, "That seems easy enough. I'll see if I can get a copy for you. What was that name again?"

I repeated the name and spelled it for him. It was clear that he did not recognize it. This concerned me, because it meant that he was not completely aware of what he was agreeing to. If the rumors I had heard about political heat and suppression of the investigation were true, it could mean trouble for him. But I did not know how to tell a gun-toting ex-linebacker like Big Mike that he should keep his head down in his own office. Anyway, I had only asked "how" I could get a copy of the report. He had volunteered to get it for me. I offered to call him back in a week, but he said that it wouldn't take that long. He told me to call him in two days. I thanked him and hung up.

Two days later, I called back. It was Friday about 3:30 in the afternoon. My plan was to call early and leave a message with his wife and then call back later that evening. I was surprised when he answered the phone himself. The stress and tension in his voice was immediately obvious. He was home early for a reason: It had been a bad day. He began with: "What *the hell* did you get me into?"

I asked naively, "Was there a problem getting the report?"

"A problem?" he said with gigantic sarcasm. "I have never seen such a shit storm in my entire life. I have done nothing for two days except field flack and try to explain why I wanted to see that file."

"I guess that means I can't get a copy of the report," I tendered.

"No, you can't! It's an open murder case, and I'm not allowed to discuss it. Don't ask again." His voice was cold. His tone was final.

I said, "Thanks for trying," waited for the click, and then slowly put the receiver down. Whatever was going on, it was clear to me that the rumors about "the heat" on this case were true. I knew that if Big Mike couldn't get a copy of the police report himself, then I wouldn't be able to through any other channel. I would have to wait for another day to find out what happened to Mary Sherman.

IN 1972 I ENTERED TULANE UNIVERSITY. It was late August of that year, and the campus was buzzing with activity of another semester preparing to begin. I went to the University Center to buy books and to register for my courses. The matriculation was held in a large cavernous room filled with folding tables stacked with boxes of computer cards. Behind the tables sat graduate students who answered questions, gave advice on professors, and signed up undergraduates for classes. I was interested in taking an anthropology course and located the right table. There I met a brilliant and beautiful young woman named Barbara.[2] She had just completed her undergraduate work at the University of Chicago and had accepted a fellowship from Tulane to get her Ph.D. Intrigued by her warmth, and her waist-length brown hair, I invited her to go to a concert being held on campus that evening. She accepted the invitation, and we discussed plans. She did not have a car, and mine was in the shop. We agreed on a convenient place and time to meet and went our separate ways.

That night Barbara and I met as planned and walked to the concert. The performance was by the New Leviathan Oriental Fox Trot Orchestra, a camp revival troupe that played dance music of the 1890-1920 period. We had a lot of fun, and I felt very comfortable with her. This was a relationship that I wanted to pursue.

After the concert she told me she lived near Louisiana Avenue. I knew the area well. While it was not far from campus, it was in a marginal area near a high-crime zone known as the Louisiana Avenue Housing Project. I did not think it was safe for a woman to be walking on the streets of that neighborhood alone at midnight, so I escorted her home on the bus.

Several days later I called her up, told her I had gotten my car out of the shop, and that I was itching to show her "my city." It was a Monday, but classes had not started. It was still early in the morning, and the weather was beautiful, so I invited her sailing. (Despite my penniless student status, I still had access to a sailboat which my older brother had left in my care when he moved out of town.) She accepted the offer and gave me her address again. I said I would be there in half an hour.

It was about ten o'clock in the morning when I turned off Claiborne Avenue into Louisiana Avenue Parkway. I remember my surprise at seeing this intriguing street for the first time in daylight. Unlike Louisiana Avenue itself, which was a broad bustling boulevard, Louisiana Avenue Parkway was a quiet oasis, isolated from the activity and noise of city life. Only three blocks long and leading nowhere, this narrow, bumpy street was shaded by massive oak trees which grew together at their tops, creating a canopy over the street and providing welcome protection from the oppressive August sun. The houses were modest, mostly two story rental units whose stucco façades made it easy to confuse one house with another. I pulled over and dug the slip of paper from my jeans to check the address: 3225 Louisiana Avenue Parkway.

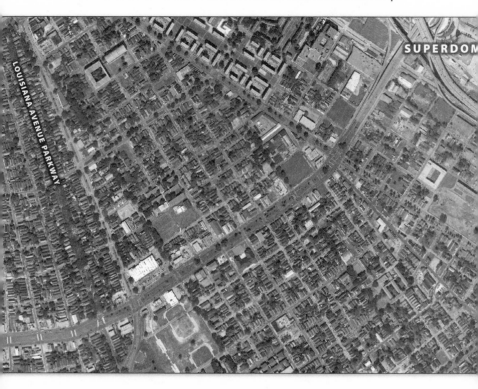

*Dr. Mary's Monkey*

When I found the faded yellow building, I made a point of memorizing some detail so I could find it more easily in the future. I settled on the two unusual columns flanking the front door, which were twisted like licorice sticks. I approached the building, found the door bell, and rang it.

Barbara came down the stairs, opened the door, and greeted me. She was dressed appropriately for sailing, in cutoff blue jeans and a baggy shirt. As I entered the stairwell, I noticed a door to my immediate left which led to a basement. It was ajar, opened about one inch. But it closed suddenly when I looked at it, and then the sound of several locks clicked away, one after another. "Who was that?" I asked.

"Oh, that's the old woman who lives in the basement," she responded as we started walking up the stairs. "I met her yesterday. She seemed like she had a really tough life." I asked her what she meant. She continued, "It's hard to describe. She looks like she might have been a stripper or maybe even a prostitute. She wears lots of make-up and has a real hard edge to her." I laughed a little and said it sounded very New Orleans, pointing out that a club owner might take care of one of his ladies after she had grown too old to be useful to his business by letting her live in a place rent-free, even if it was a basement.

One flight up we entered Barbara's apartment. Despite the weather-worn exterior of the building, it was a nice apartment and the lack of furniture emphasized its space. In fact, the only furniture in it was a waterbed mattress which lay on the floor of one of the front rooms.

I complimented her on the apartment and noted the great condition it was in. The walls were all freshly plastered and painted. The floors had been stripped and varnished. I had been in plenty of student apartments, but I had never seen one that was in such good condition. Since it was larger and in better condition that the apartment I lived in, I asked her about the rent. The rent seemed well below market value. I would have guessed about fifty percent higher based on what

I had seen. So I asked her where she found it. (Good apartments were hard to find and were hardly ever advertised in New Orleans, because landlords did not want to invite inquiries from blacks.) She said it was on a bulletin board at Tulane. "In the University Center?" I asked.

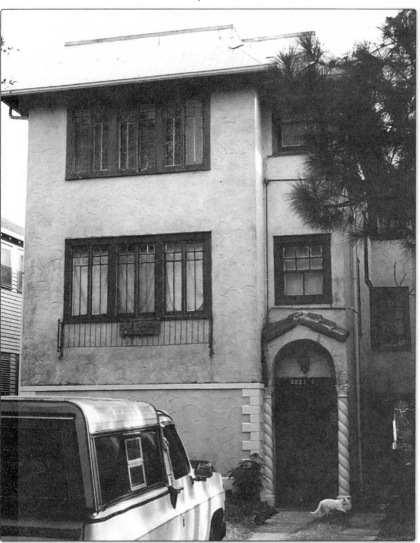

"No, in Social Sciences," she responded, referring to the building where the anthropology, sociology, and political science departments were located.

"Hmm, do you know who owns it?" I asked.

"No," she said, "I only deal with an attorney."

My thoughts now turned to the sweet smell of freshly baked bread. I had noticed it when I first came in, but had not said anything about it yet. If you have ever been in New Orleans in August, you will understand that people without air-conditioning just do not bake bread then. It is much too hot. It was, indeed, a curious activity for a hot summer morning.

"Baking bread?" I inquired.

"Yes," she said, explaining that the apartment had a "residual odor" in it and that she had heard that baking bread would help take the odor away. Then she asked if I thought it was safe to leave the windows open so the place could air out while we were sailing. I said, "Yes." As she continued to talk about the apartment, it became clear that it had an unusual history to it. It had been vacant and off the market for several years before she rented it, and during that time it had been thoroughly re-conditioned. Yet despite the fresh paint and varnish, and after years of vacancy, a musty smell remained. I asked, due to the odor, if the previous tenant had cats.

She said, somewhat mysteriously, that "they had *animals*."

I noticed the shift in the language from "cats" to "animals" and asked her, "What kind of animals?" Then her expression changed. The moment before she was a positive upbeat young woman about to go on a date; now she was suddenly serious and concerned.

"She didn't say what kind of animals."

I just looked at her for a minute, waiting for more. Then she started talking about the old woman who lived in the basement. She had been down to see her yesterday. She was stuck for words for a moment, and then releasing a tense breath, said, "It was so *weird*."

Something was obviously bothering her, and we weren't going to get to the bottom with generalities like "weird." So I asked her to be more specific. I offered, "Was the furniture weird?"

She laughed, breaking the tension for a moment. "Yes, the furniture was weird all right, but that wasn't the problem." Then she described how the old woman talked to her in a tense suspicious voice and how she was genuinely frightened of *something* or *someone*. Her fear had obviously transferred to Barbara.

Then Barbara said, "Ed, I got the feeling that something *really bad* happened here. Something terribly wrong, like maybe someone had been killed. You are from here, do you know what she might be talking about? She acted like it was something big, something *everyone knew about*. Maybe it was even on the news."

"What did she say about the animals?" I asked quietly.

Barbara continued, "She was really upset about them and kept saying 'those *terrible men* and the *horrible things* they did to those animals' over and over."

The sentence hung in the air. I took it apart in my head and studied the words. "Terrible men" do "horrible things." My mind flooded with images of laboratory animals I had seen — sad, sick, mice and monkeys suffering from horrifying diseases, their bodies covered with lesions and harboring tumors larger than their natural bodies. I was silent.

Then she asked the question again, "Do you know what she might be talking about?"

I shrugged and said, "The only thing that comes to mind is a secret laboratory that was discovered during the Garrison investigation. There was this political wacko and this woman doctor who had thousands of mice in cages. They were using monkey viruses to induce cancer in mice. Garrison thought they were trying to develop a biological weapon."

"What happened to the doctor?" she asked systematically in a serious voice devoid of any emotion.

My answer was reluctant but straightforward. I had not planned on getting into this. "She was murdered," I said as simply as I could.

"How?" she countered, knowing I was holding out.

"Cut up with a knife and set on fire," I admitted.

Her fear was now visible. She crossed her arms upon her chest and leaned up against the wall. By this point I realized that she was really frightened, and rightfully so. Her parents had warned her about living in New Orleans alone, and I had expressed my concerns about her neighborhood. And who is going to get a good night's sleep in a place if you know the previous tenant was butchered in her bed. I realized our conversation was only making matters worse for her. She broke the silence by blowing out a short breath and said, "What part of town did that happen in?"

At the time I did not know and, more importantly, I wanted to change the subject. I was getting frightened too, both for her and with her. I said that I did not know where these people had lived, but I had assumed that it was in the French Quarter, since that was where all "the weird stuff seemed to happen." It would be years before I found out where we were standing.

Our date was not going well. I had offered to take her sailing on Lake Pontchartrain, but we were standing around talking about brutal murders and monkey viruses. Knowing she was quietly wondering if her apartment was infected with a flotilla of bizarre diseases, I pointed out that viruses could not survive more than a couple of hours in the air. She shook her head in cautious agreement. It was time to shift tactics. I switched my tone to confident and our conversation to sailboats. She accepted my lead, and we left the apartment within minutes to go sailing. (How was I to know we were standing in David Ferrie's shadow?)

Classes started the next day, and we saw each other daily, exchanging comments about our classes and the people we had met. After about two weeks, we met for lunch at our usual spot in the cafeteria. Barbara said that she was really upset about something she had heard concerning Tulane's "right-wing political orientation." Specifically, she asked me if I had ever heard of Dr. Alton Ochsner. Of course, I had heard of Ochsner. Everybody in New Orleans had. An enormous hospital in town was named after him. Then she asked me what I knew about him. At the time all I knew was the standard pitch: He was one of the most respected people in New Orleans and was founder of the Ochsner Clinic, which took care of a lot of important people from Latin America. Then I added a personal comment: He was also an aggressive anti-smoking activist, which was something that I liked about him. On the other hand, rumor had it he was a Victorian moralist who held some controversial views about sex *causing cancer.*

Then she told me what was bothering her. A fellow graduate student who had lived in South America had told her that Ochsner was part of an international fascist group and had been very close to Nazi scientists who fled to South America at the end of World War II, particularly in Paraguay.[3] I did not think much of the story, quietly considering it to be a hysterical liberal rant. Yes, I had heard that he was very conservative. In fact, he was occasionally referred to as a "right-wing crackpot," but I had never heard him referred to as a fascist, and had never heard anything about his helping Nazi scientists in South America. To my ears, it all sounded like overstatement.

Anyway, it was widely known that Nazis had gone to South America at the end of the war and that the American military debriefed both German and Japanese scientists at the end of the war to find out what they were working on. Who would they ask to do that? Some Army doctor? Wouldn't they get the best scientists in America to review what Germany's top scientists were up to? I did not know if Ochsner spoke German fluently, but that would seem to be a prerequisite for the job. It's hard enough to know what scientists are saying in your own language. Who knows? Maybe the U.S. government did get Ochsner to go to South America to debrief Nazi scientists. If so, that made him an important American scientist, not a Nazi sympathizer.

She was defused. But I was curious about what she said, and made a mental note of it.

WE CONTINUED TO SEE EACH OTHER throughout the fall. Before long there emerged the subject of her other neighbor, the man who lived in the apartment above her. He was a Hispanic who spoke Spanish as his first language. I think his name was Miguel, and I do remember two incidents clearly.

In the first one, Barbara and I were at her apartment when she said she had met the man who lived upstairs. So I asked her what he was like?

"He's a Latin," she said. I shrugged a "so what" in her direction. "I mean really, really Latin." So I asked her where he was from.

She laughed a little and said, "Funny you should ask. I asked him that same question, but never got a straight answer out of him. But he did say he spent a lot of time in Honduras."

I suggested to her that his evasiveness might be a sign he was a Cuban exile. There were many of them in New Orleans, and most found it convenient to keep the word "Cuba" out of the conversation. Then I asked her what he did for a living. She said Miguel claimed he was a mechanic, but that he only occasionally worked at a gas station out in Jefferson Parish. Most of his time was spent at one particular bar. I was not surprised to hear that he invited Barbara to go to the bar with him one evening "just to see what it was like."[4] She turned him down, saying she already had a boyfriend.

Several things about Miguel did not add up. One is that it took money to pay rent and to hang out at a bar, and he did not have what you would call a visible means of support. Secondly, there were many service stations in New Orleans that could have used a good mechanic, and these were much closer to his apartment. Why would he only work occasionally at a service station in Jefferson Parish, a suburb thirty minutes away (and a cultural world apart) from uptown New Orleans?

Then I asked her if Miguel was married. "No, he's not," she said with a smirk on her face. "He's widowed." She saw me notice her half-hidden smile and turned away to hide it. "What's so funny about being widowed?" I asked.

"It's just something he said," she tentatively admitted. After a pause she added, "He said he had not been able *to come* since his wife died."

"What a great line!" I roared.

"What do you mean?" She asked, trying for an innocent voice.

"Let me ask you a question," I asked in a slow, counseling voice. "When he said that to you, did it make you wonder if *you* could make him come?"

She blushed. "Yes, as a matter of fact, it did."

"There it is. It's a line and a good one at that. The man is a cad. I'd stay away from him."

The second incident occurred several days later. Miguel knocked on Barbara's back door and called out her name in his accented voice. She motioned for me to come with her to the door, whispering, "I want him *to see* that I have a boyfriend." When she opened it, he stepped inside confidently. When he realized I was standing there looking at him, he was embarrassed. Barbara introduced me with, "Have you met my boyfriend?" Actually our relationship seemed new and tentative at the time, but I didn't argue with her. It sounded good to me.

Miguel stood about five-feet eight-inches with black hair and a stocky build. He was in his mid-thirties and was common looking. His shifty personality glistened. It was an awkward moment. Another rooster in the hen house. And to be caught coming in the back door! He was obviously uncomfortable with the situation, but that was where I wanted him. I kept my tone polite and somewhat formal. My unspoken message to him was, "I don't blame you for trying, but let's not have this happen again." His unspoken message to me was, "You lucky devil, you beat me to it." He mumbled through a couple of social courtesies trying to portray his presence as a concerned neighbor just stopping by to see if she was all right. Then as quickly as he had appeared, he said good-bye and went on his way. I never saw him again, but we heard his footsteps coming and going down the back stairwell for months.

As the fall semester progressed, Barbara and I saw a lot of each other. I was in and out of her apartment repeatedly, though we spent less and less time there and more time over at my place. Shortly after Thanksgiving, I forced myself to begin writing a term paper that I had been ignoring. It was for my Pre-Columbian Art course, and I had chosen a comparison of two Mayan carvings from Guatemala as the subject. Much of the information I needed was in the Middle American Research Institute, located on the fourth floor of the Tulane's main library. I ate an early lunch and headed to the library about noon. Little did I know what lay ahead?

As I entered the glass doors of the Middle American Research Institute, I was greeted with the unmistakable look of terror on the faces of two women.[5] Both were staring wide-eyed and slack-jawed out the window. One mumbled "My God" as she shook her head in disbelief. I turned to see what they were looking at. Out the window and across the tree tops there was an unobstructed view of the downtown skyline seven miles away. One of the tall buildings had just exploded into flames. Enormous flames were shooting out of the windows. A thick plume of dense black smoke had not yet reached more than a couple of hundred feet above the roof, indicating the fire had just started. But the forty foot flames indicated a massive sudden explosion, probably a firebomb. I recognized the building immediately, it was the

Rault Center. The top three floors of the building were the Lamplighter Club, where I had worked in the summer of 1968. The building was owned by Joseph M. Rault, Jr., an independent oil man and real estate entrepreneur. Rault was very close to U.S. Senator Russell Long, and was sitting in an airplane next to both Senator Long and New Orleans D.A. Jim Garrison when Long originally proposed the JFK investigation to Garrison. To facilitate the secret investigation, Long asked Rault to form an organization, now known as "Truth and Consequences," to finance trips so Garrison and his staff could investigate the murder of the President quietly.

I grabbed the phone and called my friend Claire, who lived around the corner from the library.[6] Her husband worked in the Lamplighter Club. Yes, she knew about the fire. Someone just called. Did she need a ride down there? Yes, she did. I ran to my car, rushed to her house, and drove her downtown.

Down at the Rault Center all hell was breaking loose. Rault had been at his normal post on the sixteenth floor,

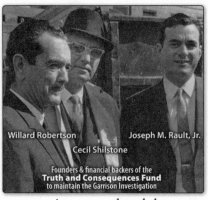

Willard Robertson      Joseph M. Rault, Jr.
Cecil Shilstone
Founders & financial backers of the
**Truth and Consequences Fund**
to maintain the Garrison Investigation

meeting and greeting local dignitaries who had come to the club for lunch. Congressman Hale Boggs, Senator Russell Long, and New Orleans Mayor Vic Schiro were just a few who frequented this club, though none were there that day.[7] Local bankers and developers congregated around this seat of power to be close to the pulse and to see the right people. At noon, the club was packed with its normal lunch crowd from the Central Business District.

Suddenly, there was a loud explosion from down below. The building shook violently. A firebomb had exploded on the fifteenth floor. Flames leapt out the window. The crowd panicked and stampeded for the exits. For some reason Rault headed for the roof. Others headed for the ground. Seven people followed Rault to the roof. As the forty-foot flames leapt up above the roofline of the building, Rault must have wondered if he made the right decision. He must have also wondered what happened to the three floors of "fireproof" paneling that he had bought for the Lamplighter Club, which was now burning like a blowtorch.[8] The concrete and steel stairwells quickly became ovens. No one could pass now. The eight people trapped on the roof knew that unless someone descended from the sky, they would either be burned alive or would have to jump to their

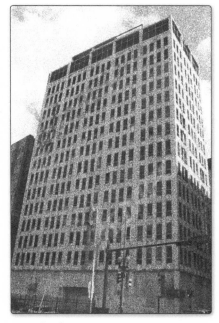

deaths from the seventeenth-floor roof. The seven women trapped in a window on the fifteenth floor faced the same situation. I got as close to the building as I could, but the roads were blocked off. Claire jumped out of the car and ran the final few blocks. I turned my car around and headed for a television set.

It was the greatest of fortunes that a helicopter carrying an oil executive happened to be flying over downtown New Orleans at the moment of the explosion. The pilot dropped his passenger on the grassy field in front of the Louisiana Supreme Court building and headed for the roof of the flaming building. Nine people were trapped there, but his small helicopter could only carry three passengers at a time. Some would have to wait for the next trip. The rest would have to wait for the third trip. So three separate times, this determined pilot landed on the roof surrounded by onyx smoke and orange flames. Rault was the last person to leave the roof. He was lucky. The women who were trapped in their beauty salon on the fifteenth floor were not. Fire investigators estimated the bomb contained five gallons of gasoline, and had exploded in the utility closet right outside the door of the salon. The hallway was immediately filled with flames, blocking the women's exit. The helicopter could not help them. Faced with certain death by fire, or jumping to their deaths, seven women jumped. There was no net. No air bag. Six died on impact. The camera crews were there. They filmed it all. That night veteran broadcaster Walter Cronkite warned his viewers that he was about to show the "grimmest footage" of his career. The nation watched helplessly. I turned off the television and went back to the library, trying to concentrate on thousand year- old hieroglyphs buried in a Mayan grave. One question has smoldered since the fire: Was the Rault Center firebombing the result of Rault's financing of Garrison's JFK investigation?[9]

When Christmas break came, Barbara gave me a key to her apartment and asked me to keep an eye on it while she flew home to see her family. A couple of days after she left, I dropped by for a routine check and found that her waterbed mattress, which was resting on the hardwood floor without a frame, had started to leak. I quickly went outside, borrowed a hose from a neighbor's lawn, and drained the mattress. But the damage had already been done. The wooden floors were severely buckled. It was hundreds of dollars of damage. The landlord would certainly flip. That night I called her at her family's farm and told her about the leak. She said that she would call the landlord in the morning and tell him.

Several days later, New Orleans woke up to yet another incredible event: Someone had set fire to the Howard Johnson Motel.[10] It was directly across the street from the Rault Center, but these arsonists were not experts. And the fire was small in comparison, one smoky hotel room. But in light of what happened at the Rault Center, the hotel guests panicked and ran to the street. And having recently been humiliated in the national news by their inability to do anything

*Dr. Mary's Monkey*

to help the seven women who jumped, the New Orleans Fire Department rushed to the scene, hoping to redeem its reputation. The longest ladder was raised to reach the fifth floor window. The bravest firemen rushed up the ladder with no other thought than trying to save someone's life. As they approached the window, a rifle barrel slid through the opening. The sniper squeezed off round after round, murdering the very men who had come to save him.

The police department broke into a fit of rage. Nearly 600 policemen swarmed to the building in pre-SWAT chaos. Two snipers were reported. The Deputy Chief of Police grabbed several men and led them into a stairwell to find the snipers. Somebody thought he saw something. Somebody fired a high powered rifle in the concrete and steel stairway. When the bullet finished ricocheting, the Deputy Chief of Police was dead.

On the roof, one of the snipers rushed to get a better position. A police rifle team in the Rault Center overlooking the roof shot him with a high-powered rifle and killed him. The second sniper was believed to be at large in the building.

Police sealed the building. As the situation developed, a police spotter thought he saw something in the blockhouse on the roof. Twelve police fanned out and approached the blockhouse like they were going to a western shootout. Standing in a semi-circle in front of a steel door cemented into a concrete wall, they opened fire. As one might expect, the bullets ricocheted off the concrete wall and steel door, right back at the very men who fired them. Yes, live on national television, they shot themselves. Several policemen fell wounded on the building's roof. One officer charged the blockhouse. It was empty.

They never found the second sniper. Some believe he walked out the front door before the building was sealed. Others think there was only one sniper. The FBI seemed to know all about these guys, and had apparently been tracking them since Kansas City. Militant black radicals they claimed.

I turned off the TV and drove to the airport to pick up Barbara, who was returning from Christmas break. It seemed like she had been gone a long time. Her flight was early and I found her entering the terminal. Knowing that I had worked at the Rault Center, she asked if I had heard anything new about the fire. I told her I had heard it was a bomb. Somebody was trying to kill somebody. As we rode the escalator leading down to the baggage claim, she noticed a big lighted sign advertising the Howard Johnson's Motel rising above our heads. She had been traveling most of the day but had heard rumors of something happening at Howard Johnson's in New Orleans.

I filled her in as quickly as possible, and then asked her if she had called her lawyer landlord about the floor damaged by her leaky waterbed. Yes, she had, but he said it was not a problem. "In fact," she continued in an astonished voice, "he didn't seem concerned about it at all."

I had seen a lot of strange things in the past months. But it all made some kind of twisted sense. In the Rault Center fire, somebody was mad. They were either mad at Rault for some reason and were trying to destroy him, or they were mad at society and chose his building and his success as a target. In the Ho-Jo Massacre, an angry and frustrated black man (or men) decided to strike back at a white racist society. He died venting his anger. Others died with him.

But this? A lawyer holding a damage deposit did not care about hundreds of dollars of damage done by a tenant to his client's building? It didn't make sense. Whatever was going on, it was clear that this was no ordinary apartment. All I could think of was "those terrible men and the horrible things they did to those animals." One month later, when she moved out of the apartment, Barbara got her full security deposit back. The person or persons pulling the strings on this building had succeeded in their objective, and that was a lot bigger than Barbara's security deposit. They got a real live human being to live in a virtually haunted apartment.

*Dr. Mary's Monkey*

And not just any human being. They had placed a naive and studious graduate student from out of town, who would not know any of the local history and who would not have the time or inclination to find it out. Now that the apartment was warmed up, they could put it back on the market for real.

I SCRATCHED MY HEAD about this apartment for years. Frankly, I was afraid to understand it. It was so close and so strange that it scared me. I could have gone back and talked to the old woman who lived in the basement, but I didn't. I was afraid of what she might tell me. I was afraid of what I might learn. I denied it. I didn't go find out where Mary Sherman lived, or where David Ferrie lived. I just went sailing, played music, and worried about things like Mayan hieroglyphs from Guatemala.

It was not until 1992, when I realized the possibility that the Ferrie and Sherman cancer experiments might have something to do with the most deadly epidemic in history, that I finally woke up. At that point my choices narrowed. It was time to find out everything I could. I started by reading everything on the shelf about AIDS and then everything that was written by or about Jim Garrison. It was then that I realized that David Ferrie had lived on Louisiana Avenue Parkway. A sick feeling came over me as Garrison described the smell of white mice in Ferrie's apartment: "The special fetid smell of hundreds of unattended white mice in the dining room added to the unique rank odor of the dwelling, making it difficult for visitors to enter."[11] Then he described Ferrie's medical books and laboratory equipment and the medical treatise he had written on the viral theory of cancer.

But Garrison did not give the exact address. For a brief time, I pondered the possibility that my girlfriend had lived in David Ferrie's apartment, perhaps on the spot where the plot to kill Jack Kennedy was hatched. It was more than I wanted to wonder about. I had to find out the exact address. So I called the library in New Orleans. Ferrie was not listed in the phone book, but they found the address in his obituary, 3330 Louisiana Avenue Parkway. For a brief moment I was relieved. That must be a block away from 3225. But what to make of everything I had seen and heard myself. What about the smell in Barbara's apartment? What about the old lady in the basement? What about "those terrible men and the horrible things they did to those animals?" What about Garrison's estimate of nearly 2,000 mice?

Now, that was worth thinking about! Nearly 2,000 mice! Say five mice per cage. That's 400 cages of mice. What would an apartment look like with 400 cages of mice in it? It would

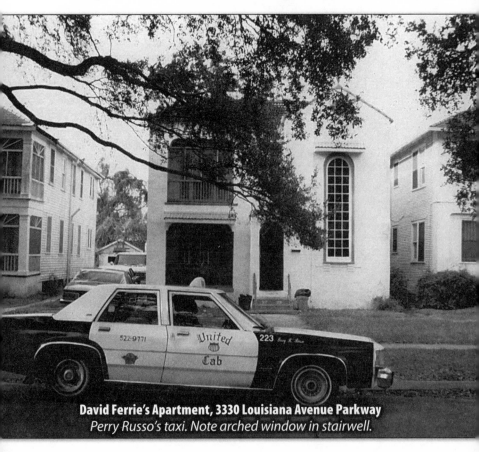

**David Ferrie's Apartment, 3330 Louisiana Avenue Parkway**
*Perry Russo's taxi. Note arched window in stairwell.*

*Dr. Mary's Monkey*

be wall-to-wall cages! And consider the mice. Consider the food. Consider the excrement. Consider the smell. Consider the diseases! No one could *live* in such a place. Let me repeat that: "No one could live in such a place." Four hundred cages would take a dedicated facility.

Then it hit me: Ferrie's underground medical laboratory was *not* in his apartment, and he did not live *in the lab*! No one could. He lived *near the lab*, so he could manage its day-to-day operations, and kept a small number of mice back at his apartment for convenience. No, I had not been in Ferrie's apartment: *I had been in his laboratory!*

---

1    I have omitted Big Mike's last name to protect his privacy.

2    I have omitted Barbara's last name to protect her privacy.

3    My research showed that many of Dr. Ochsner's financial backers were Jewish. Therefore, I believe the claim of his association with Nazis was untrue, unless he was debriefing them for the U.S. government. The comment is, however, an example of a Latin American perception of Ochsner's politics.

4    Miguel told her the bar was in the vicinity of Washington Avenue and Magazine Street. I assured her that she did not want to go to any bar in that neighborhood.

5. The date of the Rault Center Fire was November 29, 1972.

6. Claire was Claire de la Vergne Rault, wife of the building's owner Joseph M. Rault, Jr. Born Claire de la Vergne, she was a member of the de la Vergnes, one of the families that founded New Orleans. Claire died of cancer in 1999.

7. Congressman Hale Boggs disappeared on Oct. 16, 1972 when his plane went down in the Gulf of Alaska, so he was presumed to be dead at the time of the Rault Center fire. U.S. Senator Russell Long was scheduled to be at the Rault Center for a meeting later that afternoon, but had not yet arrived by the time the fire started.

8. The only place that this particular synthetic paneling proved to be "fireproof" was in the laboratory where the test conditions required the paneling to be horizontal. On walls, where it is installed vertically, it proved to be extremely flammable. Rault had no way of knowing this when he purchased the paneling, and certainly would not have headed to the roof if he had.

9. The last time I spoke to Congressman Boggs was when he visited Rault in the Lamplighter Club shortly before his death on Oct. 16, 1972. It should be mentioned that Congressman Hale Boggs who was very close to Rault had been on the Warren Commission in 1964. But by 1972 Boggs had grown increasingly uncomfortable with its conclusions and was starting to claim the J. Edgar Hoover had lied to the Commission about Oswald, the rifle, and other things. As previously stated Rault helped finance Jim Garrison's investigation into the Kennedy assassination.

10. The date of the incident at the Howard Johnson's Motel happened on the morning of January 7, 1973.

11. Garrison, *A Heritage of Stone*, p. 121.

---

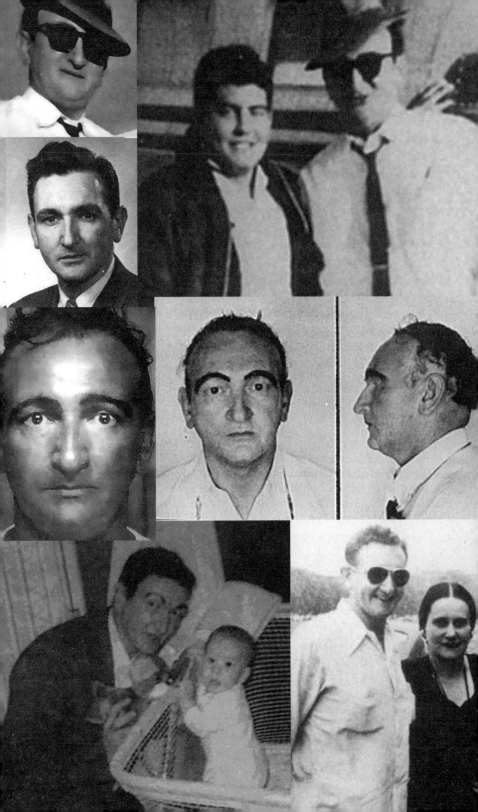

# CHAPTER 5

# A Bishop in His Heart

**D**AVID FERRIE HAS BECOME A CHARACTER of almost comic book proportions. A brilliant man rejected by society, he was a collection of contradictions. A man of high moral aspirations who was compromised by personal cravings. A respected airline pilot who became a tattered Bohemian rebel. The son of a police captain who helped defend a Mafia boss against prosecution. From his orange wig haphazardly glued to his head to his grease-paint eyebrows, to his wardrobe full of religious vestments, to his home-brewed cancer experiments, to his burning desire to help teenage boys, to his ability to land planes in jungle clearings at night, to his violent schemes against Castro, to his friendship with Lee Harvey Oswald, to his unrewarded genius, he was the most colorful figure dredged up during the JFK investigations. Today Ferrie has emerged as the keystone in several JFK assassination theories, including:

☞ **THE GARRISON CASE.** Ferrie's trip to Texas on the afternoon of November 22, 1963 triggered Garrison's suspicion that Ferrie was involved in the JFK assassination, perhaps as a getaway pilot. Next, based on additional evidence, Garrison suspected Ferrie may have been a prime

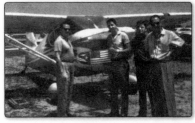

organizer of the plot. Garrison finally concluded that a high-level faction within the CIA was ultimately responsible for Kennedy's death, and that Ferrie had played a lesser role. Ferrie's relationship with the CIA is well known. He trained pilots for the CIA-sponsored Bay of Pigs invasion, and flew covert missions into Cuba.

☞ **THE MAFIA HIT.** In his book *Mafia Kingfish,* John Davis presented the theory that the Mafia killed John Kennedy in an effort to neutralize Bobby Kennedy, the president's brother and U.S. Attorney General. Bobby was prosecuting certain Mafia leaders, particularly Carlos

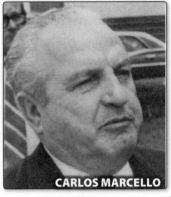

CARLOS MARCELLO

Marcello, reportedly the head of the Mafia in Louisiana, and some say the entire nation. Davis proposed that Ferrie planned and organized the plot to kill the President on Marcello's instructions. That Ferrie had some form of relationship with Carlos Marcello is beyond question, but the extent of that relationship is still unclear. Ferrie was sitting with Marcello in federal court at the moment JFK was assassinated.

Descriptions of Ferrie from those who knew him personally range from "a living god"[1] to "a sexual deviant capable of any form of crime."[2] Unfortunately, most books which reference Ferrie devote little time to examining who he was and what made him that way. What do we really know about him today? What made him tick? Why was he experiment-

*Dr. Mary's Monkey*

ing with cancer? And who was he really mad at? Castro? Kennedy? Or God?

Much of what I am about to describe comes from a report none of us were supposed to see. It was a private investigation on David William Ferrie prepared by Southern Research Company Inc. of New Orleans, beginning in the winter of 1963,[3] six months before Oswald arrived in New Orleans, nine months before the raid on the anti-Castro guerilla training camp, and eleven months before the JFK assassination. I do not know who authorized it or why, but I am told it was Eastern Airlines, which was building a case in order to dismiss Ferrie. An advertisement at the bottom of the report describes the Southern Research Company as "A firm principally staffed by former agents of the FBI."

DAVID FERRIE BEGAN HIS LONG, TWISTED JOURNEY in the middle class suburbs of Cleveland, Ohio, in 1918. His father was James H. Ferrie, a captain in the Cleveland Police Department and later an attorney. Young David was baptized, confirmed, and raised as Catholic, and he was educated in a string of Catholic schools. First, he graduated from St. Ignatius High School in Cleveland in 1935. Readers familiar with Catholicism will recognize the name St. Ignatius as referring to "St. Ignatius of Loyola," the militant crusader who founded the Society of Jesus, more commonly known as "the Jesuits." Then Ferrie enrolled at John Carroll University from 1935 to 1938, a college also run by the Jesuits. There he studied Greek, Latin, history, and government, getting A's or B's in all subjects. Despite his scholastic success, other forces were obviously churning within him, and he dropped out during his senior year to begin his quest for the priesthood.

In 1938, he entered St. Mary's Seminary in Cleveland, where he studied for the priesthood for

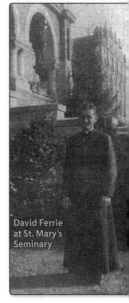

David Ferrie at St. Mary's Seminary

three years. Then, in 1940, just prior to graduating, he had a nervous breakdown.[4] This was his first failure in a long series of attempts to become a priest. Later, when he applied for re-admission, he was rejected. Having known him for three years, St. Mary's did not want him back. He seemed to have a problem with authority.

In 1940, Ferrie's objective changed from becoming a priest to becoming a teacher. He entered Baldwin-Wallace College, and did student teaching at Rocky River High School from 1940 to 1941. A department chairman summarized his performance with a tongue-in-cheek statement: "His interest in teaching students is very closely tied up with his religious faith."[5] When questioned years later about her evaluation, she remembered Ferrie clearly, but this time she was less charitable. She quickly portrayed him as having an inflated self-image when, in fact, he was "the poorest teacher they ever had." From there, she went straight after his personality describing him as "tricky, a bluffer, shrewd, and probably a liar." She added that she received "complaints about his psychoanalyzing his students," but never had "complaints involving moral problems." However, she expressed her own doubts about his moral character, advising that he be kept away from both girls and young boys. He seemed to have "a particular interest in the younger students, more than a teacher should have."

In August 1941, Ferrie made a second attempt to become a Catholic priest and entered St. Charles Seminary in Carthagena, Ohio. There he stayed for three years. During this time his father bought him a plane, and he learned to fly. In 1944, on the eve of ecclesiastical accomplishment, the faculty refused to allow him to continue his religious studies. Having spent six years of his life in seminaries studying for the priesthood, he was again formally rejected from a life of prayer. Ferrie was shattered.

An unsigned memo found in Ferrie's file at the St. Charles Seminary told the faculty's side of the story. It began, "We had serious misgivings about admitting him to our seminary

*Dr. Mary's Monkey*

after learning he had been refused re-admittance to Saint Mary's in Cleveland." Attempting to give a balanced portrayal, they described Ferrie as "a paradox," saying "many of his ways were likable." They even assumed some responsibility for their part in Ferrie's tragedy by pointing out that they had renewed his relationship for over three years, but alas "there was surely an element of instability in his character somewhere." Then they described what became a familiar pattern in Ferrie's life, initial success both socially and scholastically, the achievement of a leadership position amongst his peers, growing conflict and jealousy, back-stabbing, self-pity, exaggeration, manipulation, misuse of leadership and trust, excessive criticism, threats, and contempt of authority.

In a tone that approached apology, the anonymous author said there was no single event of magnitude, but rather a pattern of minor infractions, mostly of the rules of the house, but also "emotional instability," especially "his inclination to suspicion and rash judgement and uncharitable conclusions" that indicated "he would not fit into a religious community."

The final stroke: "When corrected, his attitude seemed to be that *the rule should be changed* rather than that he should be forced to observe it." On November 27, 1944, the Faculty of St. Charles Seminary refused to allow him to continue his quest for priesthood "due to the questionableness of his disposition." He was unfit for the Society of the Precious Blood.

In 1945, Ferrie was treated by a psychiatrist and began a period of relative stability. He lived at home, worked teaching English and Aeronautics at Benedictine High School, and began his long relationship with the Civil Air Patrol. This calm lasted through 1948, though the seven traffic violations from this stretch showed he was still having some trouble with "the rules of the house."

In 1948, he became involved in a series of serious misconduct incidents at the Civil Air Patrol which eventually drove him from Ohio. In the first case, he appropriated a squadron airplane which had been grounded by the U.S. Air

Force and flew it, after dark and without landing lights, from Columbus to Cleveland. Identifying himself as a lieutenant in the U.S. Air Force during the incident got him into even hotter water. The CAP commander tried to have Ferrie dismissed from CAP, but the paperwork was "lost." So Ferrie was still on their books in 1950, when two CAP cadets signed papers reporting that Ferrie, their instructor, had taken them to a house of prostitution in a nearby town. Ferrie was not charged with a crime, but his dismissal from CAP became imminent. Ferrie negotiated his disastrous situation into a transfer to Louisiana. When the Louisiana branch asked for his personnel file, the Cleveland office found it missing, but could not prove it was stolen.

Ferrie did have his friends and allies along the way. One was a well-known female pilot who hired Ferrie to fly her ex-husband's twin-engine plane on business trips down to Texas.[6] She considered Ferrie a near-genius whose piloting skills were above reproach. She personally felt he did much for the Civil Air Patrol, building up their squadron to one of the largest in Ohio. She blamed his problems at CAP on jealousy from other instructors and blamed them for stealing his personnel files to remove his many letters of recommendation.

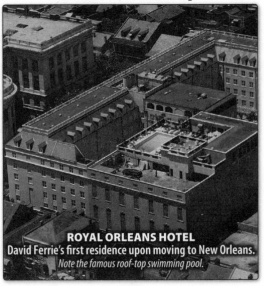

**ROYAL ORLEANS HOTEL**
David Ferrie's first residence upon moving to New Orleans.
*Note the famous roof-top swimming pool.*

In 1951, David Ferrie finally bailed out of Ohio and headed for his new home in New Orleans. There he moved into the French Quarter and before long was living on Bourbon Street. It must have been quite a change for someone who spent six years in a seminary!

Ferrie's life in New Orleans was successful for most of the 1950s. He landed a good job with Eastern Airlines and learned to fly big jets. He wore the Eastern uniform, and was eventually promoted to the rank of Captain.

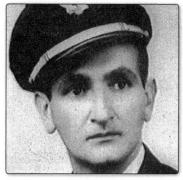

The life of a pilot is an unusual one. Hours of boredom punctuated by moments of fear and stress. When they are traveling, pilots are required to rest a certain number hours for each hour of flying time. This creates long layovers which are full of idle hours.

Ferrie appears to have made good use of his time. His ability to teach himself intellectually complex subjects proved to be his major strength. He began his study of bio-chemistry and took a correspondence course in psychology and hypnotism, albeit from an un-accredited medical school in Italy. He listed himself in the phone book as Dr. David Ferrie.

He continued his involvement with the Civil Air Patrol and reached the rank of Captain. There he met a cadet named Lee Harvey Oswald.[7]

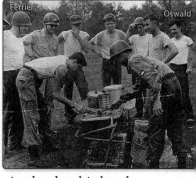

Towards the end of the 1950s another personal tragedy entangled Ferrie. His hair started falling out in clumps. Before long all of the hair on his body, including his eyebrows and eyelashes, was gone. He compensated for this by wearing a crude homemade wig glued to his head and false eyebrows painted on his face. It is unclear whether his study of bio-chemistry was related to his hair loss, as some have suggested. But what is clear is that something happened in the 1950s that set his beast of unrest in motion again. With it came the awakening of a violent and intolerant political temperament. A glimpse of this can be seen in a letter that he wrote to the U.S. Secretary of Defense, "There is nothing

I would enjoy better than blowing the hell out of every damn Russian, Communist, Red, or what-have-you. Between my friends and I, we can cook up a crew [*sic*] that can really blow them to hell … I want to train killers …"[8]

Someone in the government must have seen the value in an airline pilot who wanted to train killers, because Ferrie started moonlighting as a pilot for the CIA.[9] The precise extent of Ferrie's relationship with the CIA is not fully known. Many of the documents are still classified. But it is widely reported that he flew numerous missions in and out of Cuba, first supplying Castro with arms to fight Batista and later supplying the anti-Castro underground with weapons.

Castro came to power on January 1, 1959. Within a year he had seized American assets (casinos, factories, and oil refineries), openly embraced Communism, and militarily allied himself with the Soviet Union. Ferrie felt personally betrayed, and set out with a vengeance to destroy Castro and his Communist dictatorship. This hatred led Ferrie into a long and complex relationship with the anti-Castro Cuban underground here in the United States. He firebombed targets inside Cuba,[10] and traveled to Guatemala to train Cuban exiles to fly planes in support of the Bay of Pigs invasion.

Back in Washington, D.C., events were unfolding that would greatly impact Ferrie's life.[11] Kennedy's White House and the CIA had very different ideas about how to stop Communism, especially the expansion of Soviet influence in the Western Hemisphere. This policy dispute erupted into open conflict between the two camps. Many of the CIA's activities were untraceable even by the CIA inspector general. These "unvouchered expenditures" essentially meant that the CIA was refusing to be controlled by the White House. The situation oscillated between insubordination and treason. In 1975 when the Senate Intelligence Committee finally looked into these activities, Chairman Frank Church likened the CIA's activities to "a rogue elephant rampaging out of con-

*Dr. Mary's Monkey*

trol."[12] Actually, the problem was even deeper. The question: Who is running the government?

The stakes were enormous. The pressures unbelievable. The players believed nothing less than the destiny of the planet was at stake. The CIA's plan for keeping the Soviets at bay was to put a gun to their head. Batteries of American missiles armed with nuclear warheads sat in Turkey on the U.S.S.R.'s southern border. All major Soviet cities, including Moscow, were now ready to burst into the flames of a nuclear nightmare within thirty minutes of an order from Washington. Kennedy ordered them removed, but the Pentagon did not comply. The Soviets were very unhappy about such intimidation and were anxious for an opportunity to show the Americans just what it felt like to have someone point a nuclear missile at them. Castro gave them the opportunity.

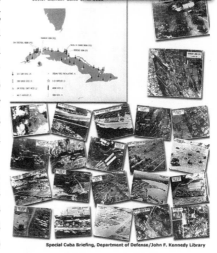

Special Cuba Briefing, Department of Defense/John F. Kennedy Library

Castro was determined to break America's grip on his island. In his words, "It is time to tell the Yankees that we are not your plantation, your gambling casino, or your whorehouse."[13] In order to discourage an American military overthrow of his government, Castro offered his island to the Soviets as launching pad for their nuclear missiles. The Soviets wasted little time in moving them into position.

In early April of 1961 American intelligence started picking up unusual radio signals from the Camaguey Mountains in central Cuba.[14] But the radio signals were too weak to analyze properly. They were simultaneously receiving reports from the anti-Castro guerillas inside Cuba that some large facility was under construction in a deep ravine in the jungle in the Camagueys. Were the Soviets moving nuclear missiles into Cuba? The CIA needed better intelligence. They needed hard evidence. The CIA decided to send a team into Cuba to collect radio signals from a mountain top in the Camagueys.

Ferrie was ordered to come to Washington, where he met with General Charles Cabell, one of the top people at the CIA. The general explained the mission to Ferrie and a young aeronautic electronics expert named Robert Morrow. They would leave from the west coast of Florida at night on April 16, 1961. Ferrie would fly the plane, with Morrow as copilot, and land in a clearing in the jungles. Guerillas would meet the plane and take them to a location to record the radio signals. At last, Ferrie was doing something really important.

The mission went as planned, until their party was discovered by Cuban army troops, who strafed the plane as it was taking off. Ferrie was wounded in the incident. The intelligence they collected did get back to Washington, just in time for the biggest debacle in the history of the CIA.

The Bay of Pigs invasion was a disaster. At the last moment President Kennedy had refused to supply U.S. military air support for the invasion, which landed at dawn on April 17, 1961. Castro won the day and solidified his control of Cuba. Hundreds of invading Cuban exiles were killed on

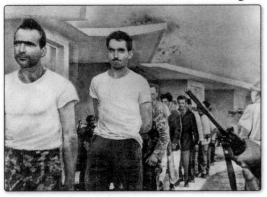
the beach. Over 1,200 were captured. Kennedy was furious at the CIA, believing they were trying to manipulate him into an act of war. He fired Dulles, Cabell, and Bissell, the top brass at the CIA, and ordered his brother Bobby, the U.S. Attorney General,

*Dr. Mary's Monkey*

to oversee the CIA, and to dismantle its system of unaccountable expenditures.

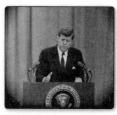

These events led Ferrie into a very complex world of covert operations where the lines between official and unofficial, between legal and illegal, became increasingly unclear.

By 1961, Ferrie lived in a three-level house near New Orleans International Airport, where he worked. Ferrie said his mother lived on the main floor, which looked like a normal middle-class house with sofas, paintings, books, and the like. Here Ferrie held air patrol meetings. The entire top floor was David's personal territory, and was strictly for his medical interests. It contained a medical library with various diplomas hung on the walls, a psychiatric couch, medical equipment like microscopes and test tubes, and about twenty caged mice for his medical experiments. In the basement sat the sawed-off remains of a World War II fighter plane, which he used as a primitive flight simulator to teach flying.[15]

This was, frankly, as good as life ever got for David Ferrie. From here we follow a descent that can only be described as tragic.

As the story was told to me by ex-CAP cadets, one night Ferrie got drunk and, in an attempt to impress a young boy, borrowed a plane and went for a joyride, buzzing the sleeping city of New Orleans at tree-top level. Some say he had sex with the boy during the flight. FAA officials were waiting at the airport when he returned. They set in motion an effort to pull his commercial license. He was also booked on "decency charges" concerning his relationship with the teenage boy.[16] About the same time, he lost his position with the Civil Air Patrol through insubordination and misconduct. Again, the basic ingredients were young boys. Ferrie insisted on sleeping in the cabin with the teenage cadets, and threw a beer party for them on the beach, both violations of CAP rules. Ferrie left the CAP and started his own flying club for teenage boys, called the Falcons, and held meetings in his home.

Ferrie's religious ambitions also re-surfaced in 1961. He became a member of the clergy of the Apostolic Orthodox Old Catholic Church of North America, an independent offshoot of the Roman Catholic Church headquartered in a house in Louisville, Kentucky. It was from this fountain of legitimacy that Ferrie sought to attain his rank as Bishop.

On November 30, 1961, wearing a wig Scotch-taped to his head and accompanied by sidekick Jack Martin, Ferrie arrived in Louisville expecting to be consecrated as a Bishop of the Church. It was not to be. The Archbishop who was supposed to perform the ceremony had heard of Ferrie's dismissal from Eastern Airlines, refused to consecrate him, and chastised him for the reports of his unnatural sexual behavior. The Archbishop's criticism went further still, telling Ferrie he intended to excommunicate him from the Church for behavior unbecoming to a Church official. Ferrie was furious and departed in anger. In January 1962, the Archbishop officially excommunicated Ferrie from the Church, advising him by letter that he had been "degraded and cast out of the clergy and Church in America."

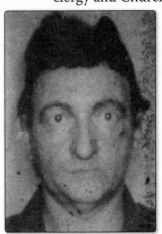

Ferrie's battle with Eastern Airlines had lasted for several years. A doctor who examined him for Eastern Airlines described him as having a "psychotic personality and no sense of responsibility."[17] He eventually lost his job. His life fell into a spiral. He moved from his tri-level house by the airport to a small apartment in town. His hair had now fallen out completely, and he began wearing a homemade orange wig which some said was made of monkey hair.[18] He replaced his natural eyebrows with dark grease paint. When combined with his newly purchased wardrobe of second-hand clothes, his appearance created an unforgettable impression on those he met.

WE ENTER 1963. Ferrie made one final try at getting someone to recognize his religious talents, his fourth attempt at the clergy. This time it was from the Orthodox Catholic Church, another offshoot Catholic sect, which split from the Church over a doctrinal dispute in 1709. The worldwide head of this church was reported to be an Archbishop in Geneva, Switzerland, who was identified in the Southern Research report as a translator at a disarmament conference.

The Chancellor of the North American Province was Bishop George A. Hyde, who lived in Washington, D.C. and ran a small seminary out of his house. Hyde had three young male novices and expected another three shortly. Each person in the house held an outside job and contributed his income to Hyde to run his house. Using the title Friar Hyde, he offered his services to the Washington D.C. Juvenile Court, which responded by placing a young boy in his home. Hyde said, "If I am successful, I would like to take in other boys like him."

Early that summer Ferrie told Hyde of his desire to become a priest and asked Hyde to ordain him. After considerable discussion, Hyde agreed to the request saying the next opportunity would be at the Bishop's conference in Kankake, Illinois. Hyde recommended David Ferrie as a candidate for ordination, but requested the hosting Bishop to ordain him, since he could not attend. Ferrie was scheduled to be ordained a priest of this church on July 19, 1963.

Just two days before Ferrie's scheduled ordination, Jack Martin, Ferrie's old sidekick in New Orleans, arrived at the Bishop's Rectory in Kankake, Illinois, and told the Bishop that David Ferrie had been arrested several times on charges of homosexuality and that he was presently appealing one such allegation in the Louisiana Court of Appeals. Martin picked up the phone, called the Clerk of Court in New Orleans, and handed the phone to one of the

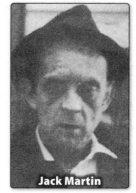
Jack Martin

priests to verify the information. The Bishop refused to ordain Ferrie.

Back in New Orleans, Ferrie's involvement with the increasingly desperate anti-Castro Cuban underground was escalating. His main employment was working as a "private investigator" for a right-wing extremist named Guy Banister, who was heavily involved in covert anti-communist activities throughout Latin America.[19] Ferrie also served as a private investigator and personal pilot for accused Mafia boss Carlos Marcello (and others). By July of 1963, Ferrie's assistance to the anti-Castro Cuban underground included the military training of a dozen Cuban exiles at a rural camp located about forty miles from New Orleans. Their target was Castro himself.[20] By this time, Kennedy had explicitly prohibited paramilitary raids on Cuba by desperate exile groups. On July 31, 1963, the FBI raided this training camp, arrested and/or detained eleven people (mostly Cubans and a few mobsters), and confiscated a large quantity of military weapons.

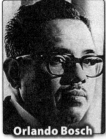
Orlando Bosch

The military weaponry included over a ton of dynamite, aerial bomb casings, detonators, and the ingredients to make napalm. It is believed that the mission of this group was the assassination of Fidel Castro and that it was one of many projects organized by the Cuban exile, Dr. Orlando Bosch, a fanatical terrorist and saboteur who began his career as a medical doctor.[21]

While there is no evidence that Ferrie was present when the FBI raided the camp, he is believed to have been closely involved and to have procured the explosives and military hardware for the operation from an explosives bunker at the Schlumberger Tool Company.

Had ordinary people been caught with that same equipment and in those same circumstances, they would have been sent to jail for years. For some reason, the FBI released these eleven saboteurs and attempted to cover up their detainment.[22] It should be noted that Ferrie-employer Guy Banister

*Dr. Mary's Monkey*

had run the FBI's Chicago office and was a close professional associate of J. Edgar Hoover.

Into this caldron walked one of Ferrie's old Civil Air Patrol cadets, who had just returned to New Orleans with his pregnant wife and baby daughter. Lee Harvey Oswald had been off in the Marines for several years, and had lived for several more years in the Soviet Union, where he had met his young bride. In New Orleans, Oswald got a job at the Reily Coffee Company, located around the corner from Guy Banister's office where Ferrie worked. Oswald was seen with Ferrie several times that summer:

- ☞ Oswald and Ferrie were seen together at Banister's office at 544 Camp St.

- ☞ Ferrie and Clay Shaw took Oswald up to Jackson, Louisiana to try to get him a job in the Southeastern Louisiana State Hospital, a mental hospital staffed with doctors from both Tulane and LSU medical schools. As part of that effort, Shaw and Ferrie brought Oswald to nearby Clinton, Louisiana, to register to vote.

- ☞ Ferrie had a party at his apartment. His guests included Clay Shaw, Lee Oswald, Perry Russo, and several Cuban exiles. Ferrie got drunk and discussed how President Kennedy could be killed if he was caught in a crossfire of high-powered rifles.

IN THE MONTHS THAT FOLLOWED, Ferrie spent his time helping Carlos Marcello defend himself against racketeering charges brought by Robert Kennedy and the U.S. Justice Department. On November 22, 1963, at the moment of President Kennedy's assassination, Ferrie was sitting in federal court in New Orleans with Marcello as the judge prepared to read the jury's "not guilty" verdict.

Later that afternoon, Ferrie made a sudden trip to Texas. Jack Martin (who had just been pistol whipped that afternoon by his employer Guy Banister) called the DA's office to say that Ferrie may have been involved in Kennedy's assassination. In response, the New Orleans District Attorney's office raided Ferrie's apartment on Louisiana Avenue Parkway. There they found aerial bomb casings, maps of Cuba, a small portion of his medical equipment and a dozen or so mice in cages. Ferrie was picked up for questioning by the DA's office when he returned to New Orleans. The New Orleans DAs found the circumstances of his trip suspicious, and Ferrie's explanation of the trip unbelievable. They turned Ferrie over to the FBI for further questioning. The FBI promptly released Ferrie with what amounted to a public apology.

At this point let me state that I cannot say if David Ferrie was involved in the assassination of President Kennedy. And more importantly, it is not critical to the issue we are discussing.

However, we *are* exploring the life and activities of a man who was running an underground medical laboratory which was said to have been using monkey viruses to develop a biological weapon. The fact that Ferrie was suspected of being involved in the Kennedy assassination is why we know as much about him as we do, and is how we know of his involvement in covert medical experiments with Dr. Mary Sherman and others. Later, in 1966, New Orleans District Attorney Jim Garrison re-opened his investigation into the Kennedy assassination at the suggestion of U.S. Senator Russell Long. Garrison found Ferrie to be central to his investigation.

Here are some comments about Ferrie from Garrison's 1967 *Playboy* interview:

> After the assassination, as a matter of fact, something psychologically curious happened to Ferrie: He dropped out of anti-Castro exile activities, left the pay of the CIA, and drifted aimlessly while his emotional problems increased to the point where he was totally dependent on huge doses of tranquilizers and barbiturates. I don't know if Ferrie ever experienced any guilt about the assassination itself, but in his last months, he was a tortured man.[23]

I had nothing but pity for Dave Ferrie while he was alive, and I have nothing but pity for him now that he's dead. Ferrie was a pathetic and tortured creature, a genuinely brilliant man whose twisted drives locked him into his own private hell. If I had been able to help Ferrie, I would have; but he was in too deep and he was terrified.[24]

For a long time afterward, Ferrie kept the remaining mice in hutches in his dining room, nursing plans for attaching small incendiary flares to them and parachuting them into Cuba's sugarcane fields.[25]

David Ferrie perennially was being defrocked, first of his priesthood, then of his hair, then of his Civil Air Patrol captaincy and then of his position as an Eastern Air Lines pilot. It is unlikely that he was unaffected by this accumulation of bitter experience. This man with a brilliant mind and a face like a clown was a dangerous man.[26]

In February of 1967, only a few days after Garrison's investigation was made public, David Ferrie was found dead in his disheveled apartment. The Coroner ruled that Ferrie died of natural causes. To this day, speculation continues about the cause of his death: Some argue that he was murdered; some argue that he took his own life. The only three names mentioned in Ferrie's handwritten will are his brother, his friend Alvin Beauboeuf, and Rev. George A. Hyde.

Considering all the things he lost during his life, it is interesting to note that his religious garments hung in his closet until the end.

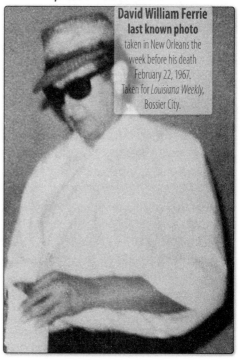

David William Ferrie last known photo taken in New Orleans the week before his death February 22, 1967. Taken for *Louisiana Weekly*, Bossier City.

IN JANUARY 1993, I FLEW TO NEW ORLEANS to assist Gus Russo in his investigation of Lee Harvey Oswald for the PBS television show *Frontline*. Before I left for New Orleans, I called Perry Russo.[27] Perry had been Garrison's key witness, who testified that he was in Ferrie's apartment when Ferrie plotted to kill Kennedy. In 1993 Perry was a cab driver in New Orleans, so I asked him to pick me up at the airport. Once in the cab I asked him to tell me everything he knew about Ferrie, starting with the first time he met him.

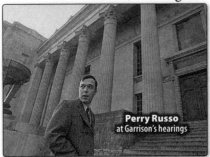

Perry Russo
at Garrison's hearings

Perry began at the beginning and talked for nearly an hour. His descriptions were detailed and insightful. His story began back in high school, when he coached a neighborhood basketball team. One of the boys on his team was the object of David Ferrie's affection. The boy had moved in with Ferrie. As a favor to the boy's parents, Perry Russo infiltrated Ferrie's group with the intention of bringing his friend home. To do this, he had to break Ferrie's considerable psychological grip on the youngster.[28] Throughout his tale, Perry Russo told me of both his successes and his failures in a balanced manner. I asked questions as we went along. He was quick to say "I don't know" when he did not know, and he struggled to remember details about the things he could. It was clear to me that Perry never really liked Ferrie, but he came to respect him. His descriptions were particularly helpful.

THE DAVE FERRIE THAT PERRY RUSSO talked about first was Captain Dave Ferrie, the successful commercial airline pilot. It was Perry who described Ferrie's house near the airport room-by-room: the middle class apartment on the main floor, the fighter plane in the basement, and his medical suite above. It was here that Ferrie was most at home, among his diplomas, reclining couches, microscopes, test tubes, medi-

*Dr. Mary's Monkey*

cal books, and mice. It was here he plotted to cure cancer and to rid the world of Communism.

When Ferrie lost his airline job in 1961, he also lost his affluent lifestyle. Perry's before-and-after descriptions contrasted a proud man who meticulously wore uniforms with a broken man who shopped exclusively at thrift stores. As Perry described Ferrie's small apartment on Louisiana Avenue Parkway, it became clear that the bulk of Ferrie's furniture, his medical equipment and his airplane-related paraphernalia did not make the transition to 3330 Louisiana Avenue Parkway. So I asked Perry about this. He said he remembered asking, "What happened to all Dave's stuff?" to either Ferrie himself or to one of the boys who hung out at his apartment. Perry was told Ferrie had stashed his extra "stuff" in another apartment nearby.[29]

TWO DAYS LATER Perry Russo picked up Gus Russo and me, and drove us over to Ferrie's apartment on Louisiana Avenue Parkway. While Gus asked Perry questions about Garrison and the Kennedy assassination, I got out of the car and walked around, checking the distance between that building and the one I knew, checking the angles, and taking pictures. When I got back in the car, Perry mentioned that Ferrie's apartment had been vacant for four or five years after his death in 1967.

Those were the same years that my girlfriend Barbara's apartment had been vacant![30] Two rental apartments, both on the same street within a dozen houses yards of each other, both with the lingering smell of animals, and both voluntarily taken off the market (without rent) for years at a time! There had to be a connection! My conclusion could only be that Ferrie had been involved in both apartments, and used 3225 Louisiana Avenue Parkway as his underground medical laboratory.

Having placed Barbara across the street from David Ferrie's known rental, let's revisit the subject of her upstairs

David Ferrie's Apartment
3330 Louisana Ave. Parkway

Ferrie's "Little Lab"
(Barbara's Apartment)
3225 Louisana Ave. Parkway

neighbor Miguel. I do not want to make too much of him. It is possible he was a real "nobody," but there are a few points worth noting.

First, consider his claim that he worked occasionally "at a service station in Jefferson Parish." From 1964 to his death in 1967, David Ferrie operated *a service station in Jefferson Parish.*

Secondly, Miguel had said he worked as "a mechanic." Within the covert operations circles in which David Ferrie ran, the word "mechanic" was a commonly used euphemism for "assassin."

Thirdly, Perry Russo testified in court that, in September 1963, he heard David Ferrie, Clay Shaw, and *several Cubans* discuss shooting President Kennedy with high-powered ri-fles. The location of this in-cident was David Ferrie's apartment at 3330 Louisiana Avenue Parkway. When I in-terviewed Perry Russo about David Ferrie, he said the Cubans frequently showed up at Ferrie's apartment. They just appeared. No phone calls. No cars. Always late at night.

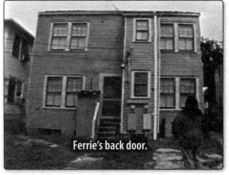

Ferrie's back door.

Always in groups. Always from the back staircase.

Ferrie's address sounds like it's in the next block from Barbara's 3225 Louisiana Avenue Parkway abode, but the numbers are misleading. There is no cross street, and both are on the same block.

How did the Cubans know *when* to show up? Were they staying in Miguel's apartment down the block? Was Miguel one of them? It is clearly stated by both Garrison in *On the Trail of the Assassins*, and by Turner and Hinckle in *Deadly Secrets* (and many other books), that Ferrie was part of the secret war against Cuba, and that these activities included an underground railroad which transported militant Cuban exiles to guerrilla-warfare training at places like Banister's camp outside New Orleans.

Now, where would you lodge a group of guerillas who had just come from a week of combat training in the swamps? At your mother's house? No, you would need to have *a safe house*. A secure place that was basically empty so it could be used as needed for a stopover. A place just like the apartment across the street from Ferrie, close to the operation, but far from high-traffic areas where it might attract unwanted attention. All of which made me wonder if our neighbor Miguel might not have been "part of the scenery," an artifact of the underground Cuban railroad left in position to keep an eye on things, and to make sure no one got too curious about the apartment building where *those terrible men did horrible things to those animals.*

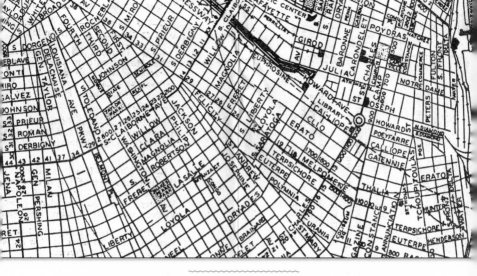

1   Southern Research Company, "Background on David William Ferrie," March 6, 1963, p. 12.

2   Comment by Jack Martin, an employee of Guy Banister and an associate of David Ferrie.

3   Southern Research Company, Inc., "Background on David William Ferrie," January 31,

1963 and March 6, 1963.

4 The fact that Ferrie, both physically able and very intelligent, did not participate in World War II supports the nervous breakdown story.

5 Mrs. Frances M. McKee, Rocky River High School, quoted by Southern Research, January 31, 1963.

6 According to Southern Research, the female pilot was Jean Naatz.

7 "Who was Lee Harvey Oswald?" *Frontline*, a television documentary, PBS, November 1993.

8 Davis, John H., *Mafia Kingfish: Carlos Marcello and the Assassination of John F. Kennedy* (New York, 1989), p. 145; also Hinckle and Turner, *Deadly Secrets*, p. 232.

9 Garrison, "Playboy Interview," *Playboy*, October 1967, p. 160.

10 Hinckle and Turner, *Deadly Secrets*, p. 233.

11 The story of Ferrie's flight to Cuba is from Robert Morrow, *First Hand Knowledge* (New York, 1992). Morrow was the electronics expert who flew with Ferrie on the mission.

12 *Baltimore Sun*, July 16, 1975.

13 I saw a film clip of this speech on network television in the mid-1970s. Unfortunately, I cannot cite the exact program. Check newsreel services for Castro speeches.

14 Morrow, *First Hand Knowledge*, p. 35-45.

15 Perry Russo, interview by author, January 1993.

16 A newspaper article on file in the New Orleans Public Library confirms the fact that "decency charges" were filed against Ferrie regarding a teenage boy prior to 1963.

17 Southern Research, March 6, 1963.

18 Davis, *Mafia Kingfish: Carlos Marcello and the Assassination of John F. Kennedy* (New York, 1989), p. 145.

19 Garrison, "Playboy Interview", p. 161-162.

20 Ibid., p. 156.

21 Hinckle and Turner, *Deadly Secrets*, p. 229.

22 For a more detailed description of this training camp incident, and other covert activities against Castro and Cuba, see Hinckle and Turner, *Deadly Secrets* (1992), previously published as *The Fish Is Red*; also see Garrison, *On the Trail of the Assassins*, p. 44.

23 Garrison, "Playboy Interview," p. 176.

24 Ibid., p. 176.

25 Garrison, *A Heritage of Stone* (New York, 1970), p. 122.

26 Ibid., p. 122.

27 Perry Russo is not related to Gus Russo.

28 Perry Russo, interview by author, January 1993.

29 Ibid.

30 This point about both apartments being vacant has been made by several people, including Barbara, who told me within days of renting her apartment in 1972 that her landlord had two properties which had been vacant, and had just rented the other unit across the street. She pointed the building out to me. It was memorable because of the arched window in the façade, which lit the stairwell by day but made it look like an aquarium at night. I am positive that this was Ferrie's apartment at 3330 Louisiana Avenue Parkway.

~~~~~~~~~~~~

# NEW ORLEANS STATES-ITEM

LARGEST AFTERNOON CIRCULATION IN LOUISIANA

Listen to The States-Item Chimes at 8, Noon and 5

**RED FLAS**

VOL. 88 — NO. 25    Associated Press, Advance News Service, North American Newspaper Alliance and AP Wirephoto    **TUESDAY, JULY 21, 1964**    Entered N. O. Post Office as Second Class Matter Under Act of March 3, 1879    PRICE 5c

# Orleans Woman Surgeon Slain By Intruder; Body Set Afi

## Guerrillas Ambush 2 Viet Units

**SAIGON, Viet Nam (AP)** — Communist Viet Cong guerrillas, using standard ambush tactics, crippled two and possibly three government units near the tip of South Viet Nam in a series of battles that continued into the night.

Reliable American sources said as many as 60 government troops had been killed and possibly 100 wounded in paddy fields and mangrove swamps of Chuong Thien province 125 miles south of Saigon. Five American advisers were wounded. He was flown to Saigon.

The battles were fought near the mud-walled fort of Vinh Chau, the center of a major engagement last week in which more than 90 government paramilitary personnel were either killed or wounded. The Communists staged two ambushes on this 10th anniversary of the Geneva accords that put the Reds in control of Communist North Viet Nam.

AT LEAST 50 troops were wounded in the ambush of a battalion-sized truck convoy wending its way south from ...

See VIET—Page 9

## French Vessel Carrying 28 Burning at Sea

**NEW YORK (AP)** — The French freighter Marguerite radioed today that she was afire about 775 miles east-southeast of Cape Race off Newfoundland, the Coast Guard reported.

The ship was en route from Montreal to Lisbon with about 28 men aboard, the Coast Guard added.

The "Mayday" (help) signal was picked up by a fishing vessel, the Campbell, about nine miles from the freighter, but headed for the area.

The Coast Guard said its merchant vessels were within a 100-mile radius of the stricken freighter.

A Coast Guard plane on base patrol also was headed for the area.

## WEATHER
### Afternoon Showers

(U. S. Weather Bureau) Sunset today, 7:00 p.m.; sunrise tomorrow, 5:13 a.m. New Orleans and vicinity: Partly cloudy today, tonight and tomorrow with widely scattered mostly afternoon showers.

**TEMPERATURES**

| A.M. | | P.M. | |
|---|---|---|---|
| 5 A.M. | 76 | 12 Noon | 89 |

Thundershowers. Variable to 10 mph. Highest temperature today, 94 to 96. Lowest tonight, 76 to 78. Louisiana — Partly cloudy, tonight and tomorrow with widely scattered mostly afternoon and evening thundershowers. Little change in temperatures. Highest today, 94 to 96. Low tonight, 70 to 76. Highest yesterday, 90; lowest today, 76.

Humidity, 57 per cent; barometer, 30.08, rising.

(Story, details on Page 36.)

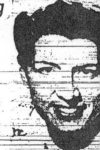

DR. MARY STULTS SHERMA

## Clues Lacking In Killing of Dr. Sherman

By KERMIT TARLETON

An intruder forced his way into a fashionable St. Charles ave. apartment early today, stabbed a prominent woman orthopedic surgeon to death and set fire to her body.

Police apparently had virtually no clues to the identity of the slayer of Dr. Mary Stults Sherman, whose body was found about 4:10 a. m. on the floor of her smoke-filled bedroom in the Patio Apartments, 3101 St. Charles

The 51-year-old cancer research specialist had been stabbed eight times in the left arm, left chest and stomach, police said, and her body was badly burned.

HOMICIDE DETECTIVES said the front door to her apartment had been forced open, her wallet was empty and her 1961 automobile was ...

Dr. Sherman was an orthopedic surgeon at the Ochsner Clinic and was director of the bone pathology laboratory of the Ochsner Foundation Hospital.

Police said apparently the body was set on fire in the bed, but rolled over onto the floor where it was found lying on the left side.

Juan Valdez, who occupies another apartment on the second floor of the apartments complex, reported that he smelled smoke and turned in the alarm.

Firemen arriving at the scene said the room was so filled with smoke they were not immediately able to enter the bedroom.

SAM MORAN, SPECIAL INVESTIGATOR for the Orleans Parish Coroner's office, said the front door had been forced open and an unsuccessful attempt made to open a jewelry box. Some rings and a watch were found inside the box, he said.

Mrs. Elinor Peterson, Negro, a maid who had been employed by Dr. Sherman for the past 13 years, said the doctor's apartment had been burglarized several times in recent years and a burglar alarm had been installed.

Police said the alarm was set off and it may have been disarmed.

**MRS. PETERSON SAID BURGLARS** stripped Dr. Sherman's apartment of jewelry some while she was on a visit to England.

The maid said that when she left Dr. Sherman about 4:30 p. m. yesterday she was in good spirits and talked of a woman friend who was expected here for a visit.

Hospital attaches said Dr. Sherman worked in her laboratory yesterday morning, but was off duty yesterday afternoon. She kept a medical appointment in the afternoon and was soon returning home at 6 p. m.

Police were not able to immediately determine whether Dr. Sherman left home after the departure of the maid.

Valdez, who said he knew Dr. Sherman for about three years, described her as being a quiet, pleasant person who kept to herself and did very little entertaining.

He said she gave a great deal of her time in work for medical groups and for the benefit of crippled children.

**DR. SHERMAN WAS A WIDOW** who came to New Orleans from Chicago, 4 years ago. Miss Barbara Stults, lived in Chicago. Her father is a resident of Boston, Tex.

Lt. Frank Hayward of the Homicide Division said police are looking for Dr. Sherman's 1961 Valiant two-door gray automobile which was reported missing. They urged anyone who may notice it to call police at once and the public is asked not to touch the vehicle.

Taking part in the investigation in addition to Hayward were Homicide Detectives Robert Townsend and Frank Hayward, and Sgt. Allen Heltner and Pts. Eugene Knight.

## Police Slaying Bulletin

Here is the text of the police bulletin on the slaying of Dr. Mary Sherman:

"Victim: White female identified as Dr. Mary S. Sherman, 3101 St. Charles ave., Apt. J; Time of Occurrence: Between the hours of 4:30 p. m. 7-20-64, and 4:10 a. m., 7-21-64; Weapon used, undetermined at present time; wanted subject of unknown."

Here is a message on Dr. Sherman's missing automobile:

"Attempt to locate the following described vehicle involved in a homicide. 1961 Valiant two-door gray, bearing 1964-65 Louisiana license, 100N894, serial number, 1112470605.

"This car was purchased from Howard Motors in New Orleans.

"Any information of it located do not touch this vehicle. Notify homicide division of detective bureau immediately."

— Maj. L. J. Cassanova

## Disarm Conference Holds 200th Meet

**GENEVA (AP)** — The 17-nation disarmament conference met for the 200th time today and reported no progress.

The delegates met for two hours. The subject under discussion was the proposed treaty on general and complete disarmament on which East and West have been deadlocked since the talks opened March 14, 1962.

### CHECKING THE SPOT WHERE THE BODY of Dr. Mary Stults Sherman was found beside her smouldering bed are Detectives FRANK HAYWARD and ROBERT TOWNSEND JR.

NEIGHBORS—REPORT—PREVIOUS INTRUDERS

## Scene of Slaying Reveals Interrupted Busy Routine

By ROSEMARY POWELL

In Dr. Mary Stults Sherman's kitchen a single place setting of china and silver, with a tea bag in the cup, were laid out on the serving bar this morning in readiness for a busy orthopedic surgeon's breakfast.

Just across the hall was the evidence of a well-organized schedule interrupted suddenly. A neatly covered bedroom explained the charted tempers of the bed where Dr. Sherman's body was set afire, after an unknown assailant stabbed her eight times.

Dr. Sherman's neighbors in the Patio Apartments, 3101 St. Charles, who described her ...

## Fired Warning Rockets Across U.S. Ship-Reds

**MOSCOW (AP)** — The Soviet Union denied today that Soviet patrol cutters fired shots across the bow of an American grain ship in the Black Sea.

The denial of the government newspaper Izvestia said only warning rockets were fired at the ship, the S. S. Sister Katingo, in order to stop her last week. The paper said the Soviet Union reported a protest of the United States to the Soviet embassy in Washington.

The cutters chased the ship after it left the port of Novorossiysk where it had been unloading a cargo of U.S. grain without getting further clearance.

The skipper of the ship, Capt. William H. Perkins, claimed the Soviets fired across his bow.

The Soviet news ministry called in the No. 2 man of the U.S. embassy, Walter Stoessel, and said Fortescue and said Perkins was forbidden to re-enter a Soviet port.

## RAUL CASTRO URGES TALKS

## Ready to Bargain, Cuban Tells U.S.

**SANTIAGO, Cuba (AP)** — Cuba is ready to meet the United States at the bargaining table "anywhere, anytime" and discuss whatever would be necessary, its iron-out problems between the two countries, Armed Forces Minister Raul Castro said today.

But for such a possible reconciliation move to succeed, Castro said, "there must be demanded by both countries"—

Castro was asked at news conference if this meant Cuba would abandon the five points set forth by his brother, Prime Minister Fidel Castro, in the October, 1962 missile crisis, as essential conditions to be met prior to any negotiations.

RAUL ANSWERED at this point that if he would have any negotiations, they would have to be without any previous conditions.

Fidel has demanded American withdrawal from Guantanamo Naval Base, suspension of "all surveillance flights," suspension of aid to "internal ..."

See CUBA—Page 4

## BULLETINS

**WASHINGTON (AP)**—President Johnson ordered today a full FBI investigation of race rioting in Harlem, declaring that "violence and lawlessness cannot, must not and will not be tolerated." (Earlier details Page 3.)

**WARSAW (AP)**—Premier Khrushchev said today Soviet Premier Nikita S. Khrushchev said today Communist leader Wladyslaw Gomulka—who also joined Goldwater. (Earlier details Page 12.)

**CASTRO TOOK THE** occasion to a mineral fizz a Cuban cocktail. But later the Cuban government announced the Marines on ninety duty at the Guantanamo border fumble ...

Later the group tried to ...

### Today's Chuckle

One of the dubious things about using a credit card: You spend what you don't think you owe, were paying at the time.

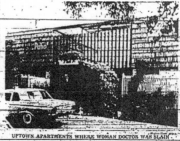

UPTOWN APARTMENTS WHERE WOMAN DOCTOR WAS SLAIN

# CHAPTER 6

# Mary, Mary

THE WOMAN ENTERS OUR STORY as an enigma. Considered "absolutely brilliant" by her medical colleagues, Mary Sherman rose rapidly to the very top ranks of the male-dominated hierarchy of American medicine in bone and joint surgery, a field that to this day has extremely few female physicians. Self-made, financially successful, and professionally respected, Dr. Sherman was a sophisticated and powerful woman during an era when the future feminists of the 1960s were still sitting at home watching *Leave it to Beaver*. Yet the glimpses we see of her very private personal life show a complex and sensitive woman who loved theater, literature, music, wine, flowers, and international travel, and who carried with her some terrible personal burdens. But we see no discernible political interest.[1] None of this seems to explain, or even hint at, her involvement with a politically violent, emotionally unstable, drug-addicted social outcast like David Ferrie, who had no formal medical training.

Most of what we know about Mary Sherman comes from newspaper articles, an unusual police report, and her will. To that we add insights from a few medical articles, and a handful of interviews with people who knew her, to produce a sketch of an unusually talented woman who met an unusually horrible end.

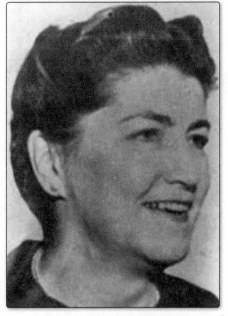

Born "Mary Stults" in Evanston, Illinois in 1913, she was one of several daughters of a musical voice teacher.[2] At the age of sixteen, Mary went to France for two years to study at L'ecole de M. Collnot, and later taught French while working on a masters at the University of Illinois. Marrying Thomas Sherman, she became Mary Sherman.[3]

The pattern of an academic superstar is immediately obvious from her Phi Beta Kappa membership to her graduate work at the University of Chicago. For those unfamiliar with this institution, please note that within academic circles, the University of Chicago is an intellectual powerhouse which rivals Harvard, Stanford, and any other famous university one might name. It was founded by a grant from the Rockefeller Foundation, and was designed on the model of the European research university, rather than the American teaching college. This was done at a time when the Rockefeller fortune was heavily involved in the drug companies, and their sponsorship of biochemical research helped develop new commercial drugs. Today, the University of Chicago continues on the leading edge of genetics and cancer research.

As an outgrowth of this biochemical medical research, the University of Chicago became one of the first major centers of nuclear research. The landmark event of this nucle-

*Dr. Mary's Monkey*

ar effort was the construction of the first "atom smasher," a huge nuclear accelerator hidden in the bowels of UC's sports stadium. In 1937, it produced the first sustained nuclear reaction for UC physicist Enrico Fermi. This is where Mary Sherman did her post-graduate work. She was trained at the headwaters of nuclear, bio-chemical, and genetic research in America.

Before she became involved in human medicine, Mary did ground-breaking research into botanical viruses which lived in soil. Her early articles were so profound and so insightful that they were frequently quoted in the 1940s, 1950s, 1960s, 1970s, and 1980s. Though she had been dead for thirty years, the *Scientific Citation Index* shows ten medical articles published in 1993 which contained references to her scientific writings published between 1947 and 1965. The names of the journals tell the story of her state-of-the-art use of radiation for the treatment of bone cancers:

| | |
|---|---|
| *Radiology* | *Acta Radiologia* |
| *Skeletal Radiology* | *Histopathology* |
| *Pathologic Research* | *Bone* |

From this, we can see the evidence of her breakthrough thinking. This young woman, who studied in France at the time when Madame Curie's name was at the top of the scientific heap, was one of America's most promising minds. With the proper training, encouragement and opportunities, she could be within striking distance of the legendary Curie herself, and could possibly become the most important woman in science. Maybe it would be Mary, who at such a young age had understood the basic life of viruses better than anyone before her, who would break through "the cancer barrier." The great minds at UC saw her potential and brought her along. During the 1940s she became Associate Professor of Orthopedic Surgery, and practiced medicine at UC's Billings Hospital.[4]

In the early 1950s, Mary Sherman's life changed. Her cancer work at the University of Chicago had attracted the attention of a famous and wealthy doctor who was president of the American Cancer Society, president of a famous medical clinic which bore his name, and Chief of Surgery at Tulane Medical School, one of the most respected medical schools of the day. The doctor was Alton Ochsner, M.D., of New Orleans.

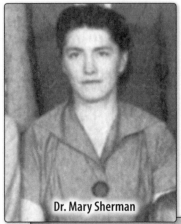

Dr. Mary Sherman

Ochsner's offer to Dr. Sherman was considerable. She would be a partner in Ochsner's clinic, the head of her own cancer laboratory, and, to keep her place in the academic side of medicine, she would be an Associate Professor at Tulane Medical School. Additionally, she would also have the personal support of one of the most politically powerful and well-connected doctors in America, a conduit for a constant flow of research funds.

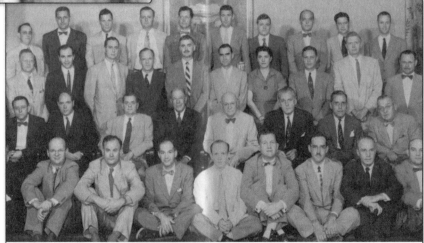

Dr. Sherman with members of the Ochsner Foundation hospital staff in May, 1953

*Dr. Mary's Monkey*

Again single, Mary moved to New Orleans in 1952, and took up residence on historic St. Charles Avenue, near the corner of Louisiana Avenue. There she lived until her death in 1964, juggling her jobs at Tulane and Ochsner's, doing surgery at Charity Hospital, and working on the medical staff of several children's hospitals. But as doctors went, she was always more comfortable in a laboratory than an operating room.

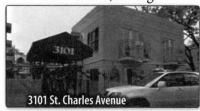
3101 St. Charles Avenue

Mary's career prospered. One of the clear marks of professional success for an orthopedic surgeon is to be elected to the American Academy of Orthopedic Surgeons. It takes years, if not decades. Some never make it. Once in the academy, the ladder continues. The bright stars get put on Committees which make the rules about science and ethics. They establish what is acceptable and who is accepted. The brightest of the stars chair these Committees. One of the most prestigious is the Pathology Committee, which reviews the state of the art on disease itself, particularly bone cancers.

Mary Sherman was Chairman of the Pathology Committee of the American Academy of Orthopedic Surgeons. Her position took her around the world. When the great wizards of medicine realized the very language which they used to describe and categorize cancers of the bone and soft tissue needed to be re-examined, they chose six of the nation's leading experts to tackle the task, including Dr. Mary Sherman.[5] When the front page of the newspaper had the sad task of announcing her death, it described her as "an internationally known bone specialist" whose main area of interest was "bone cancer treatment and research."[6]

So our question remains: What would motivate an accomplished medical professional to risk her reputation by getting involved in an underground medical laboratory with a violent political zealot owning a criminal record of sexual misconduct and with no medical credentials? Was she led there by her own ambition? Was there a dark side to her concealed from public view? Was she simply manipulated by more powerful forces? Or was there a medical problem brewing that was so serious that it was worth the risk?

## The Press Reports

IT IS IMPOSSIBLE TO DESCRIBE THE DEATH of Dr. Sherman without appearing both sensational and mysterious. This is because it was a sensational event, and much of it is still shrouded in mystery.

For nearly thirty years, the only information the world would see concerning her murder were articles published by two New Orleans newspapers, the *New Orleans States-Item* and the *Times-Picayune.*

Both papers covered the story for several weeks with overlapping reports and language, each with a slightly different editorial perspective. The coverage began with a banner headline on the front page on July 21, 1964. The *States-Item* announced:

### Orleans Woman Surgeon Slain by Intruder; Body Set Afire

*Clues Lacking in Killing of Dr. Sherman*

The lead article read,

> An intruder forced his way into a fashionable St. Charles Ave. apartment early today, stabbed a prominent woman orthopedic surgeon to death and set fire to her body. Police apparently had virtually no clues to the identity of the slayer of Dr. Mary Stults Sherman ...

The basic storyline went like this: At approximately four o'clock in the morning a neighbor smelled smoke and called the police. His name was Juan Valdez. The police checked the building and found one apartment filled with smoke. The police called the fire department. When the firefighters arrived, they removed a smoking mattress from the apartment. Within minutes the police searched the apartment and found the badly burned body of a woman that had been stabbed repeatedly. An investigator from the Coroner's office arrived and checked the scene. Then the NOPD homicide team arrived. No murder weapon was found, but a large knife was missing from the knife rack in the kitchen. Her body was removed to the Coroner's office, where it was identified by another doctor.

The *States-Item* reported,

> Homicide detectives said the front door to her apartment had been forced open, her wallet was empty, and her 1961 automobile was missing... Sam Moran, Special Investigator for the Orleans Parish Coroner's office, said the front door had been forced open and an unsuccessful attempt had been made to open a jewelry box.

Between the two papers, each of which ran three articles on their first day of coverage, the burglary motive was stated or referenced about twenty times, including several references to the fact that Dr. Sherman's apartment had been burglarized before. The burglary angle is so strong that the NOPD precinct captain complained to the press about "the departmental manpower shortage" in response to criticisms of "inadequate police protection in the neighborhood." It would not be until the next day, after a horrified city had literally millions of word-of-mouth discussions about the sensational murder/burglary, before the newspapers stated that the front door had *not* been forced open and her burglar alarm had been *turned off.* The press now reported that the homicide department, impressed by these facts, and the facts that "the intruder" knew which car belonged to Dr. Sherman and that a box full of jewelry which could have easily been carried off was left behind, *ruled out burglary as a motive.*

The first-day coverage continued with the standard biographical information about education and employment. Additionally, we learn that Dr. Sherman was a widow living alone, that she loved flowers, that her neighbors described her as "wonderful" and "thoughtful," and that her housekeeper said she was expecting a lady friend for a visit that evening.

Both papers take time to describe an unusual painting hanging in her living room:

> The most striking thing about the living room, however, is a pastel painting hung in a prominent position. In the foreground of the painting is the fear-gripped face of a woman clutching her throat. A series of smaller sketches in the background depict a Roman warrior stabbing a woman with his sword.

Deeper into this first-day coverage, we also learn that none of the neighbors, including those who were used to hearing even casual sounds from her apartment, heard a thing that night.

> Mrs. Levy [a neighbor who lived beneath Dr. Sherman for 12 years] ... usually heard Dr. Sherman when [she] came in at night, but last night she went to bed early and didn't hear anything.... "If there had been a loud commotion, I know I would have heard it," Mrs. Levy said. "The doctor was quiet, but I always heard her come in and take off her shoes, then padding around in her slippers. Sometimes I remarked to my husband, 'Doc's home again.'"

That day Dr. Sherman had come home early and washed her hair. She was seen by the building maintenance man about 4:00 P.M., and was last seen by her housekeeper at 4:30 P.M.

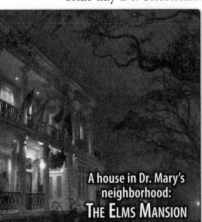

A house in Dr. Mary's neighborhood:

THE ELMS MANSION

On the second press day the case was referred to as "a mutilation slaying," to which NOPD Captain Stevens added, "Obviously some perverted mind was involved." The police were looking for a psychopath, perhaps one of her patients. The newspapers reported a "mysterious telephone caller" who had called several of Dr. Sherman's close friends to say, "You're next." The voice was male. Other developments were reported: Her car was found eight blocks away. A palm print was recovered from the car, but could not be identified. The car key was recovered from a neighboring lawn. Partial results of the autopsy leaked to the press: "Though Dr. Sherman's body had been mutilated, there was no evidence that she had been raped." Her body was held for ten days at the morgue and was then sent out of town for cremation.

Having now ruled out burglary as a motive, homicide officers proceeded "on the presumption that the killer was an acquaintance of the fifty-one-year-old widow." The press said, "Neighbors, relatives, and friends are being questioned, and police are ruling out no possibility as to the identity of the killer, the motive, or his method of entering the apartment." Police told reporters they suspected "Everybody and nobody." Over the next two weeks, "professional associates and social acquaintances" were interviewed by the police. The reported number grew to over 100 by August 3 and topped off at 150. On August 5, the *Times-Picayune* announced,

### No Leads Found in Slaying Case

… and dropped the story.

The *States-Item* continued coverage with eight more articles. On August 11, the front page of the *States-Item* announced a *press blackout* by police:

### Information in Sherman Case Halted

Information on the status of the police investigation of the mutilation-murder of Dr. Mary Stults Sherman was shut off today, as all questions on the probe were referred to Chief of Detectives Lawrence J. Cassanova, who is out of town.

Police say questioning scores of the bone specialist's professional associates and social acquaintances has turned up no lead to her killer.

The following day the front page story explained:

### Blackout Continues On Murder

Police say they have no clue on the murder ...

Dectective Chief Cassanova was still out of town, at a homicide seminar at LSU in Baton Rouge.

An exasperated police department responded by presenting the newspaper with an "if-it's-murders-you-want-it's-murders-we've-got" portfolio of unsolved murders, four male and four female, which the *States-Item* published on August 15 under the headline:

### Medic Slaying Still Baffles N.O. Police:
### One in 10 Murders Unsolved.

The papers had used a lot of colorful language to describe the murder:

| | |
|---|---|
| savage slaying | gruesome slaying |
| brutally slain | charred and mutilated |
| gruesome murder | hacked to death |
| grisly mutilation-murder | partially burned body |

But it is only in two sentences from the last column of the last article that we find any detail of the fire itself, or of the burns to Mary Sherman's body. We read,

The murderer set fire to her bed and piled underclothing on her body, setting it afire. The fire smoldered for some time — long enough to denude an innerspring mattress and burn away the flesh from one of the doctor's arms.

This article also tells us that:

Dr. Sherman had been away for two weeks prior to the weekend before the murder.

This raises another question: "Where was she?" I am told she was in Boston. Why was she there?

It would be nearly thirty years before anyone, other than the tight circle of people involved in the autopsy and the investigation, would know what the police and autopsy reports really said about Mary Sherman's murder.

Concurrent with the newspaper articles, rumors spread like wildfire, and influenced the public's perception of Mary Sherman's murder. By nine o'clock on the morning of the murder, the word had already spread throughout the offices of the New Orleans newspapers that there had been a lesbian sex killing in the uptown area. This is interesting, since the autopsy, which determined the cause of death and which discovered the laceration to her sexual organs, did not even begin until 9:15 A.M.[7]

Six weeks after the murder, in early September 1964, I personally heard another rumor about a female orthopedic surgeon killed over the summer. The source of this was a teacher welcoming our class back from summer holiday. In his version, she had been murdered by Communists. This was a head-scratcher, even in 1964. "What is the world coming to?" he asked us.

I couldn't understand why the Communists would want to kill an orthopedic surgeon. And since my father was an orthopedic surgeon, I wondered if the Communists had any interest in killing him, too. While researching this book, I wrote that teacher a letter about his comments made decades ago. He remembered the incident, and talked about the doctor's "dark side" and her association with "gay Mexicanos." Such was the word-of-mouth on the streets of New Orleans in 1964.

In 1992, I set out to get copies of the police reports. With the help of the NOPD item number (G-12994-64), I found them in the City Archives of the New Orleans Public Library. There were two reports. One was the Precinct Report, promptly written and filed by the street cops who first arrived at her apartment that July morning; the other was a Supplementary Report written by the Homicide Department months after the investigation had subsided. The Precinct Report was signed and approved by all parties. The Homicide Report was not. It was only signed by the officer who prepared it and was then filed without being co-signed or approved. I consider this violation of basic procedure extremely unusual for such a high-profile case.

## The Precinct Report

FROM THE PRECINCT REPORT we get a straightforward view of the post-call events at the crime scene. The police arrived and were met by Juan Valdez, who told them he thought the smoke was coming through the ventilation ducts from another apartment. A search of the various apartments found the door to the patio of Apartment J ajar, and the sliding door entrance to the apartment open one to two inches. Inside, the living room was full of smoke. The police called the fire department. Valdez told the police it was Mary Sherman's apartment, and brought them a wet towel to use as a gas mask, but they were unable to penetrate the smoke of the apartment. They waited for the fire department to arrive, and to remove the smoldering mattress using oxygen masks. When the smoke cleared, they found a body lying on the floor next to the bed. Their report said,

> The feet of the white female's body was pointed towards the head of the bed ...

Soon the coroner's team and the homicide team arrived. The scene was photographed. Certain items were confiscated. The Assistant Coroner pronounced the body dead and made comments about the victim:

*Dr. Mary's Monkey*

A preliminary examination by Dr. LoCascio on the scene determined that there were several possible stab wounds of the left arm of the body, which had not been deteriorated by the fire. There also appeared to be several stab wounds in the torso. There was also a large wound of the inside of the right thigh just above the knee. From further examination of the body, it was noted by the coroner that the right arm and a portion of the right side of the body extending from the right hip to the right shoulder was completely burned away exposing various vital organs.

The body was removed from the apartment and taken to the Coroner's office. The other residents in the building were all questioned. None heard anything between the time they retired and the time the police arrived, except one who heard Juan Valdez walking around his apartment before the police arrived.

From Elmener Peterson, Mary's housekeeper, police learned that the burglar alarm was in the "off" position, that Dr. Sherman was "expecting visitors from out of town," and that she had laid out a polka dot dress, which they found lying on a chair in the bedroom. As to the issue of whether the intruder had forced the door open, the report says,

> The officers could find no signs of the door leading to the apartment patio or sliding glass door having been forced open.

It is mentioned that the body was positively identified by Dr. Carolyn Talley, and that their police captain had summarized the results of the autopsy for them.

> The cause of death was also given to Patn. Knight by Capt. Stevens as follows: 1. Stab wound of the chest, penetrating the heart, hemopericardium and left hemithorax [*sic*] 2. Multiple stab wounds of the abdomen, with incid wound of the liver. 3. Multiple stab wounds of the left upper extremity and the right leg. 4. Laceration of Labia Minora. 5. Extreme burns of right side of body with complete de-

struction of right upper extremity and right side of thorax and abdomen.

## The Homicide Report

NOW WE LOOK AT THE HOMICIDE REPORT, a baffling document written in two parts. The first half, covering the crime scene, was completed on October 29, 1964, approximately ten weeks after the police stopped their investigation. The second half was dated several days later, on November 3, 1964. The report should have been signed by both investigators, Detective Frank Hayward and Detective Robert Townsend, Jr., and their supervisor, Lt. James Kruebbe. But there is only one signature, that of Detective Robert Townsend, Jr. The extreme delay in preparing this report and this unusual violation of a basic procedure show that, for some reason, this was not an ordinary report. My guess is that it was not signed by his co-investigator and supervisor for a reason. Perhaps they refused to sign it in protest. Perhaps they filed it without signing it so they could say they never saw it. Perhaps Townsend filed it himself, just to put something in the file. Who knows? I tried to contact Townsend to find out, but he did not return the calls.

This report begins with recounting the same events as the Precinct Report, except told from the perspective of the homicide team. As they arrived, they found the firemen cleaning up debris. They instructed them to stop and to leave all debris where they had placed it, so that the homicide team could inspect it and see what was being removed from the crime scene. (This is an important detail.) Then they described what they saw:

> The undersigned entered Apt. J. from the patio, the only entrance to said apartment, into the living room area. Said apartment was composed of a living room, kitchen, bathroom, study, and a bedroom.... Located in the bedroom, was the body of a white female, apparently dead, later learned to be one Dr. Mary Stults Sherman, WF, 51

yrs., formerly residing 3101 St. Charles Ave., Apt. J., who lived alone.... The body was in a supine position, the head in the direction of the river, the feet in the direction of the lake, and both legs were outstretched and parallel to each other... The left arm was outstretched and parallel to the left side of the body. The right side of the body from the waist to where the right shoulder would be, including the whole right arm, was apparently disintegrated from the fire, yielding the inside organs of the body. There was what appeared to be a stab wound in the left arm and also in the inner side of the right leg near the knee. The body was nude; however, there was clothing which had apparently been placed on top of the body, mostly covering the body from just above the pubic area to the neck. Some of the mentioned clothes had been burned completely, while others were still intact, but scorched.

The condition of the apartment did not support the idea of a violent crime:

It appeared that no scuffle took place inside of said bedroom, and nothing appeared to be dis-arranged in the bedroom or throughout the apartment.

Soot covered the apartment and made fingerprinting nearly impossible. Part of one print was recovered from the sherry bottle near her bed. Two burnt wooden matches were found on the cedar chest. From the soot prints, the detectives were sure these matches were there prior to the fire, though no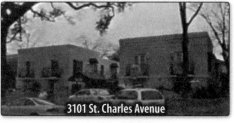

3101 St. Charles Avenue

other wooden matches of any kind could be found within the apartment, the inference being that the murderer must have brought the matches.

Sam Moran, the investigator from the Coroner's office who later erroneously told the press that the front door had been forced open and that the burglar had unsuccessfully tried to open the jewelry box, arrived, looked around, and then left with Mary's jewelry box, purse, check book and other personal items, including thirteen keys on a key ring found in the kitchen.

At the morgue, the autopsy was performed by Dr. Samuels, a pathologist, who told police (1) the victim died prior to the fire, (2) the victim had not been raped, and (3) the victim was dead before the laceration to the labia minora was inflicted. When the Coroner's officials examined the clothing piled on Dr. Sherman's body, they noted, "Most of the clothes were still neatly folded when placed on top of the body." The criminologist observed that these clothes were composed of a synthetic material which would ignite into a flame at 500 degrees Fahrenheit. At lower temperatures they would have only smoldered.

Back at the apartment, police removed approximately forty items, including two passports, two address books, one pair of white gloves with "apparent blood stains" found in the laundry hamper in the bathroom, and a copy of "Our Marriage Vows."

When Dr. Sherman's car was found, they searched a 350-foot radius of the car, and recovered numerous items common to women's handbags, none of which could be proved to be Dr. Sherman's. The key to her car, however, had been thrown over a nearby wall, and was found separately by a neighbor.

The remainder of the report (the 11/3/64 section) takes a bizarre turn. You recall the 150 professional associates and social acquaintances that the press said the police had interviewed concerning the murder? Look what we find instead!

Seven percent of the homicide report discussed John, a "Peeping Tom" who had ogled a twenty-six-year-old woman in Dr. Sherman's apartment complex six months earlier. He had since moved across town. His activities on the evening of July 20 were accounted for and supported by credible witnesses. The report clearly stated where he was employed, at a local vending machine company. The objective of this section seems to be to imply that sex crimes did occur in Mary's neighborhood.

Twenty percent of the report discussed Jane, a young woman from New Jersey with short red hair and toreador pants, who walked past Sherman's building around midnight, apparently on her way to a lesbian rendezvous in the French Quarter. The girl stopped in to see the night watchman across the street from Mary's apartment so she could make a phone call. She had nothing to do with the case, but the report clearly said where she was employed, at a theater on Canal Street. The objective of this section seems to be to point out that lesbians did live in (or at least walk through) Mary's neighborhood.

Ten percent of the report discussed Max, a social acquaintance of Mary Sherman. He was an author, and Max was his pen name. He suffered from arthritis and walked with a cane. Max only knew Mary for a year and had not

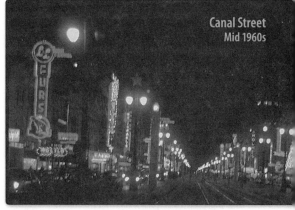

Canal Street
Mid 1960s

seen her in nine months. She used to stop by and discuss the theatre and literature with him. Due to his fondness for her, Max became depressed after one of her visits and wrote her a letter asking her not to return. Max described her as a "lesbian who lived in grand fashion." When the police asked Max how he knew she was a lesbian, he said he "had known a lesbian once in Venice," but "he did not concern himself with such matters." Speaking in a "very dramatic" voice to Detective Hayward, Max called her death a "delegated suicide." He said, "she seemed to be torn within herself; that there was something bothering her; that was destroying her," and if the investigators "would wait, it would be disclosed because this would be the 'grand finale' Mary Sherman would want."

One has to wonder how much of Max's description was based upon his own depression rather than on Mary's. We know that Max was self-employed as an author. The objective of this section seems to be to show that at least one of the 150 people interviewed called her a lesbian, though his grounds for doing so are admittedly weak.

So let's add them up: 7% + 20% + 10% = 37%. These three sections account for thirty-seven percent of the linage in the *entire* homicide report ... and have absolutely nothing to do with what happened to Mary Sherman between 4:30 P.M. on 7/20/64 and 4:00 A.M. on 7/21/64. Their only purpose appears to be to imply a sexual motive for the killing.

Since the police were careful to explain where each of these essentially *irrelevan*t people were employed, it is interesting to note that this same homicide report did not say where some *principal* players were employed. Consider these omissions:

| NAME | ROLE IN CASE | EMPLOYED BY |
| --- | --- | --- |
| Mary Sherman | Victim | Ochsner Clinic; Tulane Med. Sch. |
| Carolyn Talley | Identified Body | Tulane Medical School |
| Juan Valdez | Called police | International Trade Mart |

Another person was included in the report because he supposedly helped explain Mary's movements in the hours before her death. Here comes David Gentry, 4919 Magazine St., who sold Mary an ashtray following her dental appointment the afternoon before her murder. (The dentist's name, however, was not mentioned.) One has to wonder if the police were aware that Mr. Gentry lived next door to, and was acquainted with, Lee Harvey Oswald, when Oswald lived at

4907 Magazine during the summer of 1963.[8] But they could not have anticipated that Gentry would become a grand jury witness in 1967, when he was asked by Jim Garrison's staff to identify photos of people who attended parties at the residence of Clay Shaw, former Director of the International Trade Mart, employer of Juan Valdez.[9]

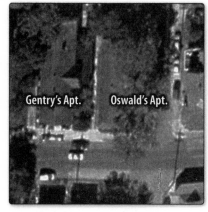

Gentry's Apt.     Oswald's Apt.

The only professional associate of Dr. Sherman that is mentioned in the report is Dr. Carolyn Talley, and that was unavoidable because she identified the body for the police, based on shape and hair color. For some reason Talley called Sherman's apartment at 5:00 A.M. the morning of the murder. No explanation of this phone call was given in the police report. My guess is that Talley, a pediatrician, was going to drive to the Crippled Children's Hospital across the lake with Dr. Sherman later that morning, and that she called at 5:00 A.M. to give her a wake-up call so they could get an early start and avoid getting stuck in the morning traffic and the July heat.

IN THE SUMMER OF 1993, a friend sent me a copy of a surprising article recalling the mystery of Mary Sherman's murder that appeared in a small alternative newspaper in New Orleans. It was entitled "A Matter of Motives."[10]

In this article, journalist Don Lee Keith challenged the lesbian angle: "From the beginning, the investigation followed but a single direction: the pursuit of a killer who was a lesbian. Police operated on the premise that the dead woman was also a lesbian."

Unable to find anyone, including gay colleagues who worked with Sherman, who had any knowledge of her sexual preferences before her death, Keith concluded that the lesbian angle was a red herring to draw attention away from the real motive.

Keith's article pointed out that the sex-murder rumor was well in place before 9:15 A.M. on July 21, when the autopsy began. Keith also considered the word "mutilation" to be "too strong" for the one centimeter cut on the victim's labia. Forensically speaking, genital mutilation would suggest the killer was a man, not a woman. Quoting from his article, "Instances in which women have mutilated the genitalia of other women are so rare as to practically be unheard of."

When he presented the murder to four medical examiners from other cities, all four said that it was "obviously a case of overkill," with all but one suggesting the fire was an attempt to call attention to the crime scene.

From my perspective, the most important point in Keith's article was calling attention to the fact that the police reports omitted the victim's place of employment. Why would the police not want to tell us the victim ran a cancer laboratory for Dr. Alton Ochsner? All of which was kind of silly, since that information was on the front page of both newspapers. This omission can only have been intentional.

Keith also observed that Warren Commission investigators started taking their testimony in New Orleans on the morning of July 21, 1964, several hours after Mary Sherman's murder. Some consider this coincidental timing suspicious, and have speculated that her death may have somehow been related to the Kennedy assassination or to her association with David Ferrie.

A few JFK assassination researchers have mentioned Mary Sherman in their writings. John Davis, author of *Mafia Kingfish*, called Mary Sherman "David Ferrie's closest female friend,"[11] and raised the possibility that her death might have been related to Ferrie's death. But Davis had the date of her death wrong, and thought that she had died shortly after Ferrie in 1967.

*Dr. Mary's Monkey*

For a more obvious error, we look at the work of Gerald Posner, who wrote a book called *Case Closed*, which argued that Oswald was the lone assassin of JFK. Posner ended his book with a chapter called "The Non-Mysterious Mystery Deaths," to supposedly dismiss a host of ill-conceived theories. There he said,

> Dr. Mary Sherman (house fire) had no connection to the case, though she was acquainted with David Ferrie ... According to the medical records, she was killed in an accidental fire ...[12]

An accidental house fire? According to the medical records? Please draw your own conclusions about Posner's "facts."

STILL, DESPITE ALL MY RESEARCH, I did not know how to *feel* about Mary Sherman.

Credentials mean little to me. I have seen terrible people carry impressive diplomas and fancy titles, and I have seen great people with neither. The few clues I had about Mary's personal life told me little. The suicide of her husband and the painting of suffering on her wall told of her emotional hurt. But how did she manifest this? In malice, or charity, or both? Was she a childless, sadomasochistic lesbian witch who tried to become a goddess by developing her own life form? Or was she a deep, sensitive, honest caring physician who struggled to find a cure for cancer? Or was she a nonjudgmental scientist who had simply been manipulated into doing things which finally brought about her own demise? I did not know. But I wanted to find out.

Courtyard of 3101 St. Charles Avenue

As I studied the 1964 newspaper articles and the police reports, I noticed the name of the maintenance man who had worked in Dr. Sherman's building. It was Alvin Alcorn, "colored, male, age 51." He had known Dr. Sherman for twelve years and was one of the last people to see her alive. At 4:00 P.M. he saw her standing on her patio talking to her housekeeper of twelve years, Elmener Peterson, also "colored," as they insisted on reporting. As Alcorn left, he noticed that Dr. Sherman's car was in the parking lot as usual, and confirmed such to police once they needed to know. Alvin Alcorn?

Quite by coincidence, I had met a man named Alvin Alcorn in New Orleans about five years before, but I had no idea at the time he was involved in any way with Mary

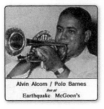

Alvin Alcorn / Polo Barnes
*live at*
Earthquake McGoon's

Sherman. He was an elderly trumpet player who led a New Orleans jazz band called the Alvin Alcorn Group. Alvin frequently played at parties and brunches around town. Not a major celebrity by any means, but a well-known musician. I had heard his name for years. In the 1950s and 1960s Alcorn played so many parties for fraternities and faculty at Tulane that many considered him "the house band." By the spring of 1987, when we met accidently at an outdoor function for the New Orleans Museum of Art, he was semi-retired and only played sporadically. His band had just finished performing, but I had missed them. I was waiting outside for my family, and he was walking about in the same area. After a while we started talking. He was warm, sensitive, perceptive, and completely devoid of any sense of "jive." I knew if this was the same Alvin Alcorn, and if he was still alive, that he could give me a clean read on Mary Sherman, at least the parts he knew about.

I grabbed my old New Orleans phone book, found his number, and called him. Yes, he was alive, now in his eighties, but still quite alert. I confirmed that he was "Alvin Alcorn the musician," and reminded him that we had met several years before. When he heard I was calling from Detroit, he insisted on reminiscing about his younger days, touring with the big bands and playing at the Graystone Ball Room in downtown Detroit. Then I changed subjects, and asked him if he had ever been to the Patio Apartments on St. Charles Avenue.

*Dr. Mary's Monkey*

Yes, he had, adding he had worked there for a real estate company. Then he paused to consider the curious question. I told him I wanted to come see him when I got to town. He agreed.

Soon I was in New Orleans and found his house, a small wooden shotgun design on the edge of town. Inside the low iron gate, six cats slept lazily on an old sofa on the porch. One moved away quietly when I entered. I knocked and knocked, but there was no answer. I had walked through fifteen blocks of low-income housing to find the house and was not anxious to walk back empty handed. After five minutes I resigned myself and started to leave.

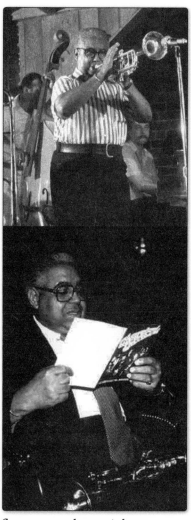

As I closed the gate, a faint "Hello" came from the screen door. Alvin was standing at the front door. Bent with age and holding a cane, he softly said, "I was in the back. Come in." His fragile steps shuffled into the front room. Each step was an effort. He balanced himself with a cane as his slippers slid across the wooden floor three inches at a time. He gestured to the sofa, and I took a seat. He negotiated into position in front of his easy chair and lowered himself into a spot where he was sure to stay for hours. The house, heated like many in New Orleans by open gas flame, was about eighty degrees. The air was stale. He was obviously quite comfortable, but I was about to melt. I figured I'd better start talking while I could. We chatted about his music career. He told his favorite stories in a gentle voice spiced with laughter. Then I asked him if he remembered Mary Sherman.

"Dr. Sherman," he corrected me with a look that said he would not tolerate any disrespect to her. The old wound was suddenly open.

"Yes, Dr. Sherman," I confirmed, seeing how difficult this was going to be for him.

"I need to know what she was like?" I said as gently as I could.

"She was a *fine* woman, a *damn fine* woman," he said without hesitation, challenging anyone to disagree. "Good hearted." That's what he meant to say the first time. "She was good to people. Good to me and good to Elmener." His head shook up and down slowly as he considered his words. Yes, they were the right ones. Then he grew still and gave me a quizzical look, asking me without any words, why, after nearly thirty years, was I asking about Dr. Sherman.

"I am trying to figure out why anybody would want to kill her."

"I don't know," he said simply, knowing that he had asked himself the same question and wished he had a better answer. "But I hope you catch the *son-of-a-bitch*." There was no hiding the hatred in his voice. He would have gladly beaten the killer with his cane. He told me all I needed to know about Mary Sherman in a few sentences.

So how does "a damn fine woman" wind up injecting mice with monkey viruses in an underground medical laboratory with a violent political extremist?

---

1  Letter from William Turner (author of *Deadly Secrets*) to Carol Hewett, April 16, 1994. Turner worked with Jim Garrison's investigators and reported the opinion of the Garrison camp on Sherman's apolitical perspective. She was not right-wing.

2  Sherman's biography was mostly compounded from several articles which ran in New Orleans' *Times-Picayune* and *States-Item* newspapers, July 21, 1964.

3  Probate Record, Mary S. Sherman, deceased July 21, 1964, State of Louisiana, New

*Dr. Mary's Monkey*

Orleans. The husband is somewhat of an enigma; after her death, friends told investigators that she had told them he had committed suicide during the 1940s, but there is no independent corroboration of this.

4  Billings Hospital in Chicago was one of the few hospitals that participated in the covert plutonium experiments of the 1940s and 1950s. Three patients were injected with plutonium without their knowledge; Welsome, "The Plutonium Experiments."

5  *Tumors of the Bone and Soft Tissue,* edited by R. Lee Clark, contains two articles by Mary Sherman, "Histogenesis of Bone Tumors" and "Giant Cell Bone Tumor."

6  "Cancer Work Slain Doctor's Main Interest," *New Orleans States-Item,* July 21, 1964, s.1 p.1.

7  Keith, Don Lee "A Matter of Motives," *Gambit,* August 3, 1993.

8  Garrison, "Playboy Interview," p. 161.

9  Who was the Juan Valdez that reported the fire in Mary Sherman's apartment? Researcher Joan Mellen in her book *Farewell to Justice* said that this same Juan Valdez worked for Clay Shaw at the International Trade Mart. Further, Mellen reports that she was told that Lee Harvey Oswald was well-acquainted with a Cuban named Juan Valdez. Locating a Cuban who knew both Clay Shaw and Lee Oswald, and who lived next to Mary Sherman, might be very important. So New Orleans journalist Don Lee Keith tried to find Juan Valdez to talk to him. Keith told me that he had searched all over the country for Mary Sherman's neighbor. After interviewing 34 people without success, Keith finally gave up, and questioned whether "Juan Valdez" was really his name.

But the spelling of Juan Valdez's name has always been in question and may explain why he had been so difficult to locate. While the newspapers referred to him as "Juan Valdez," the NOPD Homicide Report used another common variation of Valdez and spelled his name as "Juan Valdes" with an "s" instead of a "z," and said that he was a 34-year-old male who lived in Apt. E. But maybe both spellings were wrong. Maybe the correct spelling was yet another variation of the common Spanish surname: "Valadez" with an "A" in the middle. We don't know that answer, but we do note that in 2001 the bulletin of The World Trade Center of New Orleans said that "on October 11, Mr. Juan Valadez, an international security consultant and retired U.S. intelligence officer… made a presentation… for international travelers and businesses."

Later the vigilant Romney Stubbs sent me a newspaper article from New Orleans about this same Juan Valadez, now of New Orleans, which listed the 30 years he worked for the CIA among his many credentials. Did this Juan Valadez work at the International Trade Mart in New Orleans in 1963 and live in the apartment complex with Mary Sherman? If "yes," it means that the man who called the police to report the fire in Mary Sherman's apartment was a CIA agent. This is such an important issue that it deserves a better determination than I can provide here. No, I have not contacted the retired CIA officer to ask him about any contact he may have had with Lee Harvey Oswald or Mary Sherman. But I wish HSCA or ARRB had. Due to the importance of this question, it would be best to get the answer under oath. Doing so would minimize speculation about the similar sounding names and the possible role of the CIA.

10  Keith, "A Matter of Motives."

11  Davis, *Mafia Kingfish,* p. 372.

12  Posner, Gerald, *Case Closed* (New York, 1993), p. 496.

~~~~~~~~~~~~~~

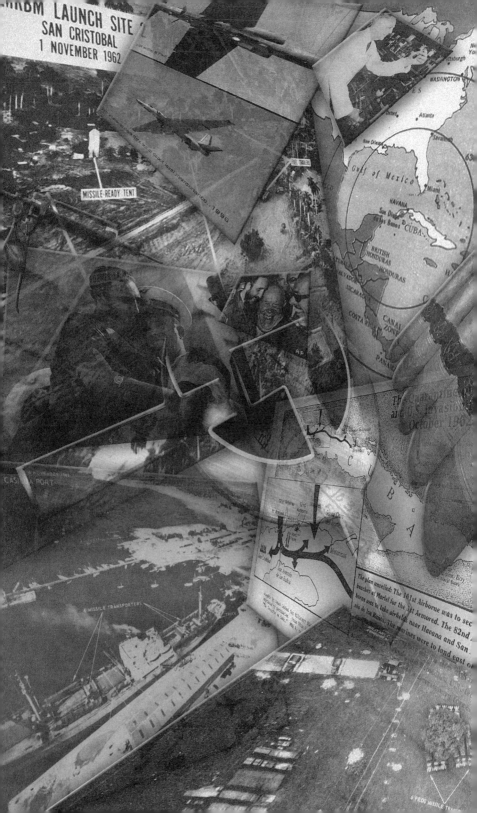

MRBM LAUNCH SITE
SAN CRISTOBAL
1 NOVEMBER 1962

MISSILE-READY TENT

FUEL TRAILERS

Gulf of Mexico

WASHINGTON

Atlanta

New Orleans

Miami

HAVANA

San Diego

CUBA

BRITISH
HONDURAS

HONDURAS

EL SALVADOR

NICARAGUA

COSTA RICA

CANAL
ZONE

PANAMA

The Quarantine
at U.S. Invasion
October 1962

C U B A

CASTLE PORT

MISSILE TRANSPORTERS

TRUCK

The plan unveiled: The 101st Airborne was to sec...
beaches at Mariel for the 1st Armored. The 82nd...
borne was to take airfields near Havana and San...
nio de los Baños. The marines were to land east of

FROG MISSILE TRAN

# CHAPTER 7

# The Cure for Communism

B Y THE FALL OF 1979, I found myself in the Graduate School of Tulane University, enrolled in its Latin American Studies Program. My "area of expertise" was Political Science. Our story picks up in a seminar called the "Urbanization of Latin America," taught by William Bertrand, Ph.D., from the faculty of Tulane University's School of Public Health.

William "Billy" Bertrand was a great professor by any measure, probably the best I encountered in my years of college and graduate school. He possessed a brilliant analytical mind, a deep commitment, a positive sociable style, and a gift for presenting the most complex subjects in simple language. Professionally, he was an epidemic fighter, thoroughly schooled in the most advanced techniques of statistics, medicine, and sociology in order to battle deadly epidemics around the globe. This ex-Marine personally travelled from continent to continent witnessing the ravages of disease, be they in Africa or Ecuador. A typical summer assignment for Bertrand would be six weeks in remote regions of Zaire trying to sort out the path of transmission of some mind-boggling illness. He occasionally suffered terrible infections from these Third World trips, all of which he seemed to take in stride. In my opinion, there's not a medical school or university in the world that would not benefit from having a professional of his caliber and character on their staff.

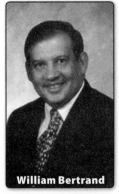
**William Bertrand**

Bertrand came from the simple, common-folk background of south Louisiana. His name "Bertrand" is a Cajun name, like Boudreaux or Bordelon. (He was not related to the infamous Clay Bertrand from the Warren Commission volumes.) Like his black hair, black eyes, and rounded features, it was proof that he was really from the core of French Acadian settlers of southern Louisiana. Bertrand used to say that he could walk from New Orleans to Houston, staying at a different relative's house every night, and that he unplugged his telephone for two weeks before Mardi Gras to keep his myriad of country cousins from calling him for a place to stay. These anecdotes were typical of his warm, personable style. He was very popular with the students.

The urbanization seminar was held in Tulane's main library, directly across the street from the law school. The seminar room itself was on a second or third floor in a windowless room toward the center of the building. It was a graduate-level course, with about eight graduate students and one or two undergraduates. About half of the students in this particular seminar were from Latin America. There were lots of affluent and well-connected Latins at Tulane. I personally knew students from Cuba (exiles), Costa Rica, Columbia, Venezuela, Ecuador, Brazil, Chile, Peru, Belize, and Panama.

I remember one of the Latins in Bertrand's seminar particularly clearly. I will call him Freckles, because his face was covered with them. He seemed younger than I, say early twenties at the time, medium height, slender build, quiet, and with a hard edge about him. He was always vague about his national origin, but he was very clear about his politics: He was an avid anti-Communist. Freckles was the only person in class who routinely let his personal political views get in the way of his academic work. Bertrand stopped him on more than one occasion, saying, "That sounds like a personal political opinion." Admittedly, it's hard to discuss the urbanization of Latin America or the dynamics of development in the Third World without discussing politics, but efforts were generally made in academic circles to stay as objective as possible.

One day Bertrand was leading the seminar's discussion on educational challenges in the Third World. He made the point that one of the problems that both socialistic and capitalistic governments faced when trying to educate their population was that education (investment in people) was ultimately "capital intensive," meaning that the investment (school buildings, books, teachers, etc.) must be paid before the benefit of the education (skilled labor, social services, etc.) can be reaped.

The point that socialists needed *capital* in order to achieve their objectives sparked a lot of discussion. It defied the black-and-white rhetoric which characterized much of Latin American political debate. As the discussion progressed, Cuba was mentioned repeatedly, since it was the only functioning socialist government in Latin America. And Cuba was a touchy subject.

To many Latins, Castro was an anti-gringo politician, and in their eyes that made him a Latin hero, which they liked. But to others, he was a thief, a murderer, and a criminal. The latter group were generally Cubans, since many of them had seen their family fortunes ruined and, in some cases, their families killed at the hands of Castro's revolutionaries.

Academically, however, the problem with discussing Cuba as a model of social development had always been more of a function of superpower relationships than one of ideology. Cuba's relationship with the Soviet Union was seen by the United States as posing a military threat to the entire Western Hemisphere, and when combined with Cuba's confiscation of American assets after the revolution, it triggered the most tenacious economic boycott in American history. This embargo crippled the Cuban economy. Add to that years of U.S.-sponsored covert warfare waged against Cuba (from blowing up Cuban oil refineries to infecting Cuban livestock with viruses), and it is amazing Castro's government survived at all.

In any event, the discussion in the seminar turned to "It's really too bad about Castro." Not only had his relationship with the Soviet Union allied him with a totalitarian Communist state and presented him as a military threat to the United States, but it also tainted his socialism. It was difficult to judge whether socialism was right or wrong for Latin America on the basis of Soviet missiles. It would be much simpler if Castro was not around — or so the discussion went. Then the inevitable discussion of how to assassinate Castro started. No one even suggested that the U.S. had not been trying, despite the fact that assassinating a foreign head of state was explicitly illegal. After all, the U.S.

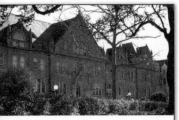

**TULANE** is a very well-respected school throughout Latin America, and is probably better known and better respected there than in the U.S. This is not accidental. Tulane has a long history in that region. This reputation is based upon a number of factors, e.g.:

Its location gave it valuable *economic interests and contacts.* New Orleans is both the mouth of the Mississippi River (the largest commercial waterway in the United States) and the northern port of the Caribbean. Until recently, it was the commercial gateway to Latin America. Lumber, sugar, coffee, and bananas flowed into the U.S. through New Orleans, while machinery, money, and medical services flowed back.

Tulane was *respected academically.* For over 100 years Tulane Medical School has specialized in fighting the diseases which plague the tropics. This ripe history is studded with major scientific accomplishments. For example, it was Tulane that helped to prove malaria was spread by mosquitoes, at a time when that defied mainstream scientific thinking. This discovery had an enormous positive impact on public health in Latin America. Consequently, Tulane was widely recognized as a top academic

CONTINUED on NEXT PAGE...

Senate Intelligence Committee had already disclosed numerous CIA attempts to assassinate Castro. The conversation covered the predictable escalating path from shoot him, to bomb him, to poison him, to the more exotic methods like blowing up his cigar. It ended with the classic exasperation, "*They* ought to be able to come up with *something* to get rid of him!"

At this point, Freckles, who was sitting directly to Bertrand's right, turned to him and said in a confidential tone, "*El Padrino* is working on a virus." Bertrand's surprise was both immediate and obvious. He was half-appalled and half-confused. Freckles had used this Spanish word for godfather in a manner that assumed Bertrand knew whom he was talking about, even if the rest of us didn't. But Bertrand did not recognize the name and paused to unravel the comment. Then he said, in an incredulous voice, "Who?"

Freckles continued, "El Padrino. You know, Ochsner. He's working on a virus to get Castro."

Bertrand was stunned and went straight into deep thought to calculate the comment. Ochsner was a very powerful man in Tulane circles. A single unthoughtful comment about Tulane's wealthiest and most powerful medical figure could

...CONTINUED from PREVIOUS PAGE

institution among educated Latins.

- It was politically correct for the Latin American elite to send their children to Tulane to be educated. Tulane had exquisite "anti-Communist" credentials. This was primarily due to the relationship between Tulane University and the United Fruit Company. Samuel Zemurray, president of the incredibly powerful United Fruit Company during the 1950s, was a New Orleans native, and became Chairman of Tulane University's Board of Directors. As Chairman, Zemurray stacked the Tulane Board with United Fruit officers. After he died, Zemurray's ornate mansion on St. Charles Avenue became the residence of the president of Tulane University. United Fruit was actually a Boston-based company which had controlled the Central American fruit business with an iron hand for nearly a century, and was at the center of the Cold War conflict in Central America. To illustrate its influence, consider Guatemala. When the democratically elected government of Guatemala purchased 250,000 acres of undeveloped land from United Fruit in 1954, the American government responded with a CIA-organized coup d'etat which ousted President Arbenz.[1] Allen Dulles (who later became CIA Director), his brother John Foster Dulles (the U.S. Secretary of State) and Sam Zemurray were all major stockholders in United Fruit.[2]

- Tulane was well promoted in the region, especially by Dr. Alton Ochsner, who was Chief of Surgery of Tulane Medical School. Ochsner travelled Latin America from Mexico to Argentina giving lectures. The implied message: If you are too sick for your local doctors, come to New Orleans, and we'll take care of you.

ruin a career. And what if this student's comment was accurate? We could see the mood on Bertrand's face change, as the idea of unleashing a designer virus on the Caribbean took hold in the mind of someone who had witnessed horrible epidemics firsthand. We all waited for him to speak. Then in a voice more serious than any I had ever heard him use, he said to Freckles, "If I were you, I'd be *very careful* who I said that to."

Freckles nodded in response to Bertrand's comment, but did not speak. Dr. Bertrand had given him good advice without questioning his honesty or his source.

Bertrand shifted our attention back to urban migration patterns in Latin America, the decline in breast feeding, the thin-ice of the Latin American middle class, the economic interests of multi-national corporations, and what, if anything, anyone could or should do about any of these things.

To this day, I wonder what mixture of fact, fantasy, and/or proximity lay behind Freckle's comment. At the time, I had seen no hard evidence which supports the claim that Dr. Alton Ochsner was involved in a medical project attempting to kill Fidel Castro.[3] Freckles' comment was, however, an indication of Latin perceptions of Ochsner's politics and evidence that *a rumor did exist* in certain Latin circles that Ochsner was (or had been) involved in a medical project which was trying to kill Castro. But was this rumor really a cover story to conceal something else?

Was there a deeper secret buried beneath the secret war against Cuba?

*Dr. Mary's Monkey*

Not long after the Freckles incident, I left Tulane University in search of a career in communications. In March 1980, I began working at Fitzgerald Advertising, Inc. in New Orleans.

Fitzgerald's offices were on historic St. Charles Avenue between the New Orleans Central Business District and the Garden District. From my sixth-floor window I could see the statue of Robert E. Lee standing on his lonely column, high above Lee Circle. The statue faced north, it was said, because Robert E. Lee would never turn his back on the South. Below, the antique green streetcars clamored down the grass median of St. Charles Avenue, clanking and hissing their way through the perpetual humidity and circling beneath his feet. A few blocks down St. Charles Avenue I could see the leafy green trees of Lafayette Square, a lush urban park flanked by large Greek Revival buildings.

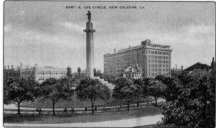

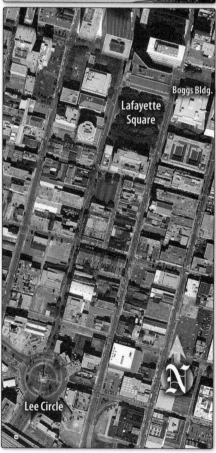

On the northeast corner of Lafayette Square stood the new Hale Boggs Federal Building, towering over an urban streetmall bordered by Camp and Lafayette Streets. This had been the site of the old Newman Building. On the sidewalk in front of the Boggs Building was a bronze plaque removed from the walls of the Newman Building. The plaque commemorated the military and financial support given by the people of New Orleans to the people of Cuba who were struggling for their freedom in the 1800s. But the plaque did not mention the military and financial support given to anti-Castro Cubans from the same building in the 1960s.

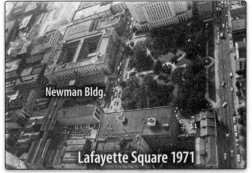

Lafayette Square 1971

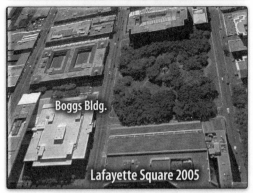

Boggs Bldg.

Lafayette Square 2005

In 1963, the Newman building held the offices of "private detective" Guy Banister, former head of the FBI's Chicago office[4] and later Deputy Chief of the New Orleans Police Department. Banister was a staunch segregationist and founded the ultra-right-wing Anti-Communist League of the Caribbean. He claimed to have the largest file system of "'anti-Communist intelligence" in the South, which he shared routinely with the New Orleans FBI office.[5] With help from his employee David Ferrie, he ran a paramilitary training camp near New Orleans to prepare Cuban exiles for covert assaults inside Cuba on Castro's government.[6]

In the blocks surrounding Lafayette Square were the local offices of the FBI, the CIA, and the Secret Service. Across the square from Banister sat Chairman Hebert of the Armed Services Committee of the U.S. House of Representatives, whose job it was to prepare the U.S. military's budget for Congress' approval and to hide the CIA's budget from both Soviet and American scrutiny.[7] One block away was the Reily

*Dr. Mary's Monkey*

Coffee Company where Lee Harvey Oswald worked. The address stamped on the famous "Hands Off Cuba" flyers that Oswald handed out that hot August day in 1963 was 544 Camp Street: the Newman Building. Banister's wife found similar flyers in her husband's office after his death. Garrison concluded that Oswald was involved with both Banister and Ferrie during the summer of 1963, and that Banister was Oswald's "handler" who arranged events,[8] such as the trip to the mental hospital, to make Oswald later appear to be a convincing political assassin.[9]

In the early 1980s Fitzgerald was the largest advertising agency in Louisiana, with impressive credentials. Among its long list of well-respected clients was the Reily Coffee Company. Fitzgerald was conservative and "old school" by all definitions of the term. Like many ad agencies, Fitzgerald was occasionally asked by clients or influential citizens to work on pet projects, and they tried to oblige when they could.

ONE DAY, IN THE SUMMER OF 1982, one of my bosses called me to his office shortly before lunch. As I entered, he asked if I knew so-and-so. The name was not familiar to me. He laughed a little and muttered: "You're one of the lucky ones." I joined him in a polite laugh, as he made light of his comment. Then he began his solicitation in earnest, explaining that he had received an inquiry from "a friend of the agency" that we had to respond to. He wanted me to check it out. He said that it was "right up my alley," and wanted me to go see whether the agency should get involved.

He handed me a small yellow slip of paper torn from an office pad with an address, but no name, written on it in pencil. He instructed me to be there at 1:45 that afternoon. "They" would explain what they wanted. He then sent me on my way, reminding me to be "on time" for the meeting. These were very "busy people." All I could tell by his tone was that he considered this to be an important courtesy call, but that he was not seriously interested in the project. Given that the advertising business depends upon clear and precise instructions, the ones he gave me that day were remarkably vague. I grabbed a quick bite to eat and caught the next streetcar to Canal Street, wondering all the time where I was going.

Canal Street was bleached white hot by the midday sun. A sweaty crowd pushed down the sidewalk into the front door of the street car. Loiterers monopolized the scarce shade. I 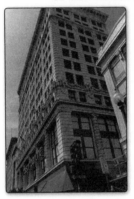 unfolded my yellow piece of paper to get my bearings. Comparing the address to the nearest storefront, I realized my destination was across the street (on the edge of the French Quarter) and in the next block. Quickly calculating the approximate location, I headed for the ornate Maison Blanche building.

Entering the brass and marble lobby of the Maison Blanche building, I savored the cool blast of air-conditioning and immediately inspected the tenant roster to figure out the identity of my mysterious destination. After a minute I realized there was no such suite. I was in the wrong building. So I went back on the street and carefully compared the numbers from my yellow paper with the numbers above the doorways. My destination was next door.

The entrance led to a small, dark, narrow, unadorned lobby. It was dark and dingy by comparison to the bright, shiny lobby of the Maison Blanche building. I felt like I was going in a side entrance. This was a building I had never been in before. I took the elevator to the top floor and started my search for the suite. As I walked the empty halls, I sensed the strange orientation of the horseshoe-shaped building. The elevators were obviously an after-thought, attached to the end of one of the horseshoe legs, rather than in the center. It was an old building, with chest-high marble walls and frosted glass doors. Many of the suites were vacant. I saw no one in the hall. Turn after turn, I looked for the number. Finally, at the farthest end of the third hall from the elevator, I found

*Dr. Mary's Monkey*

a plain windowless door. There was no identification other than the suite number. I knocked.

I was immediately greeted by an energetic young man who said, "You must be Ed!" and fired a string of questions like, "Did you have any problems finding the place?" and, "How hot is it outside?" He followed that with a barrage of small talk.

I realized that he was doing his best to control the conversation, and that he had not given me his name. But I did manage to get in a question: "What type of business is this?"

He said it was a low-wattage AM radio station. So I asked him what the call letters were. His rapid reply was, "Let's call it WNCA."[10]

Suddenly a door opened from the side of the reception area and an older man came in swiftly. He was in his sixties, with silver hair, a striped cotton suit, and a bowtie. His sudden entrance startled the younger man, who scrambled to conjure an important air in his voice to introduce him. The older man waved him off and introduced himself: "Hello, I'm Bill Fergerson. Thanks for coming." His eyes sparkled with practiced warmth. Out the corner of my eye I saw the quick jerk of the young man's head and the surprised expression on his face when the old man announced his name.

The odds were even that he had given me a false name. My immediate read on the situation was that this older man was well known in town and, for some reason, wanted to keep his real name out of the conversation. This was consistent with the secretive nature of the invitation, the virtually unmarked office, and the fact that the younger man had not given me his name either. It was obvious that they wanted to talk to me about something sensitive.

The surprise in the younger man's voice was genuine when he asked the older man, "Where did you come from?" The older man gestured casually toward the corner of the room. The younger man said, "Even I didn't know there was a room back there!"

The older man laughed underneath his breath and said, "There are lots of things about this place you don't know."

At this point I understood the pecking order pretty clearly. Whoever this younger guy was, he had been around for a long time but only in a marginal role. He obviously did not have the complete confidence of the senior members and did not really understand their operation as well as he thought. Then they had a brief conversation about what should happen next. There were some people they wanted me to meet, and they had some things they wanted to show me. They decided to show me "the operation" first and then meet the people. I remember the younger man agreeing, "Yes, *the effect* would be better." What effect? I was standing in a seedy, unmarked office that seriously needed a decorator with two men who did not want me to know their names. Was I supposed to be impressed by something? Or even astonished? I waited to see what they had up their sleeves.

As the older man left the room, he said he would be back in a minute. Curious about both my host, my location, and the reason for my visit, I turned to the younger man and said, "I'm sorry, I didn't catch your name." He said it was not important. I smiled at him and said, "Then why don't you give me *your first name*? If you're going to be showing me around, I don't want to have to say, 'Hey, you!'"

He laughed and said, "OK, that's fair. My name is Ed." I laughed back. "At least I won't have any problem remembering that," I said, wondering if he had given me his first name or mine. He suggested we start the tour and let the older man catch up.

We went back into the hall and through a door to our right. There we found a modest recording studio with an antiquated control room. The vintage microphone reminded me of something Frank Sinatra would have used. The multi-channel mixing board was the same model as the one I had used at Tulane's radio station. And there was this cheap office desk that had a huge American eagle sculpture attached to the front of it. The desk was almost comical. The eagle's wings were as wide as the desk. Whoever sat at the desk would look like they were riding on the eagle's back. What an image for a freedom writer! I was getting the picture.

Next we went to a room full of file cabinets and storage shelves. The shelves were stacked with audio and video tapes. My host described them as interviews with Cuban exiles and American political leaders. These tapes were clearly labeled and well organized. Then he started to explain what they wanted. They were trying to revive the station and were hoping our agency might help them promote it.

At this point the older man came into the room. He interrupted without hesitating and asked the younger man if he had locked the door to the hall. He said he thought so, but the older man insisted he double check it. I was left alone with the older man for a minute and took the time to observe him more closely. He was about five-feet eight-inches and moved about constantly. He was obviously very respectable, but not overly concerned about his appearance. The hair on the back of his head was messed up like it had been blown in the wind, and he had not bothered to comb it. The back of his cotton suit was badly rumpled, like he had been sitting in a chair. My guess was that he was either retired or "so important" that it did not matter. Despite his rumpled appearance, he was confident, businesslike, and obviously considered himself in control of the others. So I asked him, "What goes on here?" He said laconically, "We're trying to get the word out about Communism." I waited for more. It never came. He paced silently.

The younger man came back in the room. My curiosity was growing. I noted him in more detail. He was tall and slender, with a boyish charm about his appearance. He looked rather like a forty-year-old graduate student, with his sandy blond hair combed to the side and hanging a little in his face. He had a prep-school style from the late 1950s or early 1960s. Something about the way he wore his short-sleeved white shirt and baggy khaki pants made me think that he may have been in the military at some point. Then he started to tell me about the file cabinets. He called them "mysterious."

There were six file cabinets in a row, all black, each unit chest high. He apologized for the condition of the files, saying that they were very old and were very disorganized, but he was confident that they had "important information" in them. He started to tell me who the files had belonged to when the older man exploded, cutting him off in mid-sentence in a fit of exasperation. It was starting to get strange. The older man waved him over to the corner of the room. There they argued in tense, hushed tones about whether it was "all right to tell me" who the files belonged to. It was an awkward moment to say the least. I tried to ignore them and acted disinterested. I was uncomfortable with their whispering and did not care to be made part of the family secrets of what was obviously a right-wing propaganda mill. The older man did not want to tell me. The younger man did. The younger man suddenly broke off their discussion and said, "If he is going to work with us, he's going to find out anyway."

He marched back to the file cabinets and said to me, "Did you know Guy Banister?"

I said, "No," abruptly, in hopes that he would drop the subject.

Somewhat surprised, he said, "Are you sure? He was quite well known here in town a while back."

My reply was cautious: "If he was well known, maybe I heard the name. But I am quite sure that I didn't *know* him."

(Actually, the name was familiar to me, but my memory was vague about the details. I did remember that Garrison considered him a main figure in the anti-Castro operations in New Orleans. I had seen Banister's name in Garrison's interview in *Playboy*, and remembered Nicky Chetta discussing Banister in that memorable session at Jesuit back in 1969. But I was not going to get into all that with these people. They were obviously on the far fringe of the political right, and they were close enough to Banister to have his files! All my instincts told me to steer clear of these people.)

The older man was obviously relieved by my answer and chimed, "Then it doesn't matter. Let's just say, 'He was before your time.'"

The younger man struggled to regain his momentum and explained that the files contained "a lot of very important information," but there had been a "mysterious indexing system" which had been lost. He baited me with, "Nobody could decipher them," and offered to let me look to see if I could figure them out. I opened some drawers and inspected the file headings. I had never seen a filing system organized like this before. All the headings were typed numbers like "25-14." But without their index, they were completely unintelligible. Someone obviously wanted them that way. (Clerical staff could file and retrieve all day long without ever knowing what was in any given file.) He added, "You'd have to be an Egyptologist to figure it out."

"Well, at least hieroglyphs have pictures," I countered. "These things are completely numeric. There's no way to decode them without reading the files and reconstructing the index."

Then I looked at the contents of some of the files. What I saw were newspaper articles published in the late 1950s and early 1960s in New Orleans, Tampa, Miami, and Atlanta. Whoever put this collection together was very systematic, had subscriptions to lots of newspapers, and had adequate manpower to carefully prepare the material for orderly storage and retrieval. Then a wave of fear crashed over me. I realized that I was looking at the remains of an intelligence operation, part of the Cold War against Cuba.

And I had two people staring at me, diagnosing every expression, analyzing every word, and evaluating every reaction. I knew I'd better be careful about what I said and did. I stood frozen, staring into the files. My mind raced. I pretended to read some of the articles as I tried to sort out my situation. All I could think about was Jim Garrison. I knew he believed to his core that he had discovered the conspirators in the assassination of President Kennedy. And that he figured Banister was the pivotal man in that group.

Who were these people? And how did they get Banister's files? Garrison had been through the wringer: humiliated and hounded by a belligerent press, embarrassed with a one-hour acquittal of his accused conspirator, and harassed by the federal attorneys for years afterwards. Could he possibly be interested in the whole subject of anti-Castro groups in New Orleans thirteen years after the Shaw trial? It was easy to imagine that Garrison might want to forget about the whole tragic event that ended his promising political career. Should I contact Garrison about these files?

Then I realized that I'd better start thinking about my situation, not Garrison's. If I was standing in the viper's nest, I'd better watch my step. I emerged from my thoughts to say, "Well, it looks like you have got the complete history of Latin American Communism here, at least as reported by the American press."

They were pleased with my comments and began appealing to my interest in Latin American Political Science. The younger man said that these files would be a "great research asset if someone could take the time to go through them and make sense out of them." I said that I wished I had known about this back when I was in graduate school just a few years before. It would have made a great independent study project. And I was sincere in this lament. I could see the virtually irreplaceable library being offered to me. I would have loved to have studied it. But my life had changed since graduate school. I had moved on to other things, like building my advertising career and raising a family. My time was already over-committed back at Fitzgerald, with none to spare for any non-lucrative academic projects, regardless of how interesting they were. Of course I kept these thoughts to myself. After all, I was on a courtesy call on behalf of Fitzgerald

Advertising. My goal was to be polite to these "friends of the agency." I closed the files.

We walked back through the reception area to another office. There I was to meet the "financial backers." I remember my surprise when I entered the room. The high ceilings were emphasized by long drapes. The richly-colored carpet and the American flag hanging in the corner to my left added to the air of formality. A huge, expensive, federal-style wooden desk sat diagonally in the far corner. The objective of the decor was to look "governmental" and "authoritative." This was someone's seat of power. Suddenly, the scene struck me as tragic. It was like grown men playing dress-up. ("Let's play Oval Office. I'll be the President. You can be Secretary of State.") Two men were waiting there, both of whom were of the older man's generation and dressed in a similar manner. He introduced me to them. Both were doctors.

The doctors immediately recognized my name, and said they had known my father as a teacher of orthopedics at Tulane Medical School during the 1950s and 1960s. So I asked them if they taught at Tulane, too. Yes, they had, but it had been twenty years. I inquired about their specialty. Both were radiologists.

Trying to continue the conversation in a friendly manner, I said, "So you must have known ...," but I got no further. It was impossible for me not to notice the sudden confusion on the face of the doctor I was talking to. His eyes began darting back and forth between me and the older man, now standing slightly behind me and to my right. Curious about this untimely distraction, I turned my head to the right and saw the older man draw his finger across his throat, signaling the doctor to shut up immediately. More secrets? I had obviously stumbled upon some very sensitive territory, something having to do with doctors these radiologists might have known in the Department of Orthopedics at Tulane Medical School twenty years before.

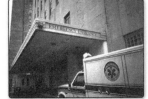

My warning lights had been flashing for some time. Now, my danger buzzers were going off. If these two were radiologists at Tulane Medical School twenty years earlier, in 1962, then they would have known every professor of orthopedic surgery in the small school, just like they knew my father.

Or to put it bluntly, both of these men knew the mysteriously murdered Dr. Mary Sherman personally. And they were experts in the medical uses of radiation, with access to x-ray machines and radioactive materials. And they were in possession of files belonging to Guy Banister, David Ferrie's employer and a suspect in the assassination of the President of the United States. And no one, except my boss, knew where I was! I pondered my situation and told myself, "Keep smiling, act relaxed, and don't mention Mary Sherman."

It worked. Fifteen minutes later, I found myself returning to Fitzgerald where I reported to my boss. I was very brief and said only that I did not think "the radio station was a business opportunity worth pursuing." He concurred and dropped the subject.

For the next ten years, I pondered the curious incident from time to time, but did nothing about it.

IN 1992, I BEGAN WORKING in earnest on this material. One of my first priorities was to find out everything I could about David Ferrie. To that end, I read *On the Trail of the Assassins*, the Jim Garrison book upon which director Oliver Stone based his movie *JFK*. There I stumbled across a section which had little or nothing to do with Ferrie, but which changed my understanding of what I had seen in New Orleans forever.

In this section, Garrison related how he had tried to find Guy Banister's files in 1966, several years after Banister's death in September 1964. His investigators sought out Banister's wife, who told them that upon her husband's death, his files had been promptly removed from his office, before she got there. She was told they were removed by federal agents.[11] For some unknown reason, these federal agents neglected to take the file-indexing system when they removed the file cabinets. Without it, no one could use the files effectively. As luck would have it, the Louisiana State Police also came to her husband's office shortly after his death and independently confiscated the abandoned file-indexing system.

Garrison immediately sent his investigator Lou Ivon to State Police Headquarters in Baton Rouge to search for Banister's index cards. When Ivon arrived, he discovered that for two years the State Police had been writing messages on the blank side of Banister's index cards and attaching them to intra-office correspondence. All that remained were a handful of index cards, none of which dealt with any so-called "private investigations." From these cards Garrison and Ivon reconstructed this partial list of Banister's files:

| | |
|---|---|
| Latin America. | 23 - 1 |
| Fair Play for Cuba Committee | 23 - 7 |
| International Trade Mart | 23 - 14 |
| B-70 Manned Bomber Force | 15 - 16 |
| Dismantling of Ballistic Missile Systems | 15 - 16 |
| Dismantling of Defenses, U.S. | 15 - 16 |
| General Assembly of the United Nations | 15 - 16 |
| Missile Bases Dismantled - Turkey and Italy | 15 - 16 |
| American Central Intelligence Agency | 20 - 10 |
| Anti-Soviet Underground | 25 - 1 |
| Ammunition and Arms | 32 - 1 |
| Civil Rights Program of J.F.K | 8 - 41 |

Note how the subjects listed in the left column could be found in the file numbers shown in the right column. These were identical in form to the numeric filing system I had seen at the radio station ten years before, when they asked me to reconstruct a "mysterious" indexing system which had been lost, and then they argued over whether to tell me that the files belonged to Guy Banister. I was sure they were the same files. Now, I had to do something about it.

I started making phone calls and writing letters. First, I tried to contact Garrison, but his publisher told me that he was already in a coma. I told her that I had seen Banister's files, and that I would be willing to try and locate them, if possible. The problem was that I did not know who had shown them to me, but I had seen them in a small radio station in New Orleans. She passed my story to Jim DiEugenio, the author of *Destiny Betrayed: JFK, Cuba, and the Garrison Case*, and sent me a copy of his book, which detailed the background of the Garrison investigation.

As I read this book, I found an interesting section on Dr.

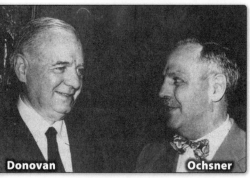
Donovan
Ochsner

Alton Ochsner. There was a photo of Ochsner with William "Wild Bill" Donovan, both elected officers of the American Cancer Society. (Donovan was a celebrity in military intelligence circles. He founded and directed the Office of Strategic Services, the WWII predecessor of the CIA. Much of the CIA's Cold War leadership was recruited from Donovan's New York law firm.) The book went on to explain that Ochsner was President and Founder of an organization called INCA (the Information Council of the Americas) which produced and distributed anti-Communist radio messages to Latin America.

This had potential. It had "radio, anti-Communist, Latin America, and doctors" all in one. After several letters and phone calls, DiEugenio brought Gus Russo into the loop. Gus had been a consultant to Oliver Stone's *JFK*, and was working on a documentary about Lee Harvey Oswald for the PBS television show *Frontline*. I gave Gus the same information, and told him what I knew about New Orleans. He was very interested in who had Banister's files, and we talked a lot.

During this string of phone calls, I found an old New Orleans phone book packed away in my Michigan basement. First, I looked up the Maison Blanche Department Store: 901 Canal. Then the Maison Blanche building: 921 Canal. Then INCA. Their address was listed simply as "Audubon Building." So I looked up the Audubon Building: 931 Canal. I told Gus what I had found. He was headed for New Orleans to do some advance work for the *Frontline* piece on Oswald, and arranged for me to meet him there to see if we could locate Banister's files. It was January 1993.

On our first day in New Orleans, we drove all over town, checking out locations for *Frontline* like Oswald's apartment on Magazine Street and the New Orleans Lakefront Airport, where Oswald had been a cadet in Ferrie's Civil Air Patrol unit.

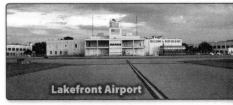
Lakefront Airport

On the second day, we went to see a man named Ed Butler, who had debated Oswald on the radio in August 1963. It was Butler who re-exposed Oswald's "defection" to the American public. Butler's job, both in 1963 and in 1993, was Executive Director of INCA.

We met him in the elevator of his office building and rode to the top floor. The entrance to INCA was a grandiose façade at the end of the hall, reminiscent of large law offices with their thick walnut doors. Upon closer inspection, it became obvious that this was not thick walnut. The façade was made of thin plywood panels nailed to a wooden frame erected in front of the old door. Screw-mounted brass letters from the local hardware store spelled out INCA. But we did not enter through this august entrance. Butler took us to a side door on the north side of the hall. There we entered a small functional office. A Frank Sinatra-era microphone sat on his desk like a paper weight. Audio and video tapes were neatly organized on the shelves. We sat down and exchanged business cards. He looked at Gus Russo's *Frontline* card, then at mine.

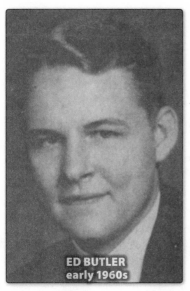
ED BUTLER
early 1960s

"Haslam," he mused. "Where do I know that name from?"

I offered some mumbo-jumbo to distract him. I did not want him to remember who I was at that moment. He might clam up. He furrowed his brow in concentration and stared at my card.

"No, that's not it. The word 'Egyptologist' keeps coming to mind," he mulled. I shrugged aimlessly, while Gus started questioning him about Oswald.

This brought Butler to life. He started banging on the desk with his fist, calling Oswald one of the "world's great revolutionaries," the "first New Leftist," the "first hippie," the "spearhead of world revolution" who set in motion a chain of events that led to the collapse of the Iron Curtain. He even called Oswald an "avatar," a Hindu word for a deity who becomes a human to accomplish some divine purpose. In the middle of his Oswald theories, he took time to criticize the Warren Commission critics for grasping at straws, and ridiculed all the reports connecting Oswald to Banister as meaningless speculation. Gus and I listened.

Then Butler proudly told us how, immediately after the assassination, he carried a reel-to-reel tape player over to Congressman Hale Boggs's office and played the tape of his radio debate with Oswald, so that Boggs could hear Oswald say, "I am a Marxist." As Butler told it, upon hearing the recording, Boggs called Lyndon Johnson to tell him he had just heard evidence that Oswald was a Communist. If this story is true, it means that President Johnson knew Boggs' position on Oswald before appointing him to the Warren Commission. Is this prejudicial? Or manipulative? Think how hard it would be for a Congressman to change his position on a subject of this magnitude after he had staked it out with the President of the United States.[12]

As Butler talked, I studied him closely. His tweed jacket and cardigan sweater. His ivy-league haircut parted to the side, hanging slightly in his face. Was this the same man who showed me Banister's files ten years before? He looked about fifty years old now. Ten years before he would have been forty. This was likely the same man, but I could not be absolutely sure.

Gus finished his questions, and Butler walked us to the hall to say good-bye. INCA occupied about seven rooms, but Butler had handled the whole interview in one small office. What about the rest of INCA? What about the files? Was INCA really WNCA?

Gus and I kept at him in the hall to keep him talking, hoping that something else would happen. Finally, in a surprise gesture, he offered to show us inside INCA. First, he took us to a room across the hall to find a record album that INCA had produced on the radio debate with Lee Harvey Oswald. It was called *Oswald: Self-portrait in Red*. Butler gave Gus and I each a copy, assuring us it was a collector's item. He was right.

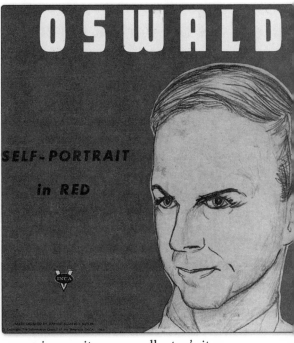

On the front of the album was a drawing of Oswald depicting him as an angry young revolutionary. On the back of

the album the headline at the top read, "I am a Marxist," with
a signature line from Lee Harvey Oswald, dated August 21,
1963. Below were three photographs: Hale Boggs, Dr. Alton
Ochsner and Ed Butler. Beneath the photo of Ochsner it said,
he was "perhaps the only listener who knew of Oswald's defection *before* the debate" [my emphasis].

# "I AM A MARXIST"

### —Lee Harvey Oswald, August 21, 196

## With these words, a few weeks before President Kennedy' assassination, Lee Harvey Oswald sketched the indelible ou line of this Self-Portrait in Red.

## HEAR OSWALD'S OWN VOICE AND LEARN:

*What did Oswald really think of President Kennedy?*
Hear the only recorded statement in existence, as Oswald gives his own opinion of President Kennedy.

*Was Oswald alone?*
Listen to this record, as Oswald defends the Fair Play for Cuba committee. Then decide for yourself.

*Was Oswald insane?*
Listen to this record . . . then judge for yourself.

*What did Oswald call his enemies?*
Hear Oswald pin a label on people he dislikes, and smear the State Department and the C.I.A.

*Whom did Oswald admire?*
Hear Oswald's own suggestion, that the United States should have dropped weapons "into the Sierra Maestra where Fidel Castro could have used them."

*How did Oswald explain his three years in Russia?*
Listen to this record, and hear his revealing reply.

This Album cointains the authentic, unedited recording of the now famous "C versation Carte Blanche" interview, origin broadcast live on Radio Station WDSU New Orleans, just a few weeks before P dent Kennedy's assassination.

This is a 33.1/3 r.p.m. high fidelity recording playback R.I.A.A. characteristic.

*Introduction by . . .*

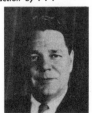

Hon. T. Hale Boggs, Congressman from Louisiana and House Majority Whip, in whose District the debate was held, and who supported the INCA TRUTH TAPES program from the outset.

*Impression by . . .*

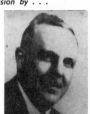

Dr. Alton Ochsner, world famed surgeon and President of both the Alton Ochsner Medical Foundation and the Information Council of the Americas (INCA), who was perhaps the only listener who knew of Oswald's defection before the debate.

*Analysis by . . .*

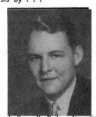

Edward Scannell Butler, Executive President of INCA and panelist on the fa evening, who has interviewed scores of ref from communist colonies, and who was the propaganda specialist ever to confront Oswa person.

## *This is the original Oswald Self-Portrait in Red. Accept no substitutes*

Narration by Marshall Pearce          Mastering by Cosimo Recording Studios          © Copyright The Information Council of the Americas (INCA)

*Dr. Mary's Monkey*

Butler gave us a quick walking tour. The place was a mess. Every conceivable space was stacked with dust-covered boxes. It had obviously not been anything but a storage area for years, but it did make me wonder who had been paying the rent for all those years. The desk with the eagle on the front was there. The high ceilings were there. The American flag was there. The expensive wooden desk was not. And the rooms seemed smaller than I remembered. Then we saw a bank of black file cabinets.

Butler continued his narration about his study of revolutions around the world, gesturing toward the file cabinets as he talked. Gus was about to climb out of his shoes. Butler opened a file cabinet. The files had obviously been worked over. The hanging files were gone. All that was left were manila file folders with hand-written names on their tabs. Butler commented that they had gotten some volunteers to update the files. He flashed some articles in front of us. Some had the aged, yellow look of thirty-year-old newspaper clippings. Others were more recently photocopied on clean white paper. Were these the remains of Banister's files? And if so, what did this mean?

Gus and I walked back to his hotel just a few blocks away. There he started pressing me: Was that the same man? Were those the same files? I realized that my answer might be used to implicate someone in a conspiracy to assassinate the President. The scale of the accusation confounded me. I wanted to make sure my answer was right. I told Gus Russo that I had to check out one more bit of information before I said anything definitive.

The next morning I stopped by to see Ron Thompson, President of Fitzgerald Advertising, Inc., the man who had sent me on the courtesy call ten years before. I told him I was in town working on a *Frontline* documentary about Oswald and that we had just interviewed a man named Ed Butler. I asked him directly if Ed Butler was the man he had sent me to see ten years before. Ron said, "Yes," adding that he had been a childhood friend of Butler's brother.[13] The brother had called and asked him, as a favor, to take a look at the operation. "They were doing some Voice of America-type work," Ron added. "I don't think they were involved in anything illegal." Since I never told Ron Thompson anything about the files, either in 1982 or in 1993, my assumption is that no one at Fitzgerald was ever aware that Butler had them.

Later that morning Gus and I went to see Boatner Reily, President of the Reily Coffee Company. Russo wanted to talk to him about Oswald, and I tagged along because I was still looking for the older man I had met at INCA. Reily received us promptly despite the surprise visit. We talked to the tall, slender, athletic Reily for about fifteen minutes. He was charming and sophisticated, which is not surprising, considering he was Chairman of the Board of Tulane University for twelve years. He was definitely not the older man I saw at INCA. He did, however, acknowledge that his uncle had contributed financially to Ochsner's political activities, and he asked us how he might get his company's employment records of Oswald back from the FBI.

To this day, I do not know who the older man at INCA was. But what is clear to me is that there was a right-wing medical-political alliance at work in New Orleans in the 1960s, and that Dr. Alton Ochsner was at the center of it.

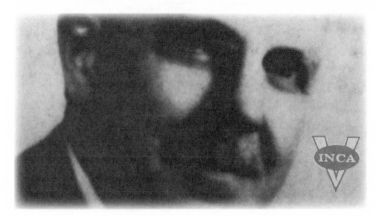

*Dr. Mary's Monkey*

1   The purchase of the United Fruit land has always been presented in the U.S. media as socialists nationalizing foreign owned assets. To the contrary, the Guatemalan government paid United Fruit exactly what the company had declared the value of the land to be for tax purposes. This was a case of eminent domain, not nationalization. United Fruit felt "cheated" because they had deliberately under-valued the undeveloped land to avoid paying taxes on it.

2   The 1954 coup d'etat in Guatemala was engineered by CIA officer Howard Hunt, who later master-minded the Watergate burglary. It has always amused me to read that John McCloy (Chairman of the Chase Manhattan Bank, architect of the Japanese internment program, target selector for the World War II bombing of German cities, and member of the Warren Commission) said, "The Warren Commission must show the American people that we are not a banana republic." The Dulles brothers' stock position in United Fruit is discussed by Hinckle and Turner, *Deadly Secrets*, p. 40.

3   It has been reported that the Ochsner Medical Center treated wounded Contra soldiers for free (Carpenter, "Social Origins," p. 163) as part of a commitment to fight Communism in Latin America, but that should not be confused with Freckles' comment, which referred to a deliberate attempt to develop a biological weapon to assassinate a foreign head of state.

4   DiEugenio, *Destiny Betrayed*, p. 38. Numerous other references in JFK assassination literature point to the FBI's Chicago office. For example, in *Deadly Secrets* Hinckle and Turner discussed Robert Maheu (p. 31-32) and William Harvey (p. 136-137), both of whom worked there before joining the CIA. Maheu was the CIA's contact with the Mafia, and later joined Howard Hughes' organization. Harvey headed the CIA's assassination squad. Guy Banister headed that same Chicago FBI office.

5   Hinckle and Turner, *Deadly Secrets*, p. 231.

6   Ibid., p. 233.

7   The Honorable F. Edward "Eddie" Hebert (last name pronounced A-BEAR). I knew where his New Orleans office was because I went there once in 1968. From his window you could see the line at the unemployment office.

8   Espionage field work is divided into two primary roles, spies and spymasters. The spymaster "handles" the spy, giving him or her assignments, rewards, and/or money.

9   Garrison, *On the Trail of the Assassins*, p. 40.

10   I remembered his precise answer because it contained a W̲, which is the FCC prefix for "east of the Mississippi," plus the first letter of each of the major networks, NBC, CBS, and ABC. Since New Orleans straddles the river, it has both "K" and "W" stations.

11   Garrison, *On the Trail of the Assassins*, p. 41.

12   Hale Boggs was House Majority Whip, the third most powerful member of that chamber, and helped pass LBJ's Great Society budget. One of two U.S. Representatives appointed to the six-man Warren Commission, he was one of the only members of the Commission to raise substantive questions during their sessions. When the theory was proposed that the bullet which entered Kennedy's back exited through his throat and then hit Connally, Boggs asked about the earlier medical reports which said that bullet path only went a few inches into Kennedy's back. Years later, Boggs is said to have expressed his doubts about the Commission's conclusions. He became Majority Leader in 1971. In October of 1972, as he campaigned for a colleague, his plane and the entire entourage disappeared over the Gulf of Alaska; no trace of it was ever found.

13   Frankly, I do not remember now if Thompson said that he knew Butler's brother or that Butler knew Thompson's brother, but a brother was a bridge between them.

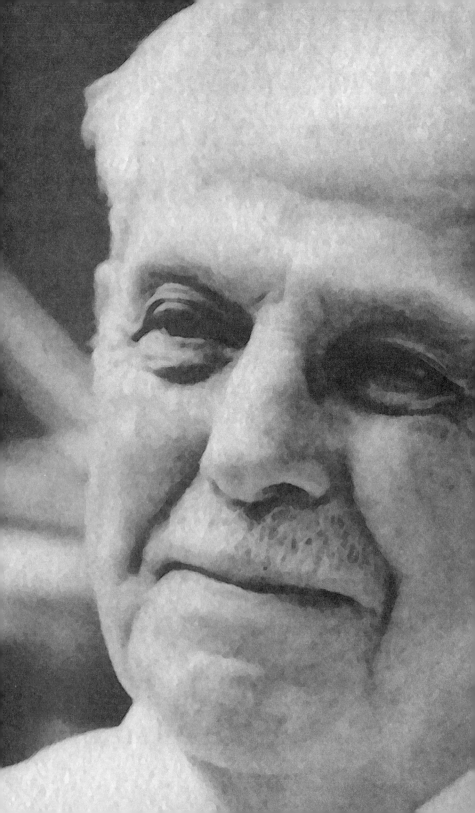

# CHAPTER 8

# Dr. O

**P**EOPLE TEND TO RESPECT both medical reputations and financial success. Dr. Alton Ochsner had plenty of both. Before his life was over he had been President of the American Cancer Society, President of the American College of Surgeons, President of the International Society of Surgeons, the Chairman of the Section on Surgery for the American Medical Association, and President of the Alton Ochsner Medical Foundation, one of the largest medical centers in America, with annual revenues approaching $300,000,000 per year. As a recognition of his contributions, he received the Distinguished Service Award of the American Medical Association in 1967, and he also received honorary awards from Ireland, England, Greece, Spain, Nicaragua, Columbia, Honduras, Ecuador, Panama, Venezuela, and Japan.[1]

As all could see, he was a highly respected man of medicine, clearly above suspicion as it is commonly known. But there was another side of Alton Ochsner which the public

Statue in front of
the Ochsner Medical
Foundation

did not see as clearly. He used his position and contacts to advance his right-wing political philosophy, and in the process developed a long complex relationship with powerful political figures and agencies of the U.S. government.

Ochsner was born in Kimball, South Dakota, in 1896,[2] towards the end of the era of sod houses and Indian massacres. The only son with five older sisters, Alton grew up the product of his German ancestry, and became what might be called an over-achiever. He attended the University of South Dakota and did his medical training at Washington University in St. Louis. His advanced medical training and many of the pivotal moves in his career were arranged by his uncle A.J. Ochsner, a famous surgeon who was chief of surgery at two hospitals in Chicago.

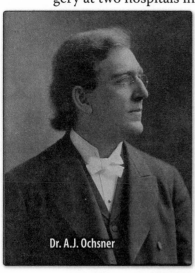

Dr. A.J. Ochsner

A.J. Ochsner's influence cast a long shadow. He was founder and later president of the American College of Surgeons, as well as head of surgery at the University of Illinois Medical School. His international contacts were considerable. A.J. saw to it that Alton trained under the leading surgeons of the day. A.J. Ochsner's best friend was William J. Mayo, founder of the famous Mayo Clinic in Minnesota, and when it was time for Alton Ochsner to start his own clinic, the Mayo Clinic was used as a model.[3]

In 1921, Alton Ochsner headed to Chicago to train at his uncle's elbow. He fainted at his first sight of surgery, and at his second, and at his third. His uncle told him to get a grip if he wanted to be a surgeon. He did. A.J. worked Alton hard and taught him his own set of medical standards, like "Don't operate on anybody who is not going to get well." Anxious to begin surgery of his own, Alton practiced by performing sur-

*Dr. Mary's Monkey*

gical procedures on dogs in an outbuilding on the grounds of his uncle's hospital.[4]

Then in 1922, again thanks to his uncle's influence, Alton Ochsner headed to Europe for a two-year residency in Switzerland and Germany. The first big medical success of his career was bringing blood transfusions to Europe. Or should we say "back to Europe." Early attempts at blood transfusions had failed miserably. It was not until an Austrian physician named Karl Landsteiner developed techniques for blood typing that blood transfusions became safe. Landsteiner's original work had been ignored in Europe, so he came to the U.S. in 1912, and introduced the technique at A.J. Ochsner's hospital in Chicago.[5] Alton Ochsner learned to type blood while working in his uncle's laboratory. His uncle provided him with blood transfusion equipment to take with him to Europe.

There, Swiss doctors refused to perform blood transfusions because of the terrible results of earlier attempts. They were skeptical of young Ochsner's claim that the techniques which he had been taught in Chicago were safe. They first let him attempt a transfusion on what they considered to be an expendable patient, a criminal who had been shot by the police. If he died, it was no great loss to society. He survived.

Several days later the president of a Swiss bank entered the hospital suffering from heavy blood loss due to a ruptured ulcer. The Swiss doctors were unable to help the banker and feared the embarrassment of such a prominent person dying in their hospital. They asked Ochsner to do what he could. When the banker pulled through, Ochsner was proclaimed the blood transfusion expert of Europe. He lit up the European scene with his first medical article, telling of the magic of blood transfusions. It was written in German. He was an American medical celebrity in Europe at the age of twenty-seven.[6] A.J. was pleased.

In 1923, while still in Switzerland, he married the daughter of a wealthy American family whom he had met in

Chicago. Soon they departed on a kind of victory tour, visiting first European and then American medical clinics for several months. In Europe he got his first exposure to politics and witnessed epidemic inflation first hand. When he arrived, the exchange rate in Germany was four marks to the dollar; when he left, the rate was four million marks to the dollar.

In 1924, at the age of twenty-eight, he returned to the United States. Educated, trained, traveled, and connected, he was prepared to take full advantage of the dawning of the golden age of medicine.[7] Before long, he landed a full-time teaching position at the nearby University of Wisconsin. His stay was brief.

The hand of his uncle's influence can be seen again, when, in 1927, at the age of thirty-one and after just one year of teaching at the University of Wisconsin, Alton Ochsner was appointed Head of Surgery at Tulane Medical School, replacing Dr. Robert Matas, an internationally-known surgeon who had headed Tulane's surgery department for years.

During Ochsner's get-acquainted visit, Matas invited him to witness a spectacular display of the older physician's own surgical skill. Even if Ochsner did not accept the position, at least he could return home with a great story about Matas. In Ochsner's presence, Matas removed a 92-pound tumor from a 182 pound patient. The tumor was so large that it had to be impaled with ice tongs and lifted with a block-and-tackle pulley system bolted to the ceiling of the operating room. The remaining 90 pounds of patient died the next day from lack of blood. The technology of blood transfusions had not yet made it to New Orleans.[8]

The appointment of a young outsider over the heads of several well-qualified, older doctors, who were waiting in the wings to get the position, raised eyebrows and set in motion a camp of anti-Ochsner sentiment in the medical community which followed Alton throughout his career. But Ochsner's success in New Orleans was so complete that this has been dismissed as jealousy.

Ochsner soon gained public recognition by stumbling into an incident with the powerful Louisiana Governor Huey Long over the management of the 1,732 bed Charity Hospital which Long had built. Ochsner's supporters character-ized the situation as the competent Ochsner in-censed over the appoint-

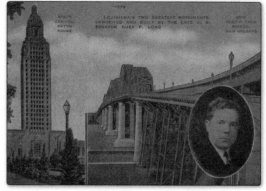

ment of an unqualified upstart. Actually Dr. Vidrine, whom Long appointed as Superintendent of Charity Hospital, was both a graduate of Tulane Medical School and a Rhodes Scholar. Both men were young. Vidrine was twenty-eight, and Ochsner was thirty-one. And both had their own agen-das for improving the hospital and advancing their careers.

Vidrine had the support of the governor and was winning. Ochsner was ready to bail out of New Orleans, and wrote a letter describing his bitterness to a friend. The letter, which Ochsner claimed he never mailed, was lost in the halls of Charity Hospital and wound up in the hands of Huey Long him-

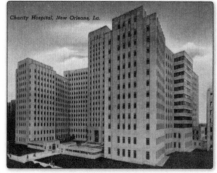

self. Long, who was battling with Tulane for other reasons, used it as an excuse to throw Tulane Medical School, and Ochsner personally, out of the Charity Hospital. The inci-dent gave Ochsner public notoriety and credibility with the elements of Louisiana which opposed Huey Long's populist agenda, which was just about everybody with money. This facilitated Ochsner's successful penetration of the elite social circles of New Orleans.

During the 1930s and 1940s, Ochsner's skill as a laboratory researcher grew. Clever and solution-oriented, he prided himself in developing practical medical innovations. As researchers go, Ochsner was a pragmatist, "the type of researcher who wasted no time in the laboratory."[9] He was fascinated by "the idea of serendipity," which is defined as "a gift for discovering valuable or agreeable things by accident,"[10] and it influenced his research. As a result of his research activities, he joined the *Society for Experimental Biology and Medicine*, and became an officer in its southern chapter. His biographers flirted with the idea that Ochsner might have even received a Nobel Prize, if he had been able to devote more time to his research efforts, but there is no evidence that the Nobel committee ever considered him for such.

However, if Ochsner should have received a prize for any of his medical work, his crusade against cigarette smoking would be my candidate. In 1936 he made a serendipitous observation, and became one of the first people to conclude that cigarette smoking was a cause of lung cancer. Noting that lung cancer was virtually non-existent in non-smokers,

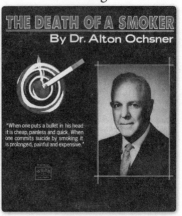

THE DEATH OF A SMOKER
By Dr. Alton Ochsner

"When one puts a bullet in his head it is cheap, painless and quick. When one commits suicide by smoking it is prolonged, painful and expensive."

and that incidences of lung cancer increased with the number of cigarettes smoked per day, he constructed a case that he took to the American Cancer Society. Here we see one of Ochsner's strengths at work: The clarity and certainty with which he saw medicine was comforting to everyone around him. And he was always willing to take action if he thought he could accomplish something positive. In Ochsner's words: "Of course, everybody thought I was crazy, but now the evidence is so overwhelming that only the tobacco people disagree."

Ochsner went on to become President of the American Cancer Society in 1949 and sat on their Board of Directors with fellow elected-officer William "Wild Bill" Donovan, the celebrated founder and head of the U.S. Office of Strategic Services (covert warfare and intelligence during World War II, and predecessor to the CIA).[11]

As a medical school professor, Ochsner was notorious for his demagogic tactics, the best known of which was "the bullpen." Here, in an amphitheater full of hundreds of medical students, Ochsner conducted an intimidating hybrid of quiz-show and psychodrama, screaming questions at medical students and berating them over their answers. He justified these tactics by saying medicine was stressful. Diagnosis was a matter of common sense,[12] and medical students had to be taught to think under pressure. Many students were humiliated by the experience. One even fainted. When his own son was in the bullpen, Ochsner grabbed him by both lapels, shook him in front of his classmates, and yelled, "You're not going to treat it any different than I would treat it."[13]

Ochsner carried his philosophy of harsh discipline back into his home. To quote one of his sons: "My father used to beat the hell out of me." Once he even broke a leather belt

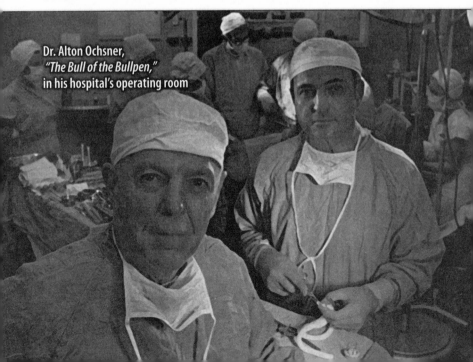

Dr. Alton Ochsner,
*"The Bull of the Bullpen,"*
in his hospital's operating room

during a beating. To quote his official biographers: "In a more tolerant time it might have been considered abuse." But Ochsner was proud to be considered "the fastest belt in New Orleans."[14]

During an interview late in his life, Ochsner blamed all of the permissiveness of modern society (all of the drugs, political unrest and promiscuity of the 1960s and 1970s, even abortion) on the ill-conceived advice of Dr. Benjamin Spock, who suggested that physical punishment and negative reinforcement were not effective means of parenting. In Ochsner's words: "...everything has to be disciplined. Even a dog has to be disciplined. A cat has to be disciplined.... You show me an undisciplined person, and I'll show you an insecure person and an unhappy person.... We now have a whole generation of insecure, unhappy persons because they don't know what discipline is, and it's a direct result of the advice of Dr. Spock."[15]

In the area of medical ethics, he was more forgiving, and conditionally embraced the concept of euthanasia: "I see no reason for keeping a person alive who otherwise has no chance of recovery."[16] Further: "I think there's nothing worse than to see a person who is a vegetable, who has no chance of ever being better... If I were in that position, I would want someone to put me out ... And, of course, the horrible thing about such situations is the tremendous cost of prolonging such cases."[17]

The backbone of Ochsner's medical reputation was his technical mastery in the operating room. He claimed 20,000 operations to his credit during his fifty-year career. Yet he was not perfect. At one point, he openly acknowledged that he had accidently killed an unidentified patient by clamping off the artery to his lungs.[18] The most legendary of his surgical feats was the successful separation of Siamese twins.[19] The most dramatic of his operating room innovations was the use of a blowtorch on a patient during a radical mastectomy.[20]

Ochsner proposed that Tulane start its own hospital. When Tulane's board turned down the proposal, Ochsner asked if he could start his own; they did not object. He gathered together five of the department heads at Tulane Medical School and organized a multi-disciplinary clinic. Other New Orleans doctors feared the encroachment of a big-business approach to medicine, protested the establishment of the multi-disciplinary clinic which would compete with independent physicians, and appealed to the AMA to stop it. The AMA refused.[21] In 1942, the Ochsner Clinic and Foundation Hospital opened its doors in uptown New Orleans. Later it moved to a decommissioned military base in Jefferson Parish, and then relocated to its current home.

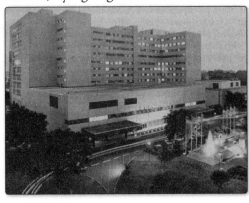

Ochsner's clinic at Aline & Prytania

Ochsner's Splinter Village

Today, the enormous medical complex stands like the Emerald City, rising high above the residential rooflines which surround its new home on Jefferson Highway. Across the front of the complex stands a string of flagpoles which welcome the elite of Latin America, flying flags from each of their countries. The idea of a medical facility which catered to the needs of Latin America's elite was integral to the concept of Ochsner's clinic,[22] and since its inception, Ochsner's medical facility has served the financial and political elite of Central and South America.

The Latin American angle was a natural for a medical clinic in New Orleans. And as we noted earlier, New Orleans was America's commercial pipeline to Latin America, and Tulane's reputation was golden in the region. For a group of Tulane doctors to form a medical clinic to serve the needs of the Latin elite was great news for those who could step on a plane in their capital city and be in New Orleans quicker than most Americans. To promote his clinic, Ochsner made over a hundred trips to Latin America during his career, and became friends with its rulers.

One event that helped jump-start his acceptance in these elite Latin circles was a phone call to Ochsner from Cordell Hull, the U.S. Secretary of State during World War II. Hull called Ochsner and asked him to take care of Tomas Gabriel Duque, the former President (and dictator) of Panama, who had helped U.S. intelligence organize a coup d'etat against pro-Nazi elements during World War II.[23] Connections within these circles grew. Before it was over, Ochsner was the President of the Cordell Hull Foundation.[24] It is hard to find information on the Cordell Hull Foundation, but those who spoke to me about it said it was politically very active, sponsoring Latin American students in American universities,

and giving scholarships to children of State Department employees.

Among his friends, Ochsner counted Anastasio Somoza, Nicaragua's former President (and dictator), who was run out of his country by revolutionaries in 1979. This relationship is what you might call a personal one, based on the letters in Ochsner's personal papers.[25] When Senora Somoza visited Tulane Medical School to investigate an exchange program between Tulane and the Nicaraguan government, a larger-than-life painting of Alton Ochsner was hung in the medical school for the occasion.[26] And Ochsner and Somoza shared mutual anti-Communist objectives. Somoza's personal physician, Dr. Henri DeBayle, sat on the Board of Directors of Guy Banister's infamous Anti-Communist League of the Caribbean.[27]

Another patient was Juan Peron, the President (and dictator) of Argentina. Ochsner flew to Buenos Aires to treat Peron for a problem in one of his legs. Peron complimented Ochsner, saying that surgeons were "men of action."[28] Peron was on the mark. Ochsner prided himself in his action orientation, saying: "Once you know what needs to be done, there is no point waiting."

Following the lead of these dictators came the oligarchies of Latin American countries which had not developed their own health care systems. By the 1980s over 10,000 patients per year were coming from Latin America to the Ochsner Clinic for treatment. There were so many, that Ochsner built a hotel on the hospital grounds to house the Latin patients' relatives, and hired a staff of Spanish interpreters to tend to their needs.

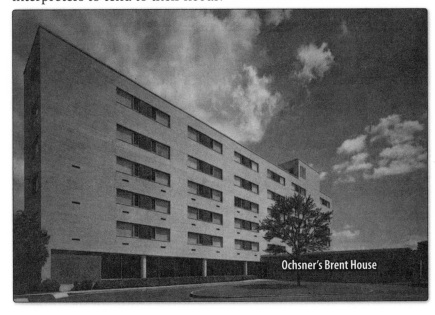

Ochsner's Brent House

On the American side, Ochsner accumulated many celebrities in his patient portfolio, from golf legend Ben Hogan to movie star Gary Cooper to the mega-wealthy Clint Murchison of the Texas oil family.

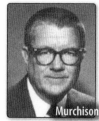
Murchison

Murchison's involvement with Ochsner seems to me to have been as political as medical. Yes, he was a personal patient of Alton Ochsner and gave him a Cadillac as a "thank you" present, but he also donated $750,000 to the Alton Ochsner Medical Foundation as seed money for Ochsner's new hospital. Meanwhile, Murchison purchased 30,000 acres of Louisiana swamp land and prepared it for a real estate development now known as New Orleans East, which covers about one-third of the land in the city of New Orleans.[29] I have always heard that Murchison bought it from Lady Bird Johnson. When LBJ announced the construction of Interstate 10 through the middle of this newly drained tract of land, plus the construction of NASA's largest facility on the same site, property values rose as fast as any in American history. Murchison made a fortune.

Ochsner was personally active in Louisiana politics. He served as campaign manager for INCA board member

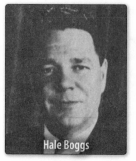
Hale Boggs

Dave Treen's successful bid for the U.S. House of Representatives and Lt. Governor Jimmy Fitzmorris' unsuccessful bid for Governor. Ochsner was always very close to Congressman F. Edward Hebert, with whom he shared an ultra-right, hard-line, anti-Communist sentiment. On the other hand, Ochsner had an off-and-on friendship with liberal Congressman Hale Boggs, whose photo appeared alongside Ochsner's on the back of INCA's phonograph album featuring the voice of Lee Harvey Oswald.

One of Ochsner's disputes with Boggs was the claim that in 1957 Boggs had assisted Ochsner in getting the multi-million dollar Hill-Burton grant from the U.S. government to build his hospital. Ochsner claimed Boggs' influence was negligible.[30] Considering that Boggs was one of the most powerful people in the U.S. House of Representatives at the time, Ochsner must have had some pretty serious connections to think that Boggs' influence was negligible. Despite all his posturing as a conservative, Ochsner was called "the most aggressive seeker and recipient of so-called federal handouts in the Second District" (Boggs' district) by a Louisiana State Representative.[31]

It is interesting to note the comments of Admiral Stansfield Turner, who testified to Congress as the Director of the CIA about the extent of the CIA's domestic activities. One of the Congressional questions was whether the CIA conducted its own medical research here inside the United States, and if so, how were they funding it? Turner said that the CIA had funded 159 medical facilities around the country for the purpose of conducting covert medical research. The funding was done in conjunction with Congress' Hill-Burton Fund. The CIA supplied seed money through blind third parties, and then the facility received matching funds as a Hill-Burton grant. When the facility was completed, the agency had access to a portion of the hospital's bed space for its purposes.[32] It has been suggested to me that the Murchison donation might have been the seed money for the project, and that Congressman Hebert's influence on the CIA budget may have been the real force that provided the Hill-Burton funding. It is probable that Ochsner's hospital was one of the 159 covert research centers which the CIA has admitted to setting up.

The FBI maintained a file on Dr. Alton Ochsner which we now have access to through the Freedom of Information Act. It shows his long relationship with the U.S. military, the FBI and other U.S. government agencies.[33] These records show that in 1941 Ochsner received an "excepted appointment" from the Civil Service Commission, and in 1946 he received a citation from the U.S. War Department recognizing the medical research he did for the government.[34] In 1955 he became a consultant to the U.S. Army, and in 1957 he became a consultant to the U.S. Air Force. Later, in 1957, the FBI cleared Ochsner for a "Sensitive Position" for the U.S. government, and J. Edgar Hoover personally approved him as an official contact for the Special Agent in Charge of the New Orleans FBI office, for whom Ochsner had already been performing discreet surgery at discounted rates.

In October of 1959, after two years of working in a "Sensitive Position," presumably with the FBI, the FBI conducted yet another "Sensitive Position" investigation on Ochsner and forwarded their findings to an unnamed U.S. government agency. Several days later, on October 21, 1959, the FBI formally discontinued Ochsner's relationship with the FBI, freeing him up to accept an assignment from the other undisclosed agency.

So what was happening in 1957 and 1959? What was this other agency? Why would they have needed the services of a doctor? And what did they need from *this* doctor that they could not get from the legions of other doctors already working for the U.S. government in one capacity or another? These are important questions.

By the late 1950s Alton Ochsner was at the pinnacle of his prestige. His clinic had grown enormously and was at its third location. His portfolio of celebrity patients and his new hospital made his name a household word. His social status in New Orleans could not have been higher. He had been King of Carnival and had won numerous civic awards.[35] In 1956 he stepped down as Tulane's Chief of Surgery, and in 1961 Tulane's Board of Directors terminated his teaching position, citing a conflict of interest with his clinic as the reason. If nothing else, it helped distance Tulane from Ochsner's increasingly covert activities. He was sixty-five years old at the time.

Having achieved considerable financial success during his career, the Tulane termination meant that Ochsner was now free to devote himself to his personal passion: politics. Basically, Ochsner was an arch-conservative with an antebellum, anti-welfare mentality. A quick glimpse of his political philosophy can be seen in the following quote from a letter he wrote in the early '60s to U.S. Senator Allen Ellender: "I sincerely hope that the Civil Rights Bill can also be defeated, because if it were passed, it would certainly mean virtual dictatorship by the President and the Attorney General, a thing I am sure they both want."[36]

One of the major news events of 1959 was Castro's revolution in Cuba. It threatened to spread to all of Latin America and to displace the nearly-free-labor economic system which American business had profited from for de-

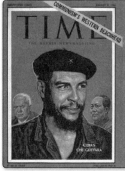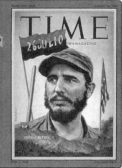

cades. Trade was New Orleans' biggest business, and seventy-five percent of it was with Latin America.[37] The entire New Orleans business community was threatened by this revolutionary trend. The reactionary sentiment in New Orleans centered around civic organizations which promoted trade with Latin America, like International House and the International Trade Mart. Ochsner himself was President of International House,[38] and he joined International Trade Mart's Clay Shaw on the Board of Directors of the Foreign Policy Association of New Orleans, which brought CIA Deputy Director Charles Cabell to New Orleans to discuss the Communist threat, a small favor for Congressman Hebert's district.

Ochsner saw the situation clearly. With revolutionaries in the capitals of Latin America, the displaced elite would no longer be able to jump on jets and fly to New Orleans for medical treatment. The medical empire he built was threatened. Ochsner did something about it. He became a fanatical anti-Communist.

In 1961, Ochsner institutionalized his anti-Communist crusade by founding an organization called INCA, the Information Council of the Americas. INCA's objective was to prevent Communist revolutions in Latin America by teaching the sordid truth about Communism to the Latin American masses. In brief, it was a right-wing propaganda mill, loosely modeled on Radio Free Europe. Ochsner served both as INCA's President and Chairman.

A typical INCA production interviewed Cuban exiles about the horrors of losing their sugar plantations or their mattress factories to Castro's forces. From these interviews, INCA produced and distributed tape recordings called "Truth Tapes" to 120 radio stations throughout Latin America. INCA's most ambitious project was a film about Castro called *Hitler in Havana*. The *New York Times* reviewed the film, calling it "the crudest form of propaganda" and a "tasteless affront to minimum journalistic standards."[39]

In a perceptive article about INCA, archivist Arthur Carpenter described anti-Communism as an ideology of convenience, which offered the ruling elite "a respectable way to discredit challenges to its power."[40] But Ochsner's conviction was deeper than that. Once I had the opportunity to ask someone who knew him personally about his political views, and got this reply: "He was like a fundamentalist preacher in the sense that the fight against Communism was the only subject that he would talk about, or even allow you to talk about, in his presence."

Financing for INCA is said to have come from Ochsner personally and from other doctors and business people in the New Orleans area. Ochsner and INCA Executive Director Ed Butler enlisted as many New Orleans business and political leaders as possible in their cause. Sears heirs Edgar and Edith Stern, owners of WDSU radio and television, were members of INCA.[41] Eustis Reily of the Reily Coffee Company personally donated thousands of dollars to INCA.[42] Of all the names on the INCA letterhead, the most interesting one is INCA's

*Dr. Mary's Monkey*

"Chief of Security," Robert R. Rainold, who was described as the "Past President of the National Society of Former Special Agents of the FBI." One must wonder if Mr. Rainold was aware that the former head of the FBI's Chicago office lived in New Orleans or that the Reily Coffee Company was managed by an ex-FBI man.

In the spring of 1963, Ochsner was quoted in a newspaper as saying, "As a surgeon, I know that in an emergency, sometimes you are forced to do things quickly or the patient will die ... We must spread the warning of the creeping sickness of Communism faster to Latin Americans, and to our own people, or Central and South America will be exposed to the same sickness as Cuba."[43]

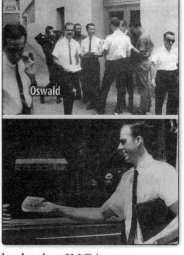

Later that summer INCA members descended upon Lee Harvey Oswald, filming his pro-Castro leafleting for television and ambushing him during a live radio broadcast with a newspaper clipping about his "defection" to the Soviet Union. The records of the Mexican consulate office in New Orleans show that when Oswald obtained his visa for his trip to Mexico, his name followed William Gaudet, who is known to have worked for the CIA and who edited an anti-Communist newsletter which Ochsner financed.[44] There is no doubt that INCA produced anti-Communist propaganda for Latin America, but one has to wonder what other activities it was involved in?

MARY SHERMAN'S MURDER happened the following summer, in July 1964. There is no mention of her in Ochsner's biography, nor of the grief or shock Ochsner must have personally felt over her tragic death. On July 22, 1964, however, *the day after* Mary Sherman's murder, Ochsner wrote a letter to his largest financial contributor saying "our Government, our schools, our press, and our churches have become infiltrated with Communism."[45] It appears the Communists must have forgotten to infiltrate "our hospitals."

Ochsner's own biographers cautioned that once Ochsner got out of his field of medical expertise, he exhibited an amazing naiveté, and even said things that could be termed as "ridiculous."[46] The problem seemed to be that he saw the rest of the world with the same clarity that he saw medicine. For example, he cited the lack of anti-war demonstrations on college campuses during the 1970-71 school year to be the result of INCA's influence.[47] In fact, this was linked to the cynical and movement-deflating initiation of a lottery system for draft eligibility, which would quickly reduce the number of college males facing potential induction by over seventy-five percent.

But none of Ochsner's monomania hindered his ability to rub elbows in increasingly powerful and wealthy circles. During one visit to Central America as a guest of the Guatemalan government, he became friends with National Airline's Chairman Dudley Swim of Carmel, California. Swim offered Ochsner a seat on National's Board of Directors.[48] There he became friends with National's largest stockholder, washing-machine baron Bud Maytag. Ochsner also sat on the Board of Directors of National Banks of Florida, courtesy of Edward W. Ball who managed the Alfred duPont Fund.[49] It was in these circles that Ochsner met William Frawley, an arch-conservative California industrialist, who headed Schick Electric and Technicolor. Frawley became INCA's largest financial contributor, and put Ochsner on his Board of Directors. Among Frawley's political friends was Richard Nixon, whom Frawley had helped in his early political career.

In the early 1960s, ex-Vice President Richard Nixon called on Ochsner in New Orleans, supposedly to discuss his future political plans. Nixon joined Ochsner and newspaper editor George Healy for a private luncheon at the exclusive Boston Club across the street from Ochsner's INCA.[50] While Nixon and Ochsner shared many political sentiments, they also shared some important medical experiences. The ill-fated polio vaccine which NIH released during Nixon's Vice Presidency (1953-61) killed one of Ochsner's grandsons and temporarily crippled his granddaughter. The publicity about the bad vaccine outraged the public and caused a political debacle, toppling the Secretary of Health, Education and Welfare and routing the leadership of NIH. Entering the office of President in 1969, Nixon promptly declared "War on Cancer," quadrupled the budget of the National Cancer Institute,[51] converted the Army's biological warfare center to a cancer research laboratory, and financed NIH's "Viral Cancer Program."[52] Were these events somehow connected? Had Nixon discussed any of his plans for his War on Cancer with the former president of the American Cancer Society?

Ochsner's second wife, whom he met at a party at Frawley's house, was even closer to Nixon than Ochsner was. Her first husband, an attorney from Los Angeles, was one of the people who helped launch Nixon's political career.[53] When problems with her passport threatened to interfere with Mrs. Ochsner's honeymoon to Greece, she called the White House and asked to speak to "Dick" Nixon. Her problems with the State Department were promptly solved.[54]

THIS IS THE LEVEL OF POLITICAL SUPPORT that Alton Ochsner enjoyed when District Attorney Jim Garrison began his investigation into the murder of JFK. And when Garrison started looking into the activities of Lee Harvey Oswald, he discovered that INCA and Ochsner were close to those events. Garrison's original intention was to arrest "the whole gang down at INCA" and squeeze them until they talked. His staff, however, felt that strategy was too risky and might backfire.[55] Garrison compromised and arrested only Clay Shaw, in the hope that Shaw's association with Oswald would be more tangible and could be proved more easily in a court of law. One has to wonder if Garrison was aware that Ochsner had been working in a "Sensitive Position" for the U.S. government.

In May 1967, as Garrison turned up the heat in his JFK investigation in New Orleans, Ochsner feared his own arrest.[56] In response, INCA's corporate records were air expressed to California, where Ed Butler put them "under lock and key."[57] Butler was in California working for one of Frawley's companies.[58] Frawley had contributed significant amounts of money to the early political efforts of Ronald Reagan who, as California governor, refused all of Garrison's extradition requests.

Needless to say, Ochsner did not take Garrison's investigation lying down. He fought back in his own inimitable manner. First, he was very vocal about his opinion that Garrison's probe was unpatriotic because it eroded public confidence and threatened the stability of the American government. (How could arresting the President's assassins threaten the stability of the American government?) Secondly, Ochsner promoted the idea that Garrison was crazy. He even managed to get a copy of Garrison's military medical records. These showed that Garrison, a frontline pilot, who flew behind enemy lines during the World War II invasion of Europe, had suffered from battle fatigue, was grounded temporarily due to mental exhaustion, and had received psychological counseling. As tenuous as it was, this could be used to assert that Garrison had some form of psychological problem at some point in his life. It was all part of the "he-must-be-crazy" tactic. Ochsner sent the file to a friend who was the publisher of the *Nashville Banner*.[59]

But that was mild compared to what came next. Garrison was being assisted by New York attorney Mark Lane, who had written *Rush to Judgement*, the first book to question the conclusions of the Warren Commission. To discredit Garrison, Ochsner attacked Lane, branding him an unscrupulous Communist and "a professional propagandist of the

*Dr. Mary's Monkey*

lunatic left," who was trying to create distrust and cause the U.S. to "crumble from within."[60] Further, Ochsner instructed Congressman F. Edward Hebert (Chairman of the House Armed Services Committee) to tell Congressman Edwin E. Willis (Chairman of the House Committee on Un-American Activities) to dig up "whatever information you can" on Mark Lane.

Hebert sent Ochsner a report on Lane extracted from the confidential government files, which cited various "Communist fronts" with which Lane had been associated.[61] Ochsner also secured a questionable second report on Lane from an unknown source. The unsigned cover memo said its information was from "the files of the New York City Police, the FBI, and other security agencies," and claimed that Lane was "a sadist and masochist, charged on numerous occasions with sodomy." Armed with these materials and a photo of a man (supposed to be Lane) engaged in a sadomasochistic act with a prostitute, Ochsner personally campaigned against Lane and the District Attorney.[62] These actions may possibly explain why Dr. Alton Ochsner was occasionally referred to as "a right-wing crackpot."[63]

And thus we have seen some of the many sides of Dr. Alton Ochsner (1896-1981), an influential doctor who helped shape the American medical system we have today, a highly-respected citizen of New Orleans who participated in civic institutions and who frequented elite social events, a businessman who promoted an enormously successful clinic and who sat on the boards of several large corporations, a crusader committed to fighting Communism in Latin America, a behind-the-scenes sponsor of Louisiana political figures, a patriot with a thirty-year history of classified assignments for the U.S. government, and, of course, Mary Sherman's boss.

What was the "Sensitive Position" Dr. Alton Ochsner held for the U.S. government? And did it have anything to do with any cancer research Dr. Mary Sherman was conducting?

1   A significant portion of the information in this chapter comes from John Wilds and Ira Harkey's "official" biography, *Alton Ochsner: Surgeon of the South* (Louisiana State University Press, 1990); AMA award: p. 195.

2   FBI file, Edward William Alton Ochsner, Freedom of Information Act, FOIPA No. 329,965, September 18,1992; on file at Loyola University Archives in New Orleans, Louisiana, 70118.

3   Wilds and Harkey, *Alton Ochsner*, p. 151.

4   Ibid., p. 24.

5   Keith, Don Lee . "Ochsner: the Surgeon, the Man, the Institution," *Times-Picayune*, June 3, 1973, s. 2, p. 8.

6   Ibid.

7   Wilds and Harkey, *Alton Ochsner*, p. 38.

8   Ibid., p. 61-62.

9   Ibid., p. 45.

10   Ibid., p. 44.

11   DiEugenio, *Destiny Betrayed*, p. 216, photo.

12   Wilds and Harkey, p. 84.

13   Ibid., p. 87.

14   Ibid., p. 90.

15   Keith, "Ochsner," s. 2, p. 9.

16   Wilds and Harkey, p. 214.

17   Keith, "Ochsner," s. 2, p. 8.

18   Wilds and Harkey, p. 104.

19   Pope, John, "Crusading pioneer Surgeon Alton Ochsner is dead at 85," *Times-Picayune/States-Item,* 9/25/81, s. 1, p. 1.

20   Ibid., s. 1, p. 4.

21   Keith, "Ochsner," s. 2, p. 8.

22   Wilds and Harkey, pp. 144-145.

23   Pope, "Crusading Pioneer Surgeon," s. 1, p. 4.

24   FBI file, Alton Ochsner, "Security Investigation Data for Sensitive Position," FBI ref. #77-60-528, October 30, 1959.

25   Arthur Carpenter, "Social Origins of Anticommunism: The Information Council of the Americas," *Louisiana History*, Spring 1989, p. 127.

26   *Bulletin of the Tulane Medical School,* Spring 1967.

27   DiEugenio, *Destiny Betrayed*, p. 216.

28   Wilds and Harkey, p. 215.

29   Wilds and Harkey, p. 158.

30   Ibid., p. 198-199.

31   Ibid., p. 199.

32   U.S. Congress, "Project MKULTRA, The CIA's Program of Research in Behavioral Modification," Joint Hearing before the Select Committee on Intelligence and the Subcommittee on Health and Scientific Research of the Committee of Human Resources, U.S. Senate, August 3, 1977 (Washington, 1977), especially letter from Stansfield Turner to Intelligence Committee Chairman Senator Daniel Inouye, Appendix B.

33   FBI file, Alton Ochsner, "Security Investigation Data for Sensitive Position," October 30, 1959.

34   FBI file, Alton Ochsner, Office Memorandum from Special Agent in Charge of FBI office

in New Orleans to J. Edgar Hoover, Director of the FBI, Re: Alton Ochsner, June 5, 1948. Cites March 25, 1946 article in *New Orleans Item*, saying, "Dr. Ochsner had received a War Department citation for his patriotic service in connection with medical research."

**35** Carpenter, p. 126.

**36** Ibid., p. 125.

**37** Ibid., p. 119.

**38** FBI file, Alton Ochsner, "Security Investigation Data for Sensitive Position," October 30, 1959.

**39** Carpenter, p. 132.

**40** Ibid.

**41** Ibid., p. 129.

**42** Ibid., p. 128-129.

**43** "Dr. Ochsner Outlines anti-Red Tape Activity," *New Orleans States Item*, April 16, 1963, p. 33; clipping found in FBI file on Alton Ochsner.

**44** Summers, Anthony and Robbyn, "The Ghosts of November," *Vanity Fair*, December 1994, p. 110.

**45** Carpenter, p. 125; letter from Alton Ochsner to R.H. Crosby, July 22, 1964, Historic New Orleans Collection. The Crosby family donated $300,000 to Ochsner Medical Foundation: Wilds and Harkey, p. 157.

**46** Wilds and Harkey, p. 189.

**47** Ibid., p. 202.

**48** National Airlines was sold to Pan American Airways, which went broke after deregulation.

**49** Wilds and Harkey, p. 203.

**50** Ibid., p. 199-200. Did Ochsner walk Nixon across the street to INCA?

**51** Shorter, *Health Century*, p. 205.

**52** These are well-known and widely-published facts, abundantly documented in NIH publications, such as *The Viral Cancer Program Progress Reports*, (National Institutes of Health, 1971-77 ); source: Richard Hatch, "Cancer Warfare," *Covert Action* pp. 14-17.

**53** Wilds and Harkey, p. 231.

**54** Ibid., p. 235.

**55** Interview with Anne Benoit, former law clerk to Judge Jim Garrison, conducted by Jim DiEugenio, 1993. Benoit reviewed JFK-related literature for Garrison during the nine years he sat on the bench, and discussed both the assassination and his investigation with him frequently.

**56** Carpenter, p. 136.

**57** Ibid.

**58** Ibid., p. 133.

**59** Ibid., p. 138.

**60** Ibid., p. 137.

**61** Ibid.

**62** I heard this "photo story" several times in both the 1960s and 1990s. I have not seen the photo which Ochsner showed around, but, while we were working on the *Frontline* piece, Gus Russo told me that he had. Therefore, I assume that the photo does or did exist, but I have always assumed that it was a fake. None of these "dirty tricks" should in any way be considered a true reflection of Mark Lane's character.

**63** Comments personally heard by the author in New Orleans from the 1960s to the 1990s.

~~~~~~~~~~~~~~~~~

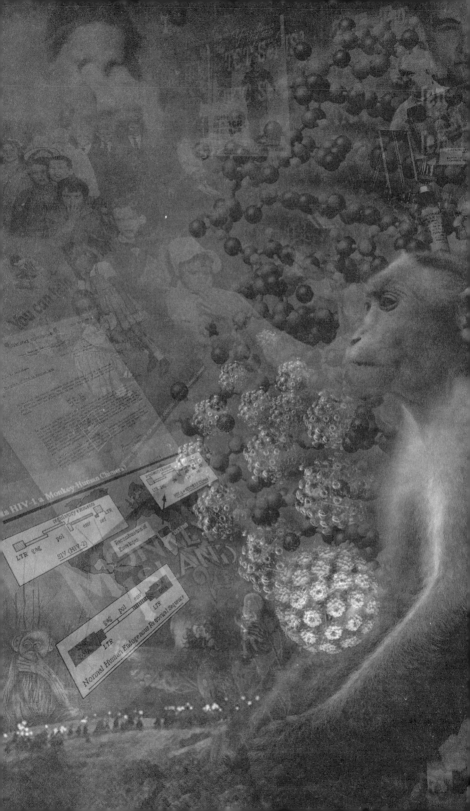

# CHAPTER 9

# The Treatise

IN THE *PLAYBOY* INTERVIEW we reviewed earlier, Jim Garrison referred to a "medical treatise" written by David Ferrie on the subject of inducing cancer virally.[1] Finding this document was a high priority for me, since it would go a long way towards verifying Garrison's claim about Ferrie's cancer research and establishing Ferrie's capability to induce cancer. The other side of the issue: What did the American medical establishment really know about cancer at the time? And how did the theories and techniques in "David Ferrie's medical treatise" relate to that leading edge of cancer research in America?

For over a year I asked many people if they knew anything about the treatise and got nowhere. I had begun to question whether it even existed. Then I got a phone call from Jim DiEugenio, the author of *Destiny Betrayed: JFK, Cuba, and the Garrison Case*, and chairman of a group of published JFK assassination authorities called Citizens for Truth about the Kennedy Assassination (CTKA), saying that one of the researchers pouring through the recently released JFK assassination materials in Washington, D.C. had found it. He sent me the document. These pages have been photocopied down several generations and are barely legible in places. They are reproduced as Document A (p. 347). Here is a brief description of their contents:

Page 1. Jim Garrison's memo describing David Ferrie's unintentional xeroxed personal notations.

Page 2. A description of a viral cancer experiment which transferred cancer tumors from animal to animal.

Page 3. A discussion of the work of a doctor who developed an experimental antibiotic for treating cancer.

Page 4. A chart showing different types of cancers and their tissue of origin.

Page 5. The first page of a bibliography.

Page 6. The second page of the bibliography.

At the top of each photocopied page we find:

**REPRODUCED AT THE NATIONAL ARCHIVES**
Collection: HSCA (RG 233)

Garrison's succesor (D.A. Harry Connick) gave this document to the U.S. House of Representative's Select Committee on Assassinations (HSCA) in 1972, and it has been at the National Archives in Washington ever since. The U.S. government released the treatise, thanks to the JFK Records Act, on October 22, 1993, nearly a year *after* I started looking for it.

The first point is that this is *a real document*. Garrison was not making up the story about the treatise in the middle of the interview, as some people had suggested to me.

Secondly, we proceed with the understanding that this document was found in Ferrie's apartment by investigators from the New Orleans District Attorney's office.

What we find upon close examination is not a complete document, but fragments of a much larger document. A reference to "Chapter Nine" of the document clearly indicates the original document had at least nine chapters.

The subject of the document is cancer research. The author appears to have compiled a state-of-the-art review of both research and literature concerning viral theories of cancer from 1901 to 1955. By simplifying the bibliography we can see both the timeframe and the subject matter clearly:

- 1901 Parasitic Theories of Cancer (Pasteur Institute)
- 1911 Transmission of Malignancy thru Cell-free Filtrate
- 1930 Metabolism of Tumors
- 1940 Breast Cancer in Mice as Influenced by Nursing
- 1944 Electron Microscopy Study of Chicken Tumor Cells
- 1948 Microscope Findings in Malignant Tissue
- 1949 Virus-like bodies in Human Breast Cancer
- 1949 Induction of breast cancer… (in)… mice
- 1950 Virus as a Cause of Human & Animal Malignancy
- 1951 Virus as the Cause of Cancer
- 1953 Is Leukemia Caused by a Transmissible Virus?
- 1955 Pathogenesis of Cancer

If we reverse-engineer for a title, it would be something like:

## The Case for the Viral Theory of Cancer:

### A Review of Research and Literature from 1901-1955

It should be emphasized that the author obviously believed that cancer was viral:

> Suffice it to say: as with Gregory's work, so here, the Koch Postulate seems fulfilled. Cancer seems caused by a virus.

So what are the contents of the original document? What did the author know about the viral nature of cancer, and of related research that was being conducted across the country? The short answer is "as much as any person in the world."

For starters, the author knew how to prepare cell-free extracts from cancerous tumors and use those extracts to transfer cancer from animal to animal:

> Extracts were made from the malignant tumors which appeared in the test group. These extracts were then injected

into other animals of the test group. A variety of malignancies appeared: leukemia, chorioepithelioma (cancer of the uterus) among them.

And the author used chemical carcinogens to induce cancer:

It was noted in the tests that the application of carcinogens does NOT always produce a malignancy. Hence, Cowdry's "final common path" seems at work. Thus the term "carcinogen" has reservations. It is to be noted that methylcholanthrene failed to give a 100% result. Of course it could be argued that there may have been a conflict since two other items were used in the carcinogenesis.

The author reviewed his/her experience with a number of experimental anti-cancer drugs:

| | |
|---|---|
| Merasptopterin | Aminopterin |
| Antivin | Magnesium Tracinate |

The last of these, he/she explained how to prepare from scratch:

1) The following is the process for manufacturing (magnesium tracinate):
2) Obtain Bacillus Subtilis, Tracy I and grow over high protein agar.
3) Catch up the culture in solution and heat at 56 degrees C for an hour.
4) Filter with a number 11 Berkfold filter for a cell-free filtrate.
5) Combine 100cc of the filtrate with 100cc of Magnesium Sulphate.
6) Place in electrophoresis for recovery.
7) Wash out the magnesium hydroxide.
8) Catch up the crystals in normal saline. 1500 mg to 50cc saline.

And the author also tells how to kill cancerous cells and viruses in the lab:

Extracts of the malignant tissue heated to 56 degrees C for one hour and then injected into animals of the control group produced no malignancies.

Since killing viruses is the foundation of vaccine development, the author takes the opportunity to prepare the reader for such a discussion later in the treatise:

This is referred to here because of a discussion, later in the paper, on the use of vaccines in cancer prevention.

This is an extremely important point for our inquiry, as we will see later. Needless to say, the scope of the original document must have been enormous.

So who wrote this document? When was it written? Where was it written? And why?

Simply stated, *David Ferrie did not write this document.* Other than Garrison's note which called the document "Ferrie's article on cancer," there is no evidence that Ferrie is the author. We do not have a title page, and the author refers to himself (or herself) in the third person. A careful reading provides numerous clues about the author. The most obvious one is that the author had daily access to x-ray machines and other professional laboratory supplies and equipment. Consider these sentences collected from disparate parts of the treatise:

Finally, the animals were subjected to small doses of x-ray over a period of three weeks.

Obtain Bacillus Subtilis, Tracy I and grow over high protein agar.

Filter with a number 11 Berkfold filter for a cell-free filtrate.

Place in electrophoresis for recovery.

Ferrie would not have had this type of equipment at his disposal.

Secondly, the author of this treatise personally performed experiments with experimental antibiotics for treating cancer, and lamented that an antibiotic had *not yet been released* to the medical community for general trials:

> Antivin is an antibiotic, developed by a mold, by Dr. John E. Gregory. This author has had the happy opportunity of using it with small laboratory animals with happy results... Antivin has not as yet been released for general trial, however.

David Ferrie would not have had access to an unreleased antibiotic developed by a top medical researcher.[2] It is clear that this document was written by a professional cancer researcher working in a well-equipped medical laboratory at the highest levels of American medicine. Minimally, someone on Mary Sherman's level. Perhaps someone even higher in the national research network.

Garrison made the assumption that finding a typewritten document in Ferrie's apartment alongside his caged mice meant that Ferrie had written it. It appears that he was wrong in that assumption. But proving Garrison wrong on this detail gives us little relief. What made Ferrie dangerous was the combination of his capabilities and his motives, not his originality. It would have been far better for the world if Ferrie had written this document based on his original theories and his home-brewed experiments. Knowing that he had access to

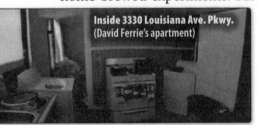

Inside 3330 Louisiana Ave. Pkwy.
(David Ferrie's apartment)

the techniques of the leading edge of cancer research makes the situation even more volatile, and raises some very serious questions about the other doctors involved in his laboratory.

When was the document written? It was not written before 1955, since it quotes articles published that year. Any review of a fast-changing field like medicine would normally concentrate on the *most recent* articles published on the subject. Since the last date on the bibliography is 1955, it is reasonable to conclude that this document was written shortly thereafter, in late-1955, 1956, or 1957. The time frame ends in 1957 because that year two researchers from the National Institute of Health announced a major discovery about viral cancer. Sarah Stewart and Bernice Eddy discovered a virus which caused multiple cancer tumors in a variety of small mammals. It was the first time one virus caused cancer in several different species. They named their virus "polyoma." This was a watershed event in cancer research, and it shifted the focus of cancer research toward viruses. It is highly unlikely that a treatise on viral cancer would have been written following the announcement of Stewart and Eddy's research without referring to it in the bibliography. Therefore, this treatise appears to have been written in 1956.

For whom was this treatise written? It was an internal document for a large organization which was heavily involved in cancer research. And it was not published. It is typewritten, but not typeset. The pages are not numbered. Despite the fact that it is written in clear and concise language by a highly educated person, there are about a dozen minor errata in the few pages we have. Any reader would have noticed this one:

*Reads:* "None of the animals developed malignancies."

*Should read:* "None of the *control* animals developed malignancies."

"Control" is a curious omission for a document written by an experimental laboratory researcher. It is hard to imagine that this error was not noticed in the author's own proofreading, since the *seven spaces* for the word "control" were left blank. Is the omission of the word "control" deliberate? Is it an indication that the researcher had some objection to the concept of control groups? This will become significant in our attempt to identify the author.

The author also recommends that his/her organization take certain actions:

> Dr. Gregory is available to come to any part of the country to demonstrate Antivin. From this writer's experience, to invite Dr. Gregory to demonstrate the antibiotic is well worth its while.

This sounds like a recommendation written by a subordinate for the explicit purpose of extending an invitation to Dr. Gregory to demonstrate his antibiotic. It is unlikely that Dr. Gregory would have traveled across the country on the invitation of David Ferrie, but he would probably have been eager to accept an invitation from a reputable medical school, a drug company, or one of the government's research laboratories. Was this document written by a frontline researcher at one of the U.S. government's laboratories which had the specific mission of battling cancer? A facility of the National Institutes of Health or National Cancer Institute?

It is there we find the mission, the equipment, the techniques, the personnel, and the budget to conduct an industry-wide review of progressive theories like virally-caused cancer, a subject that in 1956 was still on the fringe of medical knowledge. The appropriate question: How would David Ferrie have gotten his hands on an internal document from such an organization? From Mary Sherman perhaps? But how would Mary Sherman have come by the document? Just what connections did Mary Sherman (and those around her) have with the National Cancer Institute and the National Institutes of Health? And what could have motivated these contacts to send her a copy of such a document?

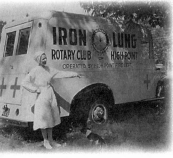

To answer these questions, we must peek behind the curtain of respect and gaze upon the mishaps of politically-controlled science, especially the enormous upheavals that rocked the National Institutes of Health in the 1950s. We begin by digging through the wreckage of the disastrous introduction of the polio vaccine in order to understand what followed.

TODAY, MANY AMERICANS DO NOT REMEMBER what a terrible curse "the polio epidemic" was upon the land. At its crest in the early 1950s over 33,000 Americans fell crippled or died slow, terrible deaths from polio each year. Most were children. The word "polio" struck fear into the hearts of parents across America. It was a casually transmitted virus that first infected the lining of the intestines, then the blood stream, and finally the nervous system, where it destroyed the victim's brain stem. The difference between crippled and dead was determined by the extent of the damage to the brain stem. Cavernous hospital wards full of hideous looking machines called "iron lungs" awaited patients who became too weak to breathe for themselves. President Franklin Roosevelt himself was crippled by polio before he entered the White House. The search for a polio vaccine became a national scientific effort supported by the most powerful political forces in the land. The problem was this: Polio was caused by a virus, not a bacteria, and viruses do not respond to antibiotics. So, despite the spectacular success of antibiotics introduced to the American clinical scene in 1942, the medical community was powerless to stop this virus from crippling and killing.

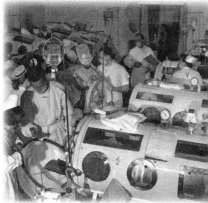

A New York City lawyer close to President Roosevelt organized The March of Dimes, and collected millions of dollars of coins from grade school children across the country to finance the research effort.[3] The progress was encouraging. By

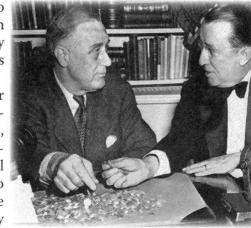

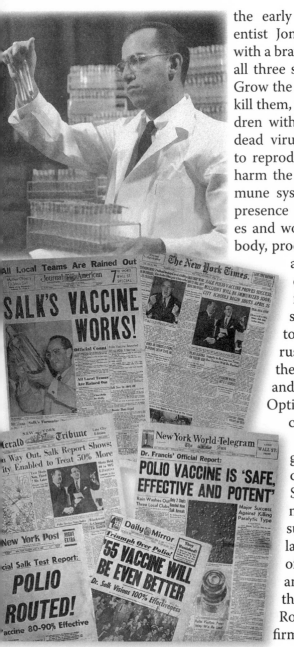

the early 1950s, American scientist Jonas Salk came forward with a brave new idea to eliminate all three strains of polio at once: Grow the polio viruses in the lab, kill them, then inject healthy children with the dead viruses. The dead viruses would not be able to reproduce, so they would not harm the children, but their immune systems would detect the presence of the invading viruses and would rally to defend the body, producing a hefty supply of antibodies in the process. Then the children's fully-armed immune systems would be ready to repel any live polio virus that attacked them in the future. His trials in 1953 and 1954 were successful.[4] Optimism about Salk's vaccine reached its peak.

Five laboratories began producing the vaccine from a procedure Salk designed, and accumulated a large enough supply for a mass inoculation beginning in April of 1955, touched off by an official ceremony on the tenth anniversary of Roosevelt's death that confirmed Salk's success. The

*Dr. Mary's Monkey*

results of years of research, millions of dollars of investment, and the fate of thousands of crippled children were ready for the most publicized and anticipated event in the history of medicine.

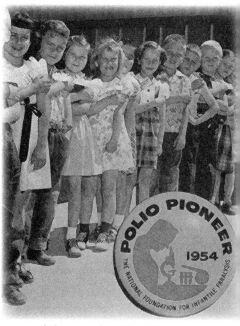

At the eleventh hour a bacteriologist at NIH was told to safety-test the new polio vaccine. Her name was Bernice Eddy, M.D., PhD.[5] When she injected the polio vaccine into her monkeys, they fell paralyzed in their cages. Eddy realized that the virus in the vaccine was not dead as promised, but still alive and ready to breed. It was time to sound the alarm. She sent pictures of the paralyzed monkeys to NIH's management and warned them of the upcoming tragedy. A debate erupted in the corridors of power. Was the polio vaccine really ready? Should the mass inoculation proceed on schedule?

A handful of prominent doctors across the country stepped into the fray to throw the weight of their reputations on the side of the vaccine. One of these doctors was Mary Sherman's boss, Dr. Alton Ochsner. To demonstrate his conviction that the vaccine was really ready, he inoculated his own grandchildren with it.

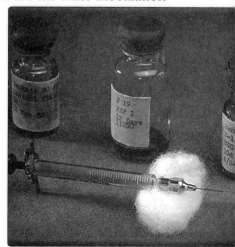

The mass inoculation proceeded on schedule. Within days, children fell sick from polio, some were crippled, some died. Estimates vary dramatically. Ochsner's grandson died. His granddaughter contracted polio but survived. An enormous lawsuit erupted. Heads rolled everywhere.[6] The Secretary of Health, Education & Welfare (Oveta Hobby) stepped down. The Director of the National Institutes of Health (Dr. William Sebrell) resigned. It was the biggest fiasco in medical history. A second, safer vaccine developed by Albert Sabin was deployed. It used a weakened live virus instead of a dead virus. It worked. Polio was history. The future was safe ... or so it seemed.

In the aftermath of the debacle, Bernice Eddy was taken off polio research and transferred to the influenza section by the thankless NIH management. She shared her frustrations with a small group of women scientists who ate brown-bag lunches on the steps of one of the laboratories. There Eddy met a tenacious scientist named Sarah Stewart, M.D., PhD., who was waging her own battle against the official paradigms of bureaucratic medicine. Bernice Eddy and Sarah Stewart became close friends.[7]

Sarah Stewart's name remains virtually unknown today, despite her huge contribution to modern medicine. Not only did she prove that some cancers were caused by viruses, but subsequent research on the virus she discovered led to the discovery of DNA recombination, which is one of the most powerful tools in medical research today.

Raised in the fertile Rio Grande Valley on the Mexican border, Stewart's educational odyssey ranged from the New Mexico Agricultural College in 1927 to a Ph.D. in bacteriology from the University of Chicago in 1939. Next, Stewart went to work for the National Institutes of Health as a bacteriologist for five years. Believing that having a Ph.D. instead of an M.D. was holding back her career advancement, she entered Georgetown Medical School and earned her M.D. in 1947. Then she joined the National Cancer Institute, and stayed there until reassigned to the U.S. Public Health Service in 1960.

*Dr. Mary's Monkey*

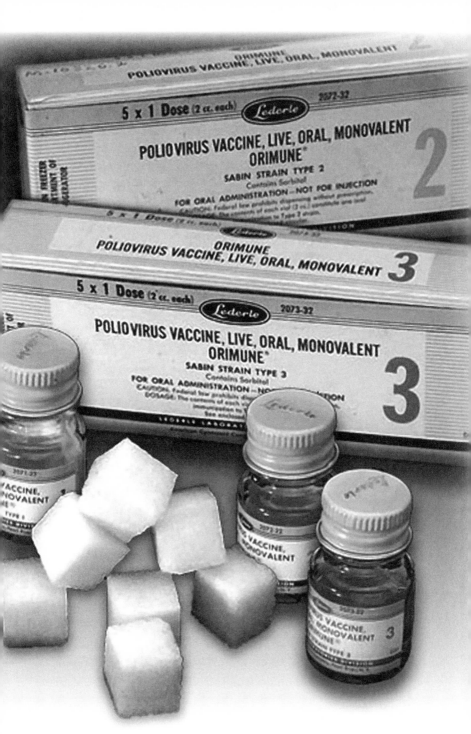

From the beginning, Sarah Stewart promoted the idea that cancer was caused by viruses. Due to this, she was not well accepted by the NIH or NCI staffs, who described her as "an eccentric lady" determined to prove her theory was right: "No one believed her ..."[8] Finally, she was given access to an NCI laboratory in Bethesda, where she could try to prove her theories. In 1953, she almost succeeded, but her work was not accepted by the ruling crowd at NIH. They found her methods sloppy, and objected to the fact that she did not culture her viruses.

In 1956 her lunch partner Bernice Eddy showed Sarah Stewart how to grow her viruses in a culture of mouse cells.[9] She now had all the ingredients she needed, and began a series of experiments which are called "classic" by modern day NIH researchers.[10]

Electron Photomicrograph of SV-40 polyoma virus

As her work progressed, she realized that she stood on the edge of an extremely important discovery and became very protective of her techniques.[11] In staff presentations, she would bewilder NIH pathologists by showing them slides of things they had never seen before. Then when they asked how she produced her results, she would giggle and say, "It's a secret." To quote her supervisor Alan Rabson: "She drove everybody crazy." One of her procedural anomalies was that *she never did control groups*, saying, "They only confuse you."[12]

In 1957 Stewart and Eddy discovered the polyoma virus, which produced several types of cancer in a variety of small mammals. Polyoma proved that some cancers were indeed caused by viruses. Her discovery officially threw open the doors of cancer virology. As Rabson phrased it: "Suddenly the whole place just exploded after Sarah found polyoma." It was the beginning of a new era of hope. But it raised some dark questions about earlier deeds. Before long Yale's laboratory discovered that the polyoma virus that had produced the cancer

Human Cancer Cel

in Stewart's mice and hamsters turned out to act like Simian Virus #40 (SV-40), a monkey virus that caused cancer.[13]

In June 1959 Bernice Eddy, who was still officially assigned to the flu vaccine project, began thinking about the polio vaccine again. This time she was worried about something much deeper than polio. The vaccine's manufacturers had grown their polio viruses on the kidneys of monkeys. And when they removed the polio virus from the monkeys' kidneys, they also removed an unknown number of other monkey viruses. The more they looked, the more they found. The medical science of the day knew little about the behavior or consequences of these monkey viruses. But times were changing. Confronted with mounting evidence that some monkey viruses caused cancer, Eddy grew suspicious of the polio vaccine and asked an excruciating question: Had they inoculated an entire generation of Americans with cancer-causing monkey viruses? She conducted her research quietly, without alerting her NIH supervisors.

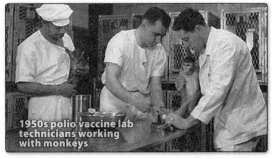

1950s polio vaccine lab technicians working with monkeys

In October 1960, one month before the Kennedy/Nixon presidential debate, Eddy gave a talk to the New York Cancer Society and, without warning NIH in advance, announced that she had examined monkey kidney cells in which the polio virus was grown, and had found they were infected with cancer-causing viruses.[14] Her implication was clear: *There were cancer-causing monkey viruses in the polio vaccine!* This was tantamount to forecasting an epidemic of cancer in America. When the word got back to her NIH bosses, they exploded. *No* suggestion of cancer-causing monkey viruses in the polio vaccine was welcomed at NIH. When the cussing stopped, they crushed Bernice Eddy professionally.

They took away her lab, destroyed her animals, put her under a gag order, prevented her from attending professional meetings, and delayed publication of her scientific papers. In the words of Edward Shorter, author of *The Health Century*: "Her treatment became a scandal within the scientific community." Later it became the subject of a Congressional inquiry.[15] In the words of Dr. Lawrence Kilham, a fellow NIH researcher who wrote a letter of protest to the U.S. Surgeon General's office: "The presence of a cancer virus in the polio virus vaccine is the matter demanding full investigation."[16] And further: "Dr Eddy's case, to many of us, represents a somewhat Prussian-like attempt to hinder an outstanding scientist."[17]

Eddy, however, was not the only one who investigated the issue. A viral specialist named Laurella McClelland, working for vaccine developer Maurice Hilleman in Philadelphia, found similar problems in the polio vaccine. The essence of the problem was that SV-40 did not cause cancer in its natural host, an Asian monkey. But what would it do in another primate that had never been exposed to it? One whose immune system had not been sensitized to SV-40?

Like Stewart and Eddy, Hilleman knew that the population of laboratory animals was hopelessly cross-infected with all sorts of viruses. Monkeys from different continents were frequently caged together. It would be impossible to guarantee that any monkey in the American laboratory population had not been exposed to SV-40 at some point in the past. Hilleman needed clean monkeys caught in the wild. To avoid any last minute contamination, he completely by-passed the commercial animal importing network. He arranged to have a group of Green Monkeys caught in Africa and sent to Philadelphia via Madrid, an airport which normally did not handle any animal traffic. His own drivers picked up the clean monkeys at the Philadelphia airport and brought them straight to his lab.

*Dr. Mary's Monkey*

When injected with SV-40, these clean African Green Monkeys developed cancer. Hilleman announced these findings at a medical conference in Copenhagen. But it was not news to the NIH staffers in the audience. The insiders already knew there was a cancer-causing virus in the polio vaccine,[18] but they had not announced it. It was the public that did not know. Should the public have been told?

It is difficult for us who have seen the enormous press coverage of AIDS to understand the indolent response of the 1960s press on *this* subject. Was it really their job to prevent public panic? Did they cower in the face of scientific authority? Were they lazy? Or stupid? Or arrogant? Or were they told not to run the story by political forces? It is hard to say. But there is evidence that the word leaked out anyway.

In the spring of 1961, one of Eddy's co-workers published a medical article which said there was live SV-40 in the polio vaccine. Eddy herself confirmed that the SV-40 monkey virus was causing cancer in hamsters as well as monkeys, proving that it was capable of crossing the species barrier. But she was not allowed to release the information until a year later. NIH notified the U.S. Surgeon General that "future polio vaccines would be free of SV-40."[19] On July 26, 1961, the *New York Times* reported two vaccine manufacturers were withdrawing their polio vaccines "until they can eliminate a monkey virus." The article ran on page 33, with no mention of cancer. Seven months later, a second article in the *New York Times* mentioned the possibility of cancer in the polio vaccine. That article ran on page 27.[20] There the story died, and the specter of an approaching epidemic of cancer silently rose on the horizon.

On the heels of the polio fiasco, the medical hierarchy feared the judgment of the masses. Their ability to destroy a painstakingly constructed scientific career overnight had been clearly proved. Another spate of bad news might shatter the public's confidence in vaccines altogether. Where would the world be then? Where would the public health establishment be then? As SV-40 discoverer Maurice Hilleman put it, the government kept the contamination of the polio vaccine secret to "avoid public hysteria."[21]

We are reminded of the scene in *Frankenstein* when a crowd of superstitious villagers gathered at the castle gate, angrily waving their pitchforks and torches in the air, demanding to know what evil was going on inside the doctor's laboratory. To quote the words of polio vaccine developer Albert Sabin: "I think to release certain information *prematurely* is not a public service. There's too much scaring the public *unnecessarily*. Oh, your children were injected with a cancer virus and all that. That's not very good!"[22]

*"Prematurely"?* Hadn't the mass inoculation already taken place? Hadn't several top scientists using carefully controlled experiments established that the problem was real? Hadn't they announced the results to their professional peers?

*"Unnecessarily"?* Wasn't there still time to try and do something about it? Shouldn't someone at least try? Sabin might as well have said, "I prefer my tombstone read, 'The Vanquisher of Polio,' and not, 'The Father of the Great Cancer Epidemic.'" His attempt to hide behind the apron of "public service" is no more than an attempt to avoid both responsibility and the unpleasant experience of facing the angry public. I am sure we would all prefer not to be held accountable for our blunders.

### Is this Dr. Eddy's forecasted epidemic?

The more important question: Was Eddy's prediction of a cancer epidemic accurate? Did the epidemic ever happen? If it did, wouldn't it show up in the cancer statistics? Wouldn't the great wizards of medicine tell us if there was really an epidemic? Wouldn't the press jump all over it? Given the times, I decided to check the numbers myself. A real epidemic should be easy to spot due to its size. So I dug out the cancer statistics published by the National Cancer Institute in 1989 and started reading related literature. Two things became clear:

1. We were *losing* the War on Cancer, and

2. We were *in the midst* of an ongoing cancer epidemic. Despite the improvements in cancer treatment which had decreased the age-adjusted, per capita death rate slightly, the hard fact remained: *Americans were getting cancer faster than ever!* Reporting on a 1994 article published in the *Journal of the American Medical Association*, the front page of *USA Today* stated, "Baby boomers are much more likely to get cancer than their grandparents were at the same age."[23] And further, "Men born between 1948 and 1957 have three times as much cancer not related to smoking as men born in the late 1800s." Why? Per *USA Today*: "The study's researchers insist the increase cannot be fully explained by smoking, better diagnosis, or an aging population." In the words of U.S. Public Health Service official Devra Lee Davis: "There's something else going on."[24]

I am not a biostatistician, but John Bailar III *was* when he worked for the National Cancer Institute. When he told these sad facts to Congress in 1991, NCI's response was "absolute rage."[25] His subsequent tenure there was brief. That "something else going on" may also help explain why the summary cancer data we have available to us ends in 1988 (Document B, p. 353).

Despite the $22,000,000,000 spent on research during the twenty-year-old War on Cancer, little progress had been made in prevention and some areas had gotten dramatically worse. The bottom line for the cancer establishment was that the NCI's initial lofty goal of a 50% reduction in the cancer rate by the end of the century had to be abandoned.[26] The "war" may have stimulated additional billions of dollars of funding in its day, but well before the end of the century, it became indefensible.

The reality is that 1988 saw a 20% total increase in cancers versus 1973! But as is true with most averages, the 20% increase does not tell the whole story. The vast majority of cancers remained relatively stable versus 1973. The 20% increase is the result of five cancers which increased dramatically: lung, breast, prostate, lymphoma, and melanoma of the skin. The rest of the cancers did not increase significantly during the same period.

Remember the dreaded polio epidemic of the 1950s with its 33,000 cases of polio each year. Compare that to these numbers from 1994: 182,000 new cases of breast cancer diagnosed; 200,000 new cases of prostate cancer diagnosed; 500,000 new cases of lung cancer diagnosed. The increase in *any one* of these diseases in the years since 1985 was greater than the entire polio epidemic at its peak!

Since 1985? Yes, 1955 + 30 years is 1985. A ten-year-old who received the polio vaccine in 1955 turned 40 in 1985! The graph entitled "The Cancer Epidemic" shows the situation clearly. It depicts the percentage increase in the incidence rate compared to the base year 1973. (The NCI age-adjusted the numbers to keep the aging baby-boomer age wave from inflating the picture.)

The first thing to notice is what didn't happen. Look at the line entitled "All other sites combined." 1988 shows a 0% increase over 1973. This includes leukemia, Hodgkin's disease, and cancers of the brain, colon, bladder, rectum, larynx, pancreas, kidney, stomach, ovary, testes, cervix, uterus, thyroid, esophagus, and liver. For some reason, bone cancers are not mentioned.

Next is the lung cancer line. Lung cancer statistics were terrible for both men and women. Both sexes showed a long, steady increase in both incidence rates and mortality rates over the 16 years from 1973 to 1988. This upward trend had been consistent ever since it began in the 1920s, when lung cancer was a virtually non-existent disease. The general consensus had been that the dramatic, but consistent, rise in lung cancer is a result of cigarette smoking, so we will isolate it from our search for Eddy's epidemic of viral cancer. But it is sobering to think that the 500,000 annual cases of this one disease consumed approximately $50,000,000,000 worth of our medical insurance premiums each year. That's twice as much money as was spent on the War on Cancer over those 20 years! If you're like most of us and have problem thinking in billions, then try this: In the U.S. alone, we were spending $137,000,000 every day on the treatment of one disease.

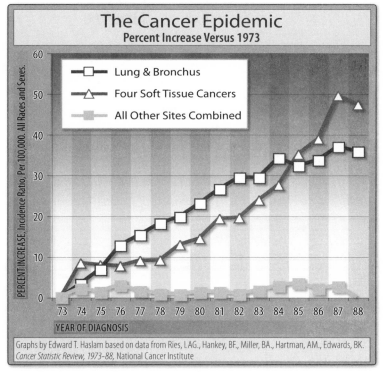

## The Cancer Epidemic
### Percent Increase Versus 1973

Graphs by Edward T. Haslam based on data from Ries, LAG., Hankey, BF., Miller, BA., Hartman, AM., Edwards, BK. *Cancer Statistic Review, 1973-88,* National Cancer Institute

The line entitled "Four Soft Tissue Cancers shows four cancers that averaged a 50% increase over this sixteen-year period. These four all show dramatic increases in their incidence rate versus 1973:

|         |      |
|---------|------|
| Skin    | 70%  |
| Lymphoma | 60% |
| Prostate | 60% |
| Breast  | 34%  |

We should note that there is no accepted explanation for what caused this!

Each of the four soft tissue cancers showed a dramatic increase in its incidence rate at the same time.[27] Is this not what we would expect to find following a mass inoculation with a virus which caused *multiple types of cancers*? This would be my candidate for Eddy's epidemic.

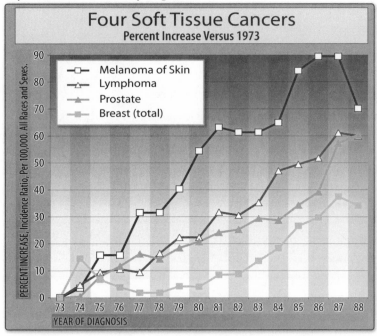

Four Soft Tissue Cancers
Percent Increase Versus 1973

Of all the cancers, none receives more press than breast cancer. Talk shows and soft-news TV features share the common burden like a giant group therapy session. *Science* magazine, which is hardly sensational, said, "The breast cancer statistics are alarming."[28]

Publicly, professionals expressed bewilderment over the breast cancer statistics. The explanations they did offer were feeble. The most commonly heard: "early detection." Early detection certainly helps treatment and the death rate, but it does not significantly affect the incidence rate. All early detection does to the incidence rate is borrow a fraction of cases from the next year or two. That lowers next year's in-

*Dr. Mary's Monkey*

cidence rate unless it too borrows from the following years with early detection. In other words, it has no long-term effect on the incidence numbers.

The "Breast Cancer" graph shows the incidence of breast cancer per 100,000 women from 1978 to 1987. There was a huge and sudden increase in the breast cancer rate around 1985. Remember: Ten-year-old girls who received the vaccine in 1955 became forty-year-old women in 1985, the age when breast cancer starts showing up in significant numbers. If the contamination of the polio vaccine was going to produce a wave of breast cancer, 1985 would be a logical year for it to show up. (Is it coincidental that 1985 just happened to be the year that my forty-year-old sister got breast cancer, when there was no history of breast cancer in our family?)

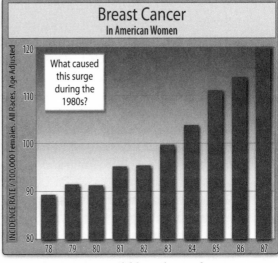

The ten year period shown in the above graph reveals an over 30 per cent increase in the rate of breast cancer. What this works out to is breast cancer in American women grew from 130,000 cases per year to over 180,000 cases per year. Is the sudden appearance of 50,000 additional cases of breast cancer per year an epidemic? Polio was considered a major epidemic with only 33,000 total cases per year! Why was breast cancer not considered an epidemic at 180,000 cases per year? These breast cancer numbers alone eclipse the polio numbers of the 1950s.

Then add the 200,000 cases of prostate cancer ... then add lymphoma ... then add skin cancer.... We should ask ourselves the obvious question: Why have we not heard more about this enormous epidemic of soft tissue cancers? Could it be because the billions of dollars which the U.S. government gave to NCI and NIH failed to produce a solution in time?

Despite the fact that the viral nature of several cancers had been proven by government scientists nearly forty years earlier, the 1994 edition of the American Cancer Society's publication *Cancer Facts & Figures* did not even mention "virus" among the possible causes of the most alarming increase in cancer ever recorded. Why?

Today, however, there is abundant evidence of a variety of simian viruses found in the human blood supply. Of particular concern is the DNA from SV-40 repeatedly extracted from several types of tumors, including brain, bone, and previously-rare chest cancers.[29] In the words of former FDA virologist John Martin, M.D., Ph.D., "SV-40 infection is now widespread within the human population almost certainly as a result of the polio vaccine."[30]

Does "almost certainly" imply some conditionality that a careful reader might object to? Does "former FDA virologist" create even the tiniest crack in seamless credibility? Am I forcing this point? Is this for real?

Did dozens of monkey viruses get into the human blood supply from the polio vaccine? Did they contaminate both the Salk and Sabin vaccines? Were these the same vaccines given to millions of children in both the United States and Europe? Consider this 1997 quote from the U.S. Government's own Journal of the National Cancer Institute: "In the 1950s, SV-40 was one of several dozen viruses that contaminated the original Salk and Sabin polio vaccines administered to millions of school children in the United States and Europe."[31] The vaccine contaminated with SV-40 was injected into trusting children until 1963. Forty-one years later, an in-depth investigation by journalists Debbie Bookchin and Jim Schumacher finally documented this same public health disaster in the detail which it deserves, including interviews with many of the scientists involved. The 2004 title speaks for itself, *The Virus and the Vaccine: The True Story of a Cancer Causing Monkey Virus, Contaminated Polio Vaccine, and the Millions of Americans Exposed*. Enough said.

BERNICE EDDY OBVIOUSLY THOUGHT the possibility of an upcoming epidemic of viral cancer was real. Why else would she have risked her career and her pension by announcing her findings to the medical community *without NIH's knowledge*? Did she fear that political interests at NIH would bury her warning, like they did when she sent them photos of the monkeys paralyzed by Salk's vaccine? Or was she just concerned that the glacially slow gears of bureaucratic science would not move fast enough to produce a solution in time? It may already have been too late. The viral damage to the genetic structure of the cell may take place very early in the infection. In 1959 Eddy explained it this way:

> It may be that the virus starts the cancerous process, but by the time we detect the tumor, there is so little virus left, —in an altered form —that we cannot detect it.[32]

In 1995, it was explained this way: If the growth-controlling *ras* gene is somehow damaged, it may become stuck in the "on" position.[33] Either way, there was no possible political benefit to be gained from telling the public about Eddy's forecasted epidemic of cancer unless a vaccine could be developed in time to prevent it. The issue was *speed*.

Developing a vaccine against a spectrum of cancer-causing monkey viruses already inoculated into millions of people in the polio vaccine was at best a long shot. But there was some evidence that anti-cancer vaccines were possible. Quoting *Time* magazine:

> Stewart and Eddy have gone a vital step farther... and made a vaccine that protects a big majority of normally susceptible animals against the polyoma virus's effects.[34]

The odds of success were slim, but the stakes were enormous: millions of Americans with cancer. They had to do something. They had to try. And they might get lucky. They might have serendipity. In a word, they were desperate.

Eddy may have underestimated the government, or she may have understood them better than any of us. Either way, it looks as if the government did spring into action, at least by bureaucratic standards, but the statistics suggest that they failed to produce a solution in time.[35]

If a vaccine were to be developed *in time* to prevent an epidemic of cancer in America, the research would need to be done *quickly, quietly, and privately*. And it would have to be directed by a competent professional. Someone with courage. Someone with resources. Someone with a reason. Someone willing to take a risk. Perhaps then, a vaccine might arrive in time to prevent a horrible and unprecedented wave of cancer among the American people.

If they succeeded, they would be national heroes, praised by the press, welcomed by a grateful public, rewarded financially and socially for demonstrating that our beloved can-do spirit of privateering really is an innate American asset, capable of triumphing even in the mysterious realms of science. And if it did not, at least no participants would have publicly stuck their necks out.

FERRIE AND THE ANGRY CUBAN EXILES may have been willing to develop a biological weapon to kill Castro, but I personally had not thought that Dr. Mary Sherman (or the other doctors) would have knowingly been party to the secret development of a biological weapon. I did, however, think that she might have been willing to be part of *a covert effort to prevent an epidemic of cancer!* Especially, if competent cancer researchers whom she personally knew and trusted thought it was possible, and if she believed that bureaucratic politics or procedures were hampering the process at the national level. The key words are "knew and trusted."

Just what were the connections between Mary Sherman (and the people around her) and the key viral researchers at NIH & NCI between 1959 and 1964? And are these connections strong enough to explain how an internal treatise on viral cancer research from NCI or NIH might have found its way to David Ferrie's apartment? And were they strong enough to support the idea that Mary Sherman (and others) may have been asked by people at NCI or NIH to be part of a covert effort to develop a vaccine to prevent a cancer epidemic caused by monkey viruses in the polio vaccine?

The most important connection between NIH and New Orleans is directly between Mary Sherman and Sarah Stewart. Both women entered the medical school of the University of Chicago as freshman graduate students in 1936. Mary, 23, had just completed her Master's at Northwestern and was working toward her M.D. Sarah, 30, had come most recently from Colorado and was pursuing a Ph.D. in Bacteriology. When Sarah received her Ph.D. in 1939, she moved to the Washington area for a job at the National Institutes of Health. Mary received her M.D. in 1941 and stayed in the Chicago area practicing orthopedic surgery until 1952, when she relocated to New Orleans.

Mary Sherman and Sarah Stewart were friends and classmates in Chicago for three years. I believe that Sarah Stewart is probably the author of the treatise found in David Ferrie's apartment, and that she may well have sent a copy of her cancer treatise to Mary Sherman.

Mary Sherman also knew Ruth Kirschstein at NIH. Kirschstein, who was thirteen years younger than Sherman, was an instructor at Tulane Medical School in 1954 and 1955. During these years Mary was an Associate Professor in Tulane's Department of Orthopedic Surgery, and that department's specialist in pathology. Sherman and Kirschstein had common interests in both pathology and cancer and taught in the same medical school. It is reasonable to assume they knew each other well. In 1957, immediately following the polio shake-up, Kirschstein went to the National Institutes of Health, where she stayed for the rest of her career.

At NIH Kirschstein began working as a pathologist in the Biologics division where Bernice Eddy worked. Her specialties were listed in the medical directories as virology, polio, and oncology.[36] But since Kirschstein was barely out of medical school when Sherman, Stewart and Eddy were already nationally recognized authorities, I do not consider their direct contact to have been very extensive. However, there are a few things about Kirschstein that should be kept in mind.

First, once at NIH, Kirschstein dated and later married Alan Rabson, who was Sarah Stewart's supervisor.[37] Therefore, she was in a position to know things about both Stewart and Eddy's research that she might not have known otherwise. And secondly, Kirschstein credits much of her professional success to the personal support and professional guidance of Tulane Medical School's Chief of Surgery, Dr. Alton Ochsner,[38] who is known to have enjoyed using his considerable contacts to help Tulane medical graduates find good professional positions.[39]

Before their careers were over, Ruth Kirschstein and Alan Rabson basically ran both NIH and NCI. The 2001 NIH telephone directory (which a friend brought me) listed Ruth Kirschstein as the Acting Director for all of NIH and the Chairperson for the Committee of the Directors from all of the various institutes of NIH. Meanwhile, her husband Dr. Alan Rabson, was Deputy Director of NCI. Do you find it interesting that a person who was so close to Sarah Stewart and knowledgeable of her research into cancer-causing virus, and who gratefully acknowledged Alton Ochsner for pivotal moves in her career, wound up in the position to control all research funding from NIH decades after Mary Sherman's death? Or that her husband, Alan Rabson, who was Sarah Stewart's supervisor wound up as the number-two person at NCI at the same time?

One can only wonder: Were these intentional moves to make sure that unwelcome research about cancer-causing viruses or the contamination of the polio vaccine did not get funded, conducted, or published?

Did Kirschstein keep Ochsner informed about the research activities at NIH and NCI? It would be hard to criticize her for keeping her mentor informed about the progress of cancer research at the national labs, especially since he was the former president of the American Cancer Society and held many important positions in the world of medicine. Additionally, as an expert in polio who lived in New Orleans in 1955, Kirschstein would also have been keenly aware of the problems that Dr. Ochsner faced after injecting his grandchildren with Salk's polio vaccine. When Eddy and Hilleman broke the news about the cancer-causing monkey virus in the polio vaccine, it would not have been unreasonable for Kirschstein to notify Ochsner about the danger his granddaughter faced.

Noting the coincidence of the time frame, we ask the question: Did the "Sensitive Position" that Dr. Ochsner was cleared for in October 1959 have anything to do with a secret attempt to develop a cancer vaccine to protect the American public from an epidemic of cancer?

And there were other connections between NIH and New Orleans. Of particular interest was Jose Rivera, M.D., Ph.D., who sat on the NIH Board of Directors in the 1960s. We will note that Dr. Rivera was really Col. Jose A. Rivera, one of the U.S. Army's top experts in biological warfare, and that in the summer of 1963 he was in New Orleans handing out research grants from NIH (its Institute for Neurological Diseases and Blindness) to Tulane Medical School, LSU Medical School, and the Ochsner Clinic.

IT IS NOT MY OBJECTIVE to pin Ferrie's possession of the treatise on any one particular person; I am trying to show that there were numerous connections between NCI and New Orleans, any one of which might explain how Mary Sherman and/or David Ferrie wound up with an internal document from NIH or NCI.

Therefore, the names contained in Mary Sherman's address books, which were confiscated from her apartment by the New Orleans Police Department, could be very helpful in understanding the exact nature of her activities.

To formalize our question: Did Sarah Stewart (or someone close to her) alert Mary Sherman (or someone close to her) to the potential of an approaching epidemic of cancer caused by monkey viruses in the polio vaccine ... *and* persuade her to try to develop a vaccine to prevent it?

If so, then the original objective of Mary Sherman's secret medical research was to develop a vaccine to neutralize the monkey viruses in the polio vaccine, not to develop a biological weapon.

So how does one develop a vaccine? There are two basic strategies. You can kill it or weaken it. The larger the virus is, the easier it is to kill. Large viruses can be poisoned with chemicals like formaldehyde. For example, the common flu vaccine is a virus grown on the yokes of chicken eggs and then poisoned with formaldehyde. But poisons are not very effective on smaller viruses like SV-40. Killing these smaller viruses was better done with radiation.[40] We are now at the heart of the matter.

Our question: Was Mary Sherman using radiation to kill or weaken the monkey viruses found in the polio vaccine?

Did Mary Sherman have access to high energy radiation equipment? We should note what equipment was being put into medical facilities at the time. In 1959 *Time* ran a cover article titled, "The New War on Cancer via Virus Research & Chemotherapy." In it, we read, "Almost daily, ways are found to give bigger radiation doses more safely to hard-to-reach

parts of the body." The list of techniques incl'
topes (cobalt-60, iridium-192, and yttrium-9(
ered x-ray machines and *linear particle ac(*
there a linear particle accelerator at one of th
Mary Sherman worked? And if so, did she h..

The real problem here is that the smallest viruses ...
(and now HIV) are so small that they are even hard to kill
with ionizing radiation.[42] So what happens if you hit one, but
don't kill it? What happens if you merely wound it with a
stream of sub-atomic particles ripping through its strands of
genetic information, mangling its molecules and scrambling
its sequence? If you do, and if it is still capable of breeding,
you now have a mutant. A new virus. One that behaves differently from the one you just mangled.

It may be more virulent; it may be less. It may even behave
differently from all other known viruses, since they evolved
naturally and this new virus did not. This is the real danger.
The moment you place a test tube full of viruses in front of

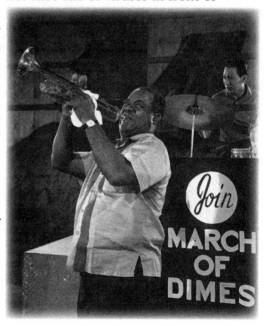

a linear-particle accelerator, you enter a brave new
world. And you become
part of the biological history of our planet.

Was Mary Sherman
using a linear particle
accelerator to kill or
weaken monkey virus-
es as part of a desperate
attempt to develop an
anti-cancer vaccine? Was
she testing the results of
those experiments in live
animals in Ferrie's underground medical labora-
tory? Perhaps this is how
good science goes bad.

Garrison, Jim, "Playboy Interview," *Playboy*, October 1967, p. 59; and Garrison, *A Heritage of Stone* (New York, 1970), p. 121.

**2** Dr. John Gregory was a Senior Instructor of Pathology at Johns Hopkins Medical School, and later an Associate Professor at Bowman-Gray Medical School.

**3** Shorter, Edward *The Health Century* (New York, 1987), from the PBS television series, p. 64

**4** Ibid., p. 67.

**5** Ibid., p. 68.

**6** Ibid., p. 69. This infamous polio disaster is known as the Cutter Incident, after Cutter Laboratories of Berkeley, California, which produced the faulty batch of Salk's polio vaccine. Dr. Alton Ochsner was a major stockholder in Cutter at the time. When Ochsner's son sued Cutter Labs over the death of his son, he was, in essence, suing his father, who had, after all, administered the lethal dose. He eventually dropped the suit.

**7** Ibid.

**8** Ibid., p. 197.

**9** Ibid.

**10** Ibid.

**11** Ibid., p. 198.

**12** Ibid.

**13** Ibid., p. 201.

**14** Ibid., p. 200.

**15** Ibid., p. 203.

**16** Congressional Record, U.S. Senate, Consumer Safety Act of 1972, Committee on Government Operations, Subcommittee on Executive Reorganization and Government Research, April 20-May 4, 1972, Title I and II of S.3419, page 520.

**17** Bookchin, Debbie and Jim Schumacher, *The Virus and the Vaccine: The True Story of a Cancer Causing Monkey Virus, Contaminated Polio Vaccine, and the Millions of Americans Exposed,* (New York 2004), p.83

**18** Ibid., p. 201, quoted from Ruth Kirschstein of NIH.

**19** Ibid., p. 202.

**20** Ibid., p. 203.

**21** Wechsler, Pat, "Shot in the Dark," *New York* magazine, November 1996.

**22** Shorter, *The Health Century*, p. 202-03

**23** Leslie Miller, "Boomers' cancer risk tops grandparents," *USA Today*, April 9, 1994, p. 1.

**24** Ibid.

**25** Marshall, Eliot "Breast Cancer: Stalemate in the War on Cancer," *Science,* December 20, 1991, p. 1719.

**26** Ibid.

**27** Ibid.: Marshall quotes the scholar-in-residence at the National Academy of Sciences as saying that only 30% of breast cancer cases are due to "identifiable causes," mostly having to do with factors, like genes or diet, which are relatively constant in any population from year to year. If we subtracted that 30% (18 points) from the annual incidence rate to exclude the identifiable causes, the remaining "unknown cause" breast cancer statistics are nearly identical to the 60% increase in prostate cancer.

**28** Ibid., p. 1719.

**29** "SV-40 like Sequences in Human Bone Tumors," by M. Carbone et al., *Oncogene*, August 1, 1996, pp. 527-35; "Evidence for and Implications of SV40-like Sequences in Human Mesotheliomas", by H. Pass, R. Kennedy, and M. Carbone, from *Important Advances in Oncology: 1996*, edited by DeVita, Hellman, and Rosenberg (Philadelphia: Lippincott-Raven Publishers); and "Natural Simian Virus 40 strains are present in human choroid plexus and ependymoma tumors," by J.A. Lednicky, R.L. Garcea, D.J. Bergsagel, and J.S. Butel, *Virology*, Oct. 1, 1995, pp. 710.

**30** "SV-40 Contamination of Poliovirus Vaccine," by John Martin, M.D., Ph.D., 1997, Center for Complex Infectious Diseases, 3328 Stevens Ave., Rosemead, CA, 91770, article available on-line at http://www.sonic.net/daltons/melissa/sv-40.html.

**31** Kuska, Bob, "SV-40: Working the Bugs Out of the Polio Vaccine," *Journal of the National Cancer Institute*, Vol. 89, No. 4, February 19, 1997, pp. 283-284. This article reported that "none of the agencies (of the National Institutes of Health) yet have new initiatives in the pipeline to bolster their current work on SV40..."

**32** *Time*, "The New War on Cancer via Virus Research & Chemotherapy," July 27, 1959, p. 54.

**33** Waldholz, Michael, "Reason for Hope," *Wall Street Journal*, March 16, 1995, s. 1 p.1. Destroying the "off" switch would have the same effect.

**34** *Time*, "The New War on Cancer via Virus Research & Chemotherapy," p. 53.

**35** The U.S. government did launch a massive research program in 1962 concerning cancer-causing monkey viruses. The project injected over 2,000 monkeys with cancer-causing and immunosuppressing viruses. See Richard Hatch, "Cancer Warfare," *Covert Action*, Winter 1991-92, p. 17. Was the Ferrie-Sherman lab racing the government labs, hoping to develop an anti-cancer vaccine in time to stop Eddy's epidemic?

**36** *American Men of Science*, 10th edition, 1960; s.v. Ruth Kirschstein.

**37** Shorter, p. 201.

**38** Comment made to Edward Shorter by Ruth Kirschstein during the tape-recorded interviews conducted for the PBS series, *The Health Century*. The quote is not in Shorter's book; source: Dr. John Roberts.

**39** Wilds and Harkey, *Alton Ochsner*.

**40** Knight, David C., *Viruses: Life's Smallest Enemies* (New York, 1981), p 109. The extremely small retroviruses are hard to kill, even with radiation. A blood cell is 100,000 times larger than SIV or HIV.

**41** *Time*, "The New War on Cancer via Virus Research & Chemotherapy," p. 54.

**42** Knight, *Viruses*, p. 109. said the National Academy of Science was working on this problem at the time.

~~~~~~~~~~~~~~~~~

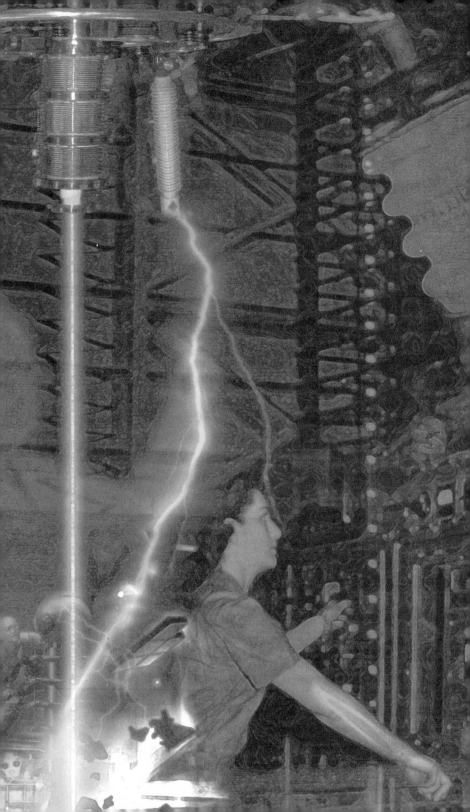

# CHAPTER 10
# The Fire

SOMETHING DIDN'T MAKE SENSE. The explanations of Mary Sherman's murder didn't add up. The press coverage focused on an "intruder," yet there was no forced entry. The police investigation failed to determine any identifiable motive, but the Homicide Report strained to imply a sexual one. And why did they not want to say where the victim worked?

The crime scene was also bizarre. How could anyone inflict such massive destruction on another person in the still of the night in a flimsy apartment complex filled with other people, and not have anyone even *hear* anything.

As I thought about these questions, I realized the single point that I was most uncomfortable about was the fire. Compared to the 40-foot flames of the Rault Center fire, Mary Sherman's fire was noticeably unimpressive. Other than the smoky mattress, a pile of half-burned clothes and some incidental furniture, the fire in Mary's apartment did not really burn anything. Yes, there was a lot of smoke and soot, but no one even reported seeing a flame. There was no structural damage to the wood-framed building. The curtains in the bedroom where her body was found did not catch fire. Even the clothes which had been piled on top of her body as fuel for the fire had not burned completely.

What about this fire? What was the temperature inside her apartment? And just how badly burned was Mary Sherman's body? My central question: Could the fire in her apartment really explain the damage to her body?

The newspapers were of no help on this. Other than generally describing her body as "charred," all the press ever said about the damage to Dr. Sherman's body was in one short line which appeared on the last day of the 1964 press coverage:

> The fire smoldered for some time—long enough to denude an innerspring mattress and burn away the flesh from one of the doctor's arms.

It is interesting to consider that this was the only detail the public heard about the actual damage done to the victim's body until the police reports were released, nearly thirty years later.

Then the following became known, from the Precinct Report:

> From further examination of the body, it was noted by the coroner that the *right arm* and a portion of the right side of the body extending from the right hip to the right shoulder was *completely burned away* exposing various vital organs [emphasis added here and following quotes].

Later in the same report:

> The cause of death was ... 5. Extreme burns of right side of body with complete *destruction of right upper extremity* and right side of thorax [chest] and abdomen.

The Homicide Report summarized these same autopsy findings, and added:

> The right side of the body from the waist to where the right shoulder *would be*, including *the whole right arm*, was apparently *disintegrated from the fire*, yielding the inside organs of the body.

*Dr. Mary's Monkey*

Further, it described the clothes which were piled on top of her body, some of which had not even burned:

> The body was nude; however, there was clothing which had apparently been placed on top of the body, mostly covering the body from just above the pubic area to the neck. Some of the mentioned clothes had been burned completely, while *others were still intact*, but scorched.

> According to the Criminologist, the mentioned clothes were composed of synthetic material which would have to reach a temperature of *about 500 F before it would ignite* into a flame; however, prior to this, there would be a smoldering effect.

Just to be clear, let me state what I think this is saying. If the temperature in the bedroom had reached 500 degrees Fahrenheit (260 degrees C) the clothes piled on top of Mary would have ignited and burned. Yet they did not. Therefore, the temperature in the room did not reach 500 degrees. The police, however, attributed the massive destruction to her body, including the disintegration of her right arm and the right side of her torso, to this less-than-500-degree fire.

Whatever burned off Mary's right arm and right torso had to be extremely hot! How hot? Who would know what temperature it took to burn a bone?

Perhaps someone who cremated bodies for a living. Since I did not know anyone in that line of work, I reached for the yellow pages and looked under "F" for funerals. After several calls, I reached a very personable and articulate man whose job it was to prepare cremated remains for burial.

"What temperature does it take to completely burn a body?" I asked promptly, expecting a quick answer with the precise number of degrees.

"Including bones?" he queried immediately.

"Well, that gets straight to the heart of the matter. Yes, including bones. I am writing a book about someone whose arm was completely burned off in a fire, and I am trying to figure out what temperature would be needed to do that."

"Burned their arm off?" he exclaimed. "How unusual! What happened to the rest of the body?"

"It was more or less still intact," I answered cautiously, concerned that he was going to get us off track.

"That's bizarre," he said. "I can't imagine that. Are you sure it wasn't cut off somehow?"

While he still had not given me the temperature number, I was impressed with how fast he got to the essence of the matter. I had not said anything about the nature of the death. It could have been a car wreck as far as he knew. But I was determined to get a cremation temperature from him before discussing any circumstantial evidence which might somehow color his answer. So I politely asked him to tell me the temperature of a cremation oven.

He said, "Well, the cremation machines are automatic nowadays so you don't have to set them, but an average cremation takes about two hours at about 1,600 degrees. But when you are finished, *there are still bones!* Depending on

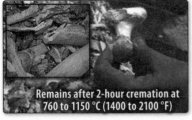

Remains after 2-hour cremation at 760 to 1150 °C (1400 to 2100 °F)

body size and fat content, some take longer. I have seen them as high as 2,000 degrees and for as long as three hours. But when you are finished, you still have bones, or at least pieces of bones like joints, skull fragments, and knuckles."

I now had my cremation number, but I was busy thinking about his answers. In the lull, he offered to give me some background on cremations and explained some popular misconceptions. The common belief, he said, is that you put a body in the cremation machine and get back ashes. No, that's not the way it works. Yes, it's true that there are some ashes produced by burning the skin and soft tissue, but that's a relatively small portion of what remains. Most of what is left after cremation is a box of dry bone parts. The next step is to grind up those remains so that they are unrecognizable. The final product is bone dust, a powdery substance that resem-

*Dr. Mary's Monkey*

bles ashes. Hence, the term and the misconception. What cremation technically does is rapidly dehydrate the bone material so that it splinters. Then it can be ground into a powder more easily. But bones do not burn. To emphasize his point he explained that even the skull cap, which is in the *direct path* of the flame during cremation, frequently survives.

While he was being very helpful and I was learning more about cremation than I anticipated, my goal was still to get a temperature figure which would explain Mary's missing right arm, so I pressed on. "Can you estimate what temperature it would take to completely burn off an arm?"

"Knuckles and all?" he countered.

"Everything," I confirmed.

"Well, it's hard to say. Before I got in this business, I saw a lot of burns. Some were military pilots who crashed their jets and got drenched in jet fuel. I would have to go get the bodies out of the wreckage. Jet fuel burns at thousands of degrees, but there were still bones left. I also saw people who had been covered with napalm and the like. But there were still bones left. I can't imagine how hot or how long it would take to completely burn a bone to the point of disintegration, but it's way up there."

I was getting his point. If Mary's entire apartment building had been burning out of control and had caved in on top of her body, it could not have produced the type of damage described in the police report. The smoky mattress and the smoldering pile of clothes with their less-than-500 degree temperature were certainly not capable of destroying the bones in Mary's right arm and rib cage. Then the critical point hit me: *The crime scene did not match the crime.* It was impossible to explain the damage to Mary's right arm and the right side of her body with the evidence found in her apartment.

Or to put it even more bluntly, the damage to Mary's right arm and thorax *did not occur* in her apartment. It had to have happened somewhere else. Her body was then quietly brought back to her apartment and deposited so it could be found there. A second fire was set to create an explanation, however tenuous, for the burns suffered earlier. It's no wonder nobody heard anything.

Something else had happened to Mary earlier that evening. It would require something much more violent than a common house fire to disintegrate her entire right arm and right rib cage. It would take something that could generate thousands, if not millions, of degrees of heat even if for only a fraction of a second, vaporizing and destroying everything in its path. Something more on the scale of lightning or a fireball from an extremely high-voltage electrical source which would destroy any tissue in its path, but leave the rest of the body which it did not hit relatively intact. Perhaps it was even an extremely powerful beam of high-energy electro-magnetic radiation just like the one that disintegrated electrical engineer Jack Nygard when he accidentally got stuck in the path of his 5,000,000 volt linear particle accelerator near Seattle, Washington.

The general outline of the explanation made sense, but the stakes were now getting to be enormous. Imagine how differently the investigation would have turned out if the initial newspaper headline had read,

**Cancer Doctor Mangled in Laboratory Mishap;**

*Secret Research Exposed*

*Monkey Viruses Roasted with Radiation*

And it put new emphasis on our question: Did Mary Sherman have access to a linear particle accelerator?

I had fairly good personal information that there was at least one linear accelerator in New Orleans in the 1960s: The Jesuit priest who taught physics in 1968 confided to our class that there was a linear accelerator being used "for research" at a medical facility in New Orleans. And I think that it is reasonable to suggest that a doctor with Mary Sherman's reputation for researching treatments for bone cancers may have had access to it. But the question remains: Did she?

My focus was on the physical evidence. Was the arm really completely burned off as suggested in the police report? What about the rest of the body? Remember that Dr. Talley identified the victim by body shape and *hair* color.

What about the proximity of charring burns to easily flammable hair? What could cause such localized damage? Did the nature of the burns on Dr. Sherman's body suggest high-powered electrical equipment? Or perhaps a powerful beam of radiation? I realized I finally had to get a copy of the autopsy report itself. I called an attorney in New Orleans and had him secure a copy for me.

## The Autopsy Report

THE AUTOPSY WAS PERFORMED on the morning of 7/21/64 by Pathologist Monroe S. Samuels, M.D., who signed the report and in the presence of Assistant Coroner Lloyd F. LoCascio, M.D. who did not. Dr. LoCascio did, however, sign the Inquest summarizing the conclusions which were reflected in the police report. Dr. Nicholas J. Chetta was actually the Coroner at the time, but his name does not appear anywhere in the newspaper articles, in the police reports, or in the autopsy report. Nor do his signature or initials appear on any related document from the Coroner's office. The only place the late Coroner's name appears in the entire file is on a pre-printed section of the Inquest which the Assistant Coroner completed and signed.

Here are the relevant sections of the autopsy report. Since many readers are unfamiliar with medical jargon, I have interpolated explanatory comments. I have also omitted the descriptions of most of the stab wounds as redundant, and have clustered related matter together for ease of reading. The full Autopsy Report is shown as Document C (p. 354).

The report summarized the general appearance of the body with the pathologist's laconic comment:

> It appears to be that of a white female.

Continuing,

> External examination of the body shows the hair over the head to be long and dark brown to black in color. It shows extensive charring and there is destruction of hair and scalp over the entire right temporal region of the head and extensive burns.

"Charring" is carbonization resulting from a high-temperature burn, as in burning a steak. The "temporal region of the head" is between the eye and the ear, in the area commonly called the temple. There were intense high-heat burns on the scalp, immediately adjacent to the unburned hair. This is evidence of an intensely focused heat source, such as a bolt of high-voltage electricity or a beam of radiation.

> There are extensive charring burns all over the right side of the face, the right thorax and the right flank.

"Thorax" is essentially equivalent to "rib cage." She was carbonized from the right side of her head down to her right hip.

> There has been complete destruction of the right upper extremity. The only portion remaining is a charred fragment of the proximal portion of the humerus.

"The right upper extremity" is of course the right arm. The "humerus" is the bone extending from the shoulder to the elbow. "Proximal" indicates the end of the bone closest to the center of the body. This confirms that her right arm was missing, and all that remained was a short piece of charred bone extending out from the shoulder. This is the critical evidence which demonstrates that these burns were not the result of the fire in the apartment. Again, such destruction could only come from an extremely high-temperature event such as a bolt of high-voltage electricity or a beam of radiation.

> There is extensive destruction of the entire right hemitho-
> rax with exposure of the lung and the pleural cavity.

The "right hemithorax" is the right half of her rib cage. The "pleural cavity" is the area inside the rib cage where the lungs and other organs are housed. Exposure of the lung means massive destruction of both the rib cage and the chest wall. Again bones were destroyed.

> There is desquamation of skin over the right thigh and also
> over the posterior portion of the left side of the body.

The skin was dehydrated and scaling on both her right thigh and her left rear torso. These burns, and the cooking of her brain, heart, liver, and lung, could have been the result of either the mattress fire in her apartment or the initial burn.

> There are extensive drying type burns over the entire face
> producing marked shrinkage of the skin, with deformity
> of the facial features and drying and shrinking of the eye-
> balls, bilaterally.

The shrunken skin, deformed face and dehydrated eyeballs sound more like a corpse from a science fiction movie than that of the victim of a mattress fire. Is it any wonder that the first two people who tried could not identify her?

There is evidence of two sets of knife wounds: one before death, and the other after.

> Examination of the left chest wall ... shows a stab wound
> to pass through the 6th intercostal space immediately ad-
> jacent to the sternum of the left side.

That is the wound that killed her. The "sternum" is the breast bone. The location is between the sixth and seventh ribs, directly over the heart.

> On removing the sternal plate the left pleural cavity is seen
> to contain approximately 1000 to 1200 cc of fluid and clot-
> ted blood. The pericardial cavity contains approximately
> 50 cc of partially clotted blood.

Upon removal of the breast bone, there was found more than one quart of variously-clotted blood near the heart, evidence that she *was still alive* when she was stabbed in the heart.

> Examination of the heart in situ shows a slit-like wound on the anterior aspect of the right ventricle immediately adjacent to the interventricular septum. A probe inserted into this wound extends into the right ventricular cavity.

A heart is composed of four chambers, two small upper chambers called "atriums," and two large lower chambers called "ventricles." The "interventricular septum" is the wall that divides the heart in half and separates the two large lower chambers. A stab wound "on the anterior aspect of the right ventricle immediately adjacent to the interventricular septum" means that *she was stabbed dead center in the middle of her heart.*

The heart is mostly muscle, and the thickest muscle in the heart is the dense wall of the powerful ventricles. The "probe" determined that this precise slit-like wound, inflicted in the exact middle of the heart, completely penetrated its thickest muscle. This would appear to be the basis for the rumor that whoever killed Mary Sherman knew what he or she was doing, and may have had medical training.

> The right side of the liver is markedly hardened and leathery and coagulated ... There is no hemorrhage noted around this particular wound.

The absence of hemorrhage around the liver wound means that the wound did not bleed, indicating that this wound to the liver was inflicted after death, during the second set of stab wounds.

> Examination of the external genitalia shows a through and through tear through the left labia majora measuring approximately 1 cm [0.4 inch] in length. There is a smaller similar tear in the right labium which does not extend

*Dr. Mary's Monkey*

through and through the structure. Further examination of the external genitalia shows it to be essentially normal. There are no areas of hemorrhage around the lacerations of the labium.

Again, no hemorrhage indicates that this stab wound was part of the second set of wounds, and occurred after death as well. The report continues its discussion with the internal genitalia, noting that the uterus had been previously removed by surgery, but it does not mention any other wounds.

The general pattern of stab wounds extends diagonally from the left shoulder across the abdomen and groin to the right thigh. These wounds appear to have been hastily inflicted immediately prior to setting the fire in her apartment. This last-minute jab to the genitals does not contribute to the idea of a sexual motive in her death. In fact, given the cuts in the clothing piled on top of the body, it indicates the body was covered at the time the second stabbing occurred; it is possible that whoever did the second stabbing was not even aware that her genitals had been stabbed. Considering this evidence, claiming "mutilation of the sexual organs," as stated in the press reports, is truly a gross exaggeration.

There were two sets of burns and two sets of stab wounds. The first set of burns was from an extremely hot and very focused heat source, and occurred somewhere other than her apartment. The total destruction of her arm is evidence of a very powerful device capable of producing thousands of degrees of heat. The partial charring of her scalp (without burning the rest of her hair) is evidence that this device focused its energy very precisely. Very few pieces of equipment would be capable of producing such a combination of burns. A linear particle accelerator is one.

The instant Mary Sherman received those initial burns her right arm was missing, her rib cage was destroyed, and she would be, from that point forward, a crippled vegetable. But her heart was still beating. She was still alive. The question at that point: Save her? Or kill her? The first stab wound (to her heart) killed her. All of the other stab wounds (all across her chest, abdomen, groin, and leg) occurred later, after her death, probably back at her apartment.

Finally it all came together for me. A perspective that explained most of the mysterious elements of the crime scene in a logical manner. *Here is one scenario:*

ON MONDAY NIGHT MARY WAS GOING TO BE WORKING on the secret project. This work had to be done at night, away from the normal daytime traffic. She took Monday afternoon off, to go to the dentist and to run an errand. Then she went home and washed her hair around 4:00 P.M., because she would not have time to do it later. She told her housekeeper, who was curious about why she was washing her hair in the afternoon, that she was expecting visitors from out of town. She asked her housekeeper to lay out her polka-dot dress for her trip to the children's hospital across the lake in the morning. The children were always happy to see her, even though they were the ones who suffered. She wanted to look happy when she saw them. It was one of the private joys of a childless widow.

After her housekeeper left, she slipped into some functional clothes and headed for the secret lab. Maybe tonight she would finally be able to neutralize the infinitesimal culprit that killed both children and adults so slowly and so painfully. Maybe this would be the step that made the dream of a cancer vaccine possible. This new machine had great potential. And it had been put in her hands. Her week of training in Boston would pay off now. Finally she stood on the leading edge of science. She went to the lab with high hopes.

That night something terrible happened in the lab. Something went wrong. There was a brilliant flash of light. Without warning an electrical arc of unbelievable magnitude leapt from the machine. A fireball of overcharged particles ran up Mary's arm and lunged through her body. The massive electrical current and intense heat literally blew her arm

Particle Accelerator

ST. CHARLES

LOUISIANA AVENUE

Dr. Sherman's Apt.

© 2007 Eurna Technologies
Image © 2007 Sanborn

off. A flashbulb of violence. Her body was destroyed almost beyond recognition in a fraction of a second. She never knew what hit her. Maimed and unconscious, she was still alive, since the path of the electricity had not crossed her heart.

Beyond their horror, the others in the lab with her now had an enormous crisis on their hands. One of America's most prominent doctors lay on the floor at their feet, maimed and mutilated by a machine most Americans did not even know existed. Maybe they could have saved her, it is hard to say. Maybe they tried. But would she have wanted that? A blind surgeon missing an arm and part of her body? And what would it do to their covert medical operation? Their secret experiments? It would be difficult to keep this one quiet.

Serious decisions had to be made fast. By dawn the die would be cast one way or another. It was time for action. Confronted with a near-dead scientist and perhaps the possibility of exposing a covert research project, the decision was made to cover up the tragedy.

Dr. Sherman would need to be terminated, her body returned to her apartment, a murder scene staged, and the investigation directed to a dead end. The plan had to be implemented immediately. There was no time to waste. Mary Sherman was terminated quickly and unceremoniously by stabbing her directly in the heart. They knew she could not recover from this. Then her body had to be returned to her apartment under the cover of darkness and in total stealth. No one could ever know.

One or two team members put on white gloves to prevent fingerprints from being left on any object. Mary's body was put into a body bag and placed in the trunk of her car. Around 3:00 A.M. they drove her car back to her apartment. Using the keys from her purse, they unlocked the gate and the door to her apartment, and turned off the burglar alarm. Once inside they quietly set her keys on the kitchen counter and dropped her purse on the sofa. Then they went back

*Dr. Mary's Monkey*

downstairs, got the body, and gently carried it up the concrete-and-steel stairs into her apartment.

When they placed Mary's body on her bed, they did not realize that the body was backwards, with the feet pointing toward the headboard. Once the body bag was removed, it did not seem to matter. A stack of neatly folded clothes was pulled from a dresser drawer and piled on top of her charred torso. Then came the hard part. They stabbed her corpse with a knife in a helter-skelter manner to create the impression of a psychopathic slashing. This left cuts in the folded clothes they had placed on her torso.

The fire was then started. The work done, they dropped the blood-stained gloves into the laundry hamper, quickly washed-up their hands, and hurriedly left the apartment, using Mary's car to flee the scene.

When the smoke from the smoldering mattress found its way through the ventilation ducts into a neighbor's apartment, he called the police. It was 4:13 A.M.

What happened in the lab that night? Secret medical experiments "under the cover of darkness" were underway. These experiments used a linear particle accelerator to mutate monkey viruses. Her euthanasic termination and the subsequent sham murder-scene were intended to preserve the secrecy of the operation, which is also the reason that the investigation into her death was sent on a wild goose chase, looking for a psychopathic lesbian butcher who never existed.

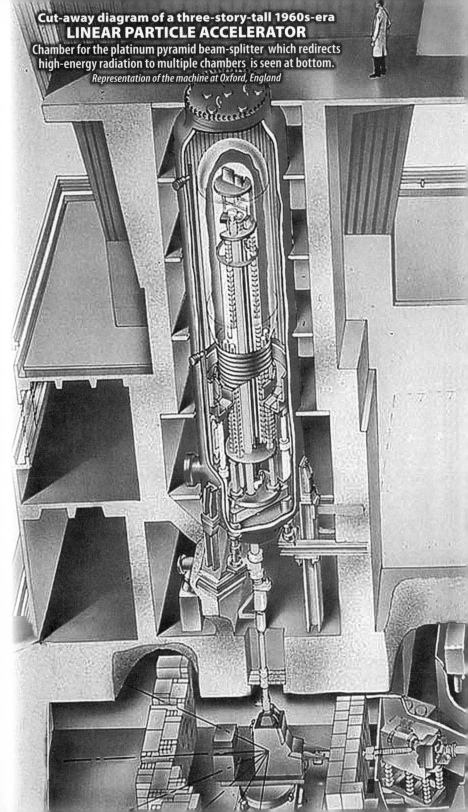

Cut-away diagram of a three-story-tall 1960s-era
**LINEAR PARTICLE ACCELERATOR**
Chamber for the platinum pyramid beam-splitter which redirects
high-energy radiation to multiple chambers is seen at bottom.
*Representation of the machine at Oxford, England*

# CHAPTER 11
# The Machine

Y THE SUMMER OF 1995, I had spent three years investigating the death of Mary Sherman, the history of monkey virus research, and the uncharted epidemic of soft tissue cancers. I was exhausted. It was a watershed point for me. Much had been done, yet much was undone. I had to make a decision about publishing. Should I publish what I had found to date, even if it was incomplete? Or should I continue researching, hoping to find more information?

On one hand, one of my major goals had been accomplished. Much of the nonsense surrounding Mary Sherman's death had been exposed. On the other, my list of unanswered questions stretched to the horizon. It was as if all my years of work were little more than clearing the brush before the real work could begin. The ultimate problem was that I had no way of knowing if additional effort would produce additional answers. Or whether a major discovery lay just around the corner.

For better or worse, I decided to publish, just to get the story out, even if there was more work to be done. Perhaps it would trigger an investigation. Perhaps someone would come forward with more information. Perhaps our Orwellian monster would stir on its own. Anyway, I needed a break and felt I had done as much as I could for the moment, and in 1995 I published the first edition of *Mary, Ferrie & the Monkey Virus.*

Ironically, it wasn't until I stopped writing and started publishing that I began to think about the set of unanswered questions from a broader perspective. My initial goal had been very general — to gather all the information into one place and look for an obvious pattern. What I found was a series of events that were both individually and collectively suspicious, but the overall pattern had not yet produced a coherent explanation.

For example, could *coincidence* adequately explain how the soon-to-be-accused assassin of the President of the United States crossed paths with the former President of the American Cancer Society, who was working on an assignment for the U.S. Government which was so "sensitive" that it required clearance from the Director of the FBI? Could *social acquaintance* explain why the Chairman of the Pathology Committee of the American Academy of Orthopedic Surgeons had been associated with a contraband pilot who flew covert operations for the CIA? Could *corruption* adequately explain the extreme manner in which the New Orleans Police Department shut down the investigation into Mary Sherman's murder and sanitized the reports?

All three seemed highly unlikely to me. I began to suspect that the individual pieces had been distorted to confuse the larger pattern. For example, if one saw Sherman's murder as *sexual*, it would be hard to see her death as a part of events which were *medical*, or as part of a larger pattern that was *political.*

But once you knew that Sherman's death was not sexual, it changed both the appearance of that individual event and the appearance of the overall pattern. And what to make of Oswald, Banister, and Ferrie? Were they colorful, albeit irrelevant, ornaments that decorated the streets of New Orleans?

*Dr. Mary's Monkey*

Or were they somehow woven into the fabric of events that ultimately produced Mary Sherman's death?

Further, the pattern of distortions begged the obvious question: What were they trying to hide? Why did people want us to think that Sherman's death was sexual? Why did they want us to think that viruses could not cause cancer? Was this in any way related to the reason that they wanted us to think that Oswald was a Communist? In short: What was the larger pattern to the events around Mary Sherman's death?

I began to see our scattered fragments like the tiles of a mosaic which would only reveal their larger pattern when arranged in exactly the right order. Perhaps there was a pivotal question, a central piece of information around which all other answers would orbit. A single question whose answer would define the pattern. The more I thought about it, the more one question came into focus. Eventually, it glared at me like a full moon on a cloudless night.

If Mary Sherman was killed by a linear particle accelerator, then the central question was clear: *Where was the linear particle accelerator located?* And then a series of related questions: Upon whose property did Mary Sherman die? Whose reputation was her masquerade-murder intended to protect? Upon whose authority was the investigation into her murder shut down? I thought about these questions every time I looked at the book, and I wondered if I would ever find the answers.

Of course, linear particle accelerators themselves were not secret. As early as July 27, 1959, the cover article in *Time* magazine bragged about the one at M.D. Anderson Hospital in Texas. However, linear particle accelerators were highly regulated. Under normal circumstances, the sale of a single accelerator would have generated a paper trail a mile long, particularly in the files of the Atomic Energy Commission. But was this a normal circumstance? My instincts said, "No."

Times being what they were, I was not about to FOIA[1] the records of the Atomic Energy Commission by myself. Their ability to sandbag, avoid, and delay was far beyond my ability to persist. So I decided to stick to my strategy of patience, and to wait for something to happen.

Six months passed with little change. Then the phone rang. It was a cold winter night in January 1996. The voice was warm and familiar. It was a medical doctor who had quietly fed me information over the past several years. His kiss-and-tell stories about radioactive medicine and medical politics had encouraged me at a time when little else did. I will call him Dr. X, for reasons that will become obvious shortly. We had spoken often, but not in recent months. During those earlier phone calls, he frequently talked about his long career and detailed many of the people and places he knew along the way. Of particular interest to me was his experience with linear particle accelerators.

As a young surgeon in the early 1960s, Dr. X had worked at a well-known cancer clinic on the East Coast. Operating on cancer patients was his business. Day after day he removed tumors and repaired organs with varying degrees of success. The daily grind was an excruciating battle between life and death. As times changed, new technology brought new hope. Chemotherapy and radiation therapy offered alternatives to radical surgery, and brought new promises to both doctors and cancer patients.

Radioactive substances, such as Cobalt-60, were injected into patients in hope of destroying their tumors. It was a desperate hope. The side effects were often terrible. None of the medical staff liked the idea of injecting patients with radioactive substances strong enough to destroy living tissue. Nor did they like the idea of standing by watching countless patients die. They all hoped that things would get better.

Considering these circumstances, it was not surprising that Dr. X and his colleagues welcomed the introduction of the linear particle accelerator as a new, improved means of

*Dr. Mary's Monkey*

destroying cancer tumors. The accelerator's main advantage was that the direction of the radioactive beam could be controlled, aimed precisely at the tumor, rather than emitting radiation in all directions and into the surrounding tissue as Cobalt had done. Fewer healthy cells would be destroyed, and less radiation would penetrate the bloodstream. It was an improvement at least, and it offered new hope. The hospital spent millions of dollars on this new technology and renovated a building to house the huge machine, which Dr. X came to use on a regular basis.

In this setting Dr. X came to know the people who designed and built his linear particle accelerator. One was Mr. Y, the manufacturer's Director of Sales, who had sold the machine and who serviced the account. Mr. Y spent so much time at Dr. X's hospital that he rented an apartment nearby. Dr. X and Mr. Y became friends, as well as professional colleagues. At one point Dr. X sublet a room in Mr. Y's apartment, so for a time they were roommates.

Mr. Y was a colorful character, a Peter Paul and Mary-vintage nonconformist with a Ph.D. in physics from Harvard. During the time Dr. X knew him, Mr. Y dated a beautiful French woman who danced with the Rockettes at Radio City Music Hall. According to Dr. X, Mr. Y's success was based both upon his brilliant mind and his father's close association with Harvard University's Board of Directors.[2] Dr. X gave me all the relevant details which I have stored safely.

That January night, Dr. X's voice was more excited than usual. He began by telling me about his recent trip to Europe, and then he updated me on a research project that he had been working on. Finally, he turned the conversation to Mr. Y.

By this time, Mr. Y and his linear particle accelerators were a familiar subject to me. He had built about 10 accelerators around the world. Each one was uniquely designed for a special application. From Israel to South Africa to New

Orleans, Mr. Y shepherded the design, sales and installation of some of the world's most mysterious machines. Dr. X had reminded me on several occasions that Mr. Y had known Dr. Ochsner.

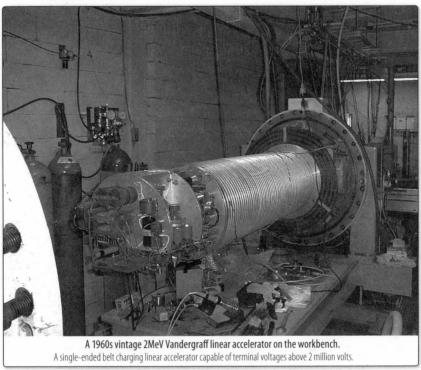

A 1960s vintage 2MeV Vandergraff linear accelerator on the workbench.
A single-ended belt charging linear accelerator capable of terminal voltages above 2 million volts.

This had been dangerous ground for me, and I had no intention of being manipulated into any accusations about Dr. Ochsner or Ochsner Clinic. Recall that my physics teacher at Jesuit had told our class in 1968 that the linear particle accelerator in New Orleans was *not* at Ochsner Clinic.[3] So I treated all these comments with caution.

Meanwhile, I had listened carefully for details which I might be able to confirm from another source. The problem was that there weren't many. Dr. X, however, kept encouraging me to look for evidence myself, evidence like a paper trail on the accelerator. At first he talked about licenses and per-

*Dr. Mary's Monkey*

mits. Since I considered this to be a covert operation, looking for an overt paper trail sounded like a giant waste of time.

Then Dr. X had reminded me that it would be difficult to hide a huge machine which required a three-story building and 5,000,000 volts of electricity. Perhaps there were records left in the files of the electric company. While this may have seemed like a reasonable route for a team of professional investigators, it sounded like a wild-goose chase down an obscured paper trail for an independent researcher like myself. And no one would leave a linear particle accelerator lying around.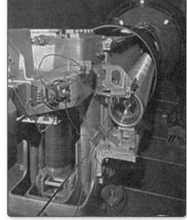

But he had persisted. There must have been some kind of evidence left, even if the accelerator itself had been removed. Perhaps there was physical evidence, like special wiring needed for the massive amounts of electricity. I told him I needed more information about the site itself. Perhaps then, I could figure out where the machine had been located. The problem had been that Dr. X had not talked to Mr. Y in years. The last he had heard, Mr. Y had burned out on the stress and secrecy of exporting nuclear machinery and had got out of the business altogether. Dr. X hadn't even been sure that he could find Mr. Y anymore.

Now, that had changed.

Dr. X said that he had stopped on the East Coast to attend a medical meeting on his return from Europe. On the spur of the moment, he decided to try and locate Mr. Y. After several phone calls from his hotel room, he located his old roommate and invited him out for a drink. They met at a local restaurant and reminisced about old times. Eventually Dr. X got his friend to talk about the accelerators he had built. Finally Mr. Y talked about New Orleans.

Here is a summary of what Dr. X said he had been told about the linear particle accelerator project Mr. Y supervised in New Orleans:

- The project was extremely secret. Mr. Y had to sign a secrecy contract with the government before taking on the project, and he could not disclose the exact location of the accelerator.

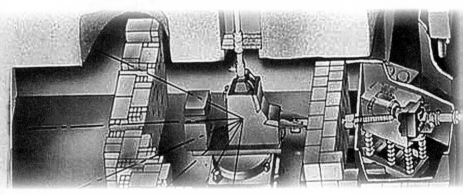

- The design of the accelerator was unusual. Normally an accelerator intended for medical use had clinical access features, like ramps for wheel chairs or beds for patients to lie down on. Here there were none. In fact, the intended use was in some form of laboratory experiments which required that the radioactive beam be split into equal portions for identical doses of radiation.
- The overall design resembled an octopus. The accelerator's particle gun was located on the top floor of the building. The beam pointed down, toward the ground, and struck a pyramid-shaped metal structure on the bottom floor. The pyramid divided the main beam into several smaller beams of equal intensity, and deflected them into series of containment chambers which encircled the pyramid. The targets were placed in the containment chambers, which were specially designed to hold heat and radiation. The metal pyramid was made out of platinum.

*Dr. Mary's Monkey*

- The financing was unusual. Since linear particle accelerators cost millions of dollars, the machines were usually purchased on long-term contracts which were paid off over many years. But this case was different, the entire amount (approximately $10,000,000) was paid in advance.

- The method of payment was unusual. Mr. Y received five or six checks in varying amounts within one week. Each check came from a different company and was drawn from a different bank. (So much for the paper trail.)

- Mr. Y went to New Orleans frequently during the construction of the machine, but once it was completed, he did not go back to the site for a long time. Suddenly there was a problem. He was sent to New Orleans to survey the situation. When he got there, something was obviously wrong. The accelerator building was guarded by soldiers with machine guns.

- Inside the building there were thousands of mice in cages. They were doing some kind of vaccine experiments. Dr. Ochsner was in charge. Mr. Y described him as tense and extremely suspicious.

- Mr. Y was particularly annoyed to discover, upon his return home, that military intelligence had been investigating his girlfriend while he was away tending to the accelerator.

What a bombshell! This was the worst-case scenario. At first, I hardly knew how to react. Needless to say, I had serious questions about the reliability of the information. Was this true? Or disinformation? Was I being handed the most important information

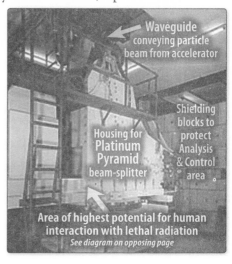

Waveguide conveying particle beam from accelerator

Shielding blocks to protect Analysis & Control area

Housing for **Platinum Pyramid** beam-splitter

Area of highest potential for human interaction with lethal radiation
*See diagram on opposing page*

of my investigation? Or was I being set up? Had I been given easily-verifiable information for over a year, only to be handed a red herring at the last minute? Or was I being lied to by someone with a hidden agenda?

It was a very perplexing situation, and I had to be very careful. On one hand, I did not even want to consider the possible implications of what could be phony information, because it might taint my view of the real information that I had fought so hard to get. On the other hand, I had seen and heard a lot of strange stuff over the past three years. And much of it pointed in this direction. It was not unusual for unsupported information to lead to supported information. So I did not reject what Dr. X said either. But the bottom line was that I could not use it if I could not confirm it. I decided to gate-keep the information, and not let it "inside" until I could verify it.

I needed an action plan to sort all this out. I created my first "information test." I decided to get Dr. X to repeat what he told me a second time. If he wouldn't repeat it, there was no point in my worrying about it. I called Dr. X back the next day and asked him to repeat everything he had said to me the previous night. He agreed. I was listening for inconsistencies. There weren't any. I recorded the phone call and made detailed notes.

Before this second phone call, I wasn't sure if I had anything real or not. Now I was sure that I either had good information or disinformation. The difference was subtle, but important. I figured the odds were 2-in-3 that I was being manipulated for some reason. My stress level doubled. Suddenly, I was back on the trail, and the stakes were higher than ever.

During my research, I had come to rely on a cadre of friends and researchers who sent me information. If I was being set up, I would be expected to rely on these same resources, any one of whom might be working with Dr. X. I needed to use a clean source, someone that nobody could an-

*Dr. Mary's Monkey*

ticipate. Not only did I need to figure out *how to confirm* the information, I would also need to figure out *whom to trust* with the assignment.

Again, the key question: Where was the accelerator?

I needed to locate it. I started to make a list of every medical related facility in the New Orleans area. If Mr. Y's information was accurate, it meant the cover was so deep that every facility in the area, even the unlikely locations like Hotel Dieu and the Children's Hospital, should be included on the potential location list. I tried to remember as much as I could about each facility. What I had heard and seen. What they looked like. Where they were located.

As I compared my location list with Mr. Y's story, the focus became obvious: the machine guns. There were very few places where soldiers with machine guns could wander about without making the patients extremely nervous. To do so would attract attention and thereby compromise secrecy. I quickly eliminated high-traffic facilities, like Charity Hospital and Ochsner Clinic, from my list. Other facilities, like the Children's Hospital,[4] were better candidates because they were low-traffic sites with sprawling campuses. I focused for a moment on the Children's Hospital. The very fact that most people would consider it an unlikely location made it an interesting possibility.

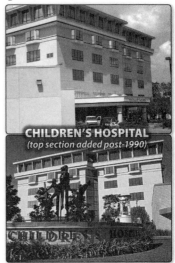

CHILDREN'S HOSPITAL
*(top section added post-1990)*

The Children's Hospital was located in the University Section, between Magazine Street and the Mississippi River near Audubon Park. I had driven by it frequently during my years at Tulane. Its shady campus was covered with old oak trees whose heavy limbs hung near the ground. I had only been inside the hospital once. My mother and I had gone there to attend a memorial service for my father, who had died the previous summer. He had been president of the small hospital, and they were dedicating a therapy room in his honor.

A nurse had given us a tour. It was a gallery of courage, and I remember the children. They were stubbornly happy, despite the fact that they could have had plenty of excuses to be sad. When the nurse explained that the hospital's name was being changed from Crippled Children's Hospital to Children's Hospital, a bed-ridden child said, "Yeah, we're *children.* Not just crippled children."

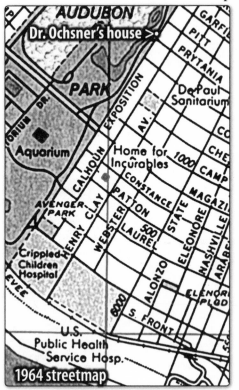

After the tour, we went outside and joined a crowd of about 100 people who had gathered near the hospital's main entrance for the dedication ceremonies. I escorted my mother. We stood in the sun and listened. Speeches from local dignitaries went on for nearly an hour. I became hot and bored, and my mind wandered.

I started looking around and noticed a group of old buildings across the street. They were surrounded by an unusually high brick wall. I studied the scene carefully. Several buildings were visible. All had pitched roofs and had been built of brick in the federal style of architecture common to the years before World War I. Fungus grew on the portions of the wall shaded by the ancient oak trees. I realized at the time that I had never seen anyone go in or out of this facility. In fact, it appeared to be abandoned, all of which made it seem rather mysterious. The windows of the building closest to the wall looked to be boarded up from the inside. The general appearance was very governmental, and very spooky. I wondered what it was.

Finally, I asked my mother. She said that it was the back entrance of the U.S. Public Health Service Hospital, and that I should be quiet and listen to the speeches. I had obliged, as

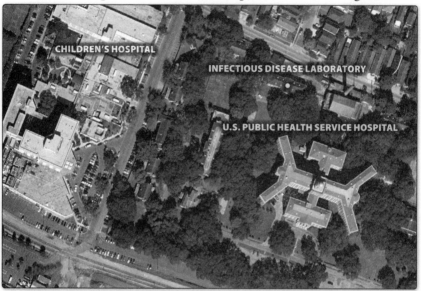

best I could, but actually was busy pondering what a great location the U.S. Public Health Service Hospital would be *for covert operations.* Trucks full of whatever could drive in through the wooden gates on one side of the campus, and cars could enter from the other. Once the gates were closed, no one on the outside would have any idea what was happening inside.

Whoa! *Covert operations! … Machine guns!* I snapped out of my reverie of recollections. The U.S. Public Health Service Hospital was operated by the U.S. military. Here was a place that could have had soldiers with machine guns. And who would go into a quarantine station unless they had to! What a great place to set up a secret laboratory!

Further, the U.S. Public Health Service had crossed my path several times during my investigation. The two most important:

- Ochsner's FBI file showed that at one point he had received covert payments from the U.S. Government at the U.S. Public Health Service Hospital.
- In 1960 Dr. Sarah Stewart left her powerful post at the National Institutes of Health to join the U.S. Public Health Service, the same year that Dr. Bernice Eddy announced that she had found a cancer-causing virus in the monkey kidney cells upon which the polio vaccine had been grown.

Finally I had a possible location: The U.S. Public Health Service Hospital. Now I needed confirmation. I had to get someone on the ground in New Orleans to look for more information. Whom to ask? Whom to trust?

There were two brothers in New Orleans whom I knew only by reputation. Both had lived in uptown New Orleans for years, and were interested in the Garrison case. I called one (Romney Stubbs) and asked him if he would help me with some research. He agreed. I did not tell him about Dr. X, Mr. Y, or any of the information I had obtained from them. I only asked him to see if he could find any information which might indicate whether or not there had ever been a linear particle accelerator on the grounds of the U.S. Public Health Service Hospital.

One week later he called back. Here is what he had to say:

In the late 1980s, the federal government had sold (or leased) the U.S. Public Health Service Hospital to the State of Louisiana for $1. The State renovated the buildings, and converted the campus into a long-term care facility for teenagers. He knew an employee and went to see her. He asked her if she knew anybody who might know about "the old days." She gave Romney the name of a building manager who had since retired. This man had been directly involved with renovating the buildings in the late 1980s. We will call him Mr. Z.

*Dr. Mary's Monkey*

Romney tracked down Mr. Z and interviewed him. No, he had not seen a linear particle accelerator, but he did see some very unusual things when he first came on board. He explained the situation. The campus had about ten buildings, one massive building which was the hospital itself, and nine or ten smaller buildings, some of which were residential in design. Mr. Z's first task was to plan for the renovation, so he had to thoroughly inspect all the buildings and inventory the situation. Mr. Z noted that all of the buildings, except one, were in comparable condition, with old desks and file cabinets full of papers scattered throughout the buildings. It was what one might expect to find in old government buildings whose funding had been gradually phased out. The only exception was a three-story building toward the back of the

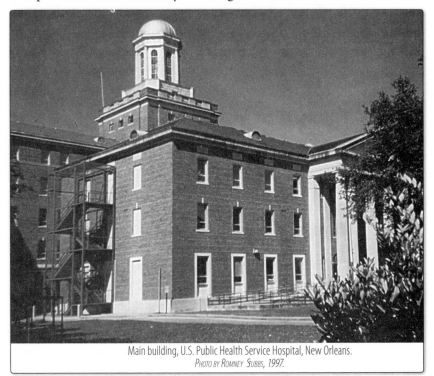

Main building, U.S. Public Health Service Hospital, New Orleans.
*Photo by Romney Stubbs, 1997.*

campus.[5] It was completely empty. There was not a single desk, file cabinet, or piece of paper in the entire building. It had been swept clean. Everything had been carried off, except two pieces of medical equipment: a large microscope and a tissue slicer used for making microscope slides. It had obviously been some type of laboratory.

Mr. Z had been trained as an engineer, and had worked with electrical systems in large buildings his entire career. He knew what to expect. He remembered the building with the microscope because the electrical wiring was very strange. In fact, *he had never seen such heavy wiring* in a building before. It had obviously been for extremely high-voltage electrical equipment, more powerful than any he had ever encountered. The equipment had been removed, but the wiring was still there. Mr. Z also noted that some of the rooms had very unusual features. One room had metal walls which were grounded by heavy cables. He described the other room as a circular shaped "operating room" on the ground floor. It was surrounded by a group of small airtight rooms which were completely lined with one-inch thick asbestos sheets on the doors, walls and ceiling.

I barely noticed that Romney had stopped talking. The silence hung in the ether. He said, "Well?"

I was speechless. Finally I mustered, "That's it."

He laughed and said, "That's it! That's what?"

"That's the building the accelerator was in."

"How do you know?"

"Because it matches the description that I was given by my source. It is *exactly* what we were looking for. It's just that I didn't really expect to find it."

The heavy gauge electrical wiring was needed to handle the huge currents required to run the 5,000,000 volt accelerator. The room with the metal walls was the control room. The metal walls were to protect the operators from the radiation. The heavy-gauge grounding wires were to reroute any errant electricity to the ground. The airtight asbestos-lined rooms

*Dr. Mary's Monkey*

were the chambers that the radioactive beams had been deflected into. What he described as the "operating room" was where the pyramid had been.

The accelerator itself and the platinum pyramid had been removed (and the building had been cleaned) when the lab was shut down. All that remained were the hard-to-remove items, like the high-voltage wiring, the metal walls and asbestos lined rooms. Romney sent a hand-drawn map of the campus and photographs of the key buildings. The accelerator had been located in the Infectious Disease Laboratory of the U.S. Public Health Service Hospital.

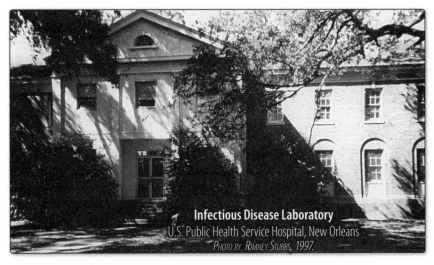

**Infectious Disease Laboratory**
U.S. Public Health Service Hospital, New Orleans
*PHOTO BY ROMNEY STUBBS, 1997.*

THE DIMENSIONS OF MY INVESTIGATION had suddenly changed. This was not a rag-tag operation run out of David Ferrie's apartment; it was a full-blown U.S. Government laboratory financed with millions of dollars from the public treasury. A state secret supported by the most powerful political forces in the land. A *medical Manhattan Project* set up in hopes of protecting the public from an epidemic of cancer which the government itself was largely responsible for. A 5,000,000 volt linear particle accelerator had been quietly placed on the grounds of the U.S. Public Health Service

Hospital so that cancer-causing monkey viruses could be roasted with radiation in secret.

Suddenly a myriad of questions surrounding Mary Sherman's mysterious murder came into focus. Is this where her near fatal burns occurred? Would the massive amounts of energy needed to operate the linear particle accelerator explain how her right arm and rib cage were burned off? Had her arm been burned off by the radiation beam itself? Or had she simply been electrocuted by operating the five mega-volt machine? Had her clothing been cut off because she received medical treatment for those third degree burns she suffered? Was she stabbed in the heart by one of the medical staff that had been treating her for those burns, to terminate her surreptitiously? Was she standing on U.S. Government property at the time of the incident? Was she relocated to her apartment to preserve the secrecy of a covert medical laboratory and prevent embarrassment to the U.S. Government?[6]

Imagine the political consequences of revealing all of this to the press. Talk about explosive! Talk about a situation that needed to be covered up! Now I understood why the police investigation into her murder had been shut down so abruptly. It was power in its purest form. The Feds told the NOPD to shut down the investigation, or else.

Now we had the answer to our pivotal question, and the incidental pieces started to fall into place. For example, I had always wondered why the damage to Mary Sherman's body was primarily in her right arm. Why hadn't the electricity traveled down her leg (to the ground) and exploded out her foot as was common in high-voltage electrocutions. The grounded steel walls provided the answer. The bolt of electricity would have likely come from something Mary grabbed with her right hand. Could it have traveled up her right arm and exploded out the back of her right shoulder into the grounded steel wall behind her? Since steel is more conductive than human tissue, the surge of electricity could go into the steel wall and then into the grounding cable, rather than

*Dr. Mary's Monkey*

down her leg into the wooden floor. I started to see the room as a giant spark plug – full of juice and ready to explode. Her arm would be the weakest part of the grounding path, "burning out" the way that the soft metal in a fuse burns out when too much electricity goes through it.

So what might she have grabbed? And could it have been loaded with electricity ready to climb up her arm?

I discussed the situation with a radiology technician. She pointed out that if you had an electrical problem with a machine, the standard safety procedure was to grab the circuit breaker by the handle and pull it down. This would shut off all the electricity to the machine. Whoever was running the accelerator would be trained to grab that handle at the first sign of trouble. If someone had wanted to sabotage the operation, or

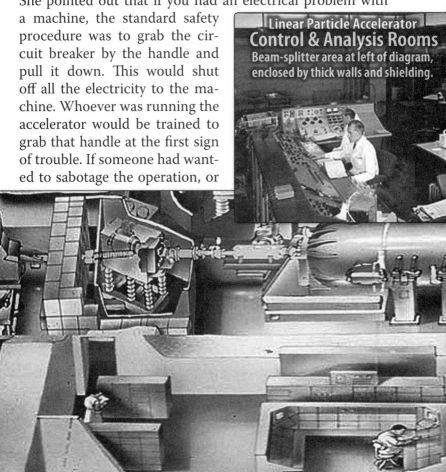

**Linear Particle Accelerator**
**Control & Analysis Rooms**
Beam-splitter area at left of diagram, enclosed by thick walls and shielding.

simply murder a key participant, a good method may have been to tamper with the machine's wiring and run the main power supply back to the circuit breaker, so that whoever grabbed the handle would be maimed or killed. Was this just an accident? Was the accident really "accidental." Was this murder? Was this sabotage?

Whatever happened to Mary that night, it required unusually large amounts of energy to damage her body in the manner reported. Amounts of energy consistent with equipment like the linear particle accelerator at the U.S. Public Health Service Hospital in New Orleans.

FINALLY, WE HAD THE LOCATION and our mosaic's elusive image had started to appear. With it came explanations ca-

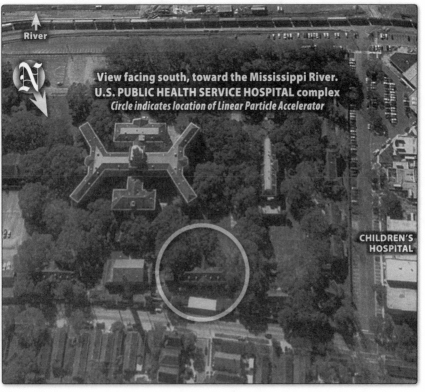

View facing south, toward the Mississippi River.
U.S. PUBLIC HEALTH SERVICE HOSPITAL complex
Circle indicates location of Linear Particle Accelerator

River

CHILDREN'S HOSPITAL

pable of sustaining our sprawling story. The trail followed the polio vaccine. It all started back in the 1950s, at the height of the polio vaccine inoculations. The moment Stewart and Eddy discovered cancer-causing viruses, top government scientists privately feared there might be a problem involving the contamination of the vaccine. By then they had already inoculated millions of children. They immediately branded the problem as National Security to keep it secret, and it is logical that they would have asked Dr. Alton Ochsner to look into it. Not only was he the former President of the American Cancer Society and a stockholder in one of the laboratories that produced the polio vaccine, but he had already lost one grandchild to that very vaccine. He understood the problem better than anyone. It was 1957, the date of Ochsner's first "Sensitive Position" for the U.S. Government.

Soon the research identified an Asian monkey as the natural host of the cancer-causing polyoma virus, and gave the virus a less hysterical name: SV-40. Then they found the same virus in the monkey kidney cells upon which the polio vaccine was being grown. By 1959 the government knew it had a problem. Vice President Nixon knew *he* had a problem.

Nixon had been given the task of rebuilding NIH in 1955, after the disastrous introduction of Salk's polio vaccine had killed dozens of children, and given others polio. He had signed off on Sabin's new polio vaccine. In fact, in terms of domestic casualties, he was holding the bag for the biggest problem in the nation. It threatened to destroy

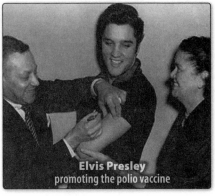

**Elvis Presley**
promoting the polio vaccine

the careers and reputations of everyone involved. The legal liabilities were astronomical. The political consequences were incalculable. It would have been the most politically sensitive secret in America. They had to do something about it, and whatever they did had to be kept super-secret. Disclosure was unacceptable.

It is likely that before long Dr. Ochsner was offered a new assignment: to develop a vaccine to prevent an epidemic of soft-tissue cancers. It was a noble cause, but an extremely dangerous project. They would be using radiation to mutate monkey viruses. What if something went wrong? What if they accidentally created a terrible new disease? Ochsner agreed on the condition that the work would be done on U.S. Government property. There could be no question about the fact that he was working on a national security assignment at the request of the highest officers of the U.S. Government. If anything went wrong, he had to be clear of personal responsibility, and there could not be any rub-off liability for either Ochsner Clinic or Tulane University. It was October 1959, the date of his second "Sensitive Position" assignment for the U.S. Government. The wheels were set in motion.

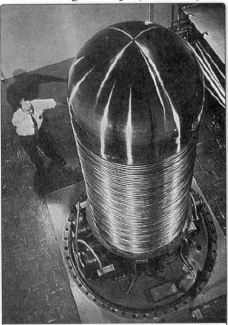

**National Institutes of Health** electron accelerator installed in the radiation wing of the US Public Health Service's Clinical Center during the late 1950s. It produced high-voltage electron energy 25 times more powerful than that from any other commercially available electron generator at the time. The 30-ton apparatus was used in research on the biological effects of high-energy radiation.
This high-voltage section on the top level of the three-story installation would be fully-enclosed in a pressurized tank of insulating gas during normal operation .

By 1960 the team was assembled. Ochsner was formally separated from Tulane.

Sarah Stewart, M.D., Ph.D., was probably recruited as the scientific director of the secret project. She was the most famous cancer researcher at the National Institutes of Health, and believed that an anti-cancer vaccine was possible. For her, it

*Dr. Mary's Monkey*

would have been a once-in-a-lifetime chance to have all the power and all the resources she needed to develop an anti-cancer vaccine. Stewart left NIH and transferred to the U.S. Public Health Service at this time. She could have secured the USPHS Hospital in New Orleans as a laboratory, with Nixon instructing the CIA to take millions of dollars from their laundered bank accounts to pay for the linear particle accelerator. By 1962 the machine had been installed, and the secret lab was fully operational. It would have been then that Ochsner and Stewart brought Sherman into the project. They both knew her well, trusted her, and respected her knowledge of the effects of radiation on cancers.

All this made me realize that there had been two underground medical labs in New Orleans in the early 1960s. I will call them the Big Lab and the Little Lab. The Big Lab was the U.S. Government's lab at the Public Health Service Hospital. It had the linear particle accelerator. It was where Mary Sherman apparently died. It started up around 1960 and continued until Mary Sherman's death in 1964. The Little Lab was on Louisiana Avenue Parkway near David Ferrie's apartment.

In the Big Lab, Mary Sherman was a high-level player who directed the medical research. Due to the security around the project, anyone involved with the lab had to have a high security clearance. Obviously they needed to find someone with a similar clearance to do the day-to-day work, like take care of the mice and prepare tissue samples for microscopic examination. David Ferrie had the right security credentials because he flew missions for the CIA, and he needed a job because he had recently lost his position with Eastern Airlines. Ferrie became a low-level player brought in to do routine lab work and oversee the mice. Ironically, our most persistent question had suddenly answered itself![7]

My guess once was that Mary Sherman's *only contact* with David Ferrie was through their covert working relationship in the Big Lab. Sherman's professional colleagues had no way of knowing she knew Ferrie, and Sherman had no reason to tell people she did. But Ferrie's situation was different. As Ferrie's life collapsed into alcohol and drug addiction, he continually "shot off his mouth" about his covert activities to impress his young friends. He used the fact that he had once worked with a famous cancer researcher (like Mary Sherman) to bolster his image, and to prove his legitimacy as a cancer researcher. This is when Ferrie listed himself as Dr. David Ferrie in the phone book.

Sherman's death demonstrated the political risk of the covert medical research at the Big Lab. Enormous political muscle had to be mobilized to shut down the New Orleans Police Department's investigation so abruptly.

The Big Lab had to be shut down. The accelerator had to be dismantled. Mr. Y was called in from Boston to survey the damage to the equipment and to make sure the accelerator could be safely removed.

Did Mary Sherman ever go to the Little Lab on Louisiana Avenue Parkway? For a long time my answer was "No." While I considered the odds to be extremely high that David Ferrie knew Mary Sherman through his custodial role at the Big Lab at the U.S. Public Health Service Hospital, I thought that Sherman had died before Ferrie brought any mice back to the Little Lab on Louisiana Avenue Parkway. Even if Ferrie planned to use the viruses as a biological weapon, I thought that Mary Sherman should not be associated with those motives, since she was already dead. In *Mary, Ferrie & the Monkey Virus*, I challenged any researcher to come forward with real evidence to support the claim that Mary Sherman was David Ferrie's closest female friend.

As we will see shortly, the evidence brought forward indicates that Sherman and Ferrie had a close working relationship. And it involved cancer and monkey viruses!

But what about INCA, Oswald, and the radio debates? Did any of that fit in? Was it part of the larger pattern?

I picked up the phone and called Carol Hewett, an attorney who had helped me during my research. When she answered the phone, I simply said, "Hello. We found the accelerator."

"Where was it?" she countered with equal brevity.

"At the U.S. Public Health Service Hospital in New Orleans."

"Hold on," she replied, as she typed "U.S. Public Health Service" into her computer.

"Here we are," she continued. "It's in Volume 19."

"Volume 19 of what?" I asked.

"The Warren Commission Volumes. The FBI went to the U.S. Public Health Service Hospital on 11/25/63[8] looking for evidence of either Lee Harvey Oswald or A.J. Hidell.[9] They went back a second time on 11/26."

The FBI was looking for Oswald at the U.S. Public Health Service Hospital! I could hardly believe my ears. "Why?"

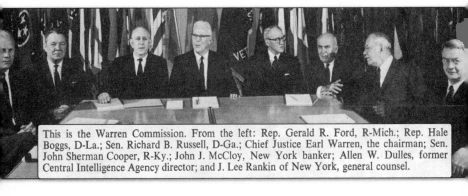

This is the Warren Commission. From the left: Rep. Gerald R. Ford, R-Mich.; Rep. Hale Boggs, D-La.; Sen. Richard B. Russell, D-Ga.; Chief Justice Earl Warren, the chairman; Sen. John Sherman Cooper, R-Ky.; John J. McCloy, New York banker; Allen W. Dulles, former Central Intelligence Agency director; and J. Lee Rankin of New York, general counsel.

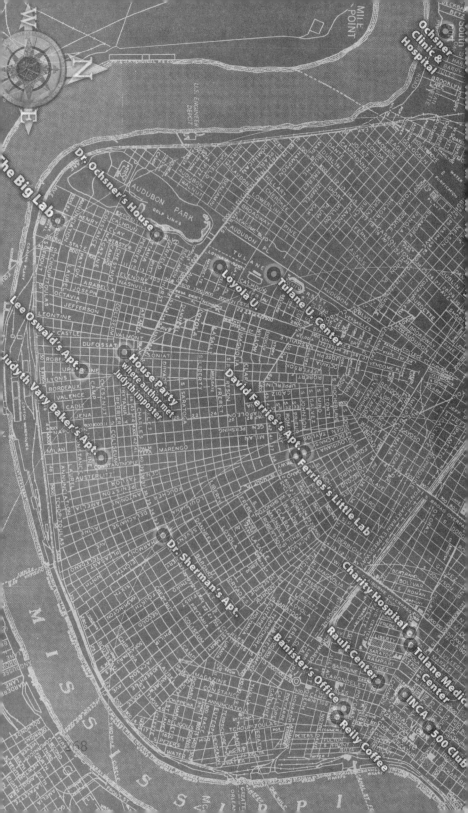

N

W    E

S

MILL POINT

Ochsner Clinic & Hospital

The Big Lab

Dr. Ochsner's House

AUDUBON PARK

GOLF LINKS

Lee Oswald's Apt.

Loyola U.

Tulane U. Center

Judyth Vary Baker's Apt.

House Party where author met Judyth imposter

David Ferrie's Apt.

Ferrie's Little Lab

Dr. Sherman's Apt.

Charity Hospital

Rault Center

Tulane Medical Center

Banister's Office

INCA

500 Club

Reilly Coffee

268

MISSISSIPPI

"According to the Dallas Police, Oswald had a vaccination card issued to him by the U.S. Public Health Service on 6/8/63, when he lived at 4907 Magazine Street in New Orleans. It was issued to Lee Harvey Oswald, and signed "Dr. A.J. Hidell." The FBI reports are in Volume 19. I'll send you the citations."[10]

Had Lee Harvey Oswald been on the grounds of the U.S. Public Health Service Hospital at the time the linear particle accelerator was there?

Take a look at the map. Does it strike you as unusual that both Lee Harvey Oswald and Dr. Alton Ochsner lived within one mile of the most secret government laboratory in America?

Here one should also consider the testimony of Dr. Adele Edisen, a Ph.D. neurologist, to the Assassination Records Review Board in the 1990s. She stated that she had been given Lee Harvey Oswald's name and his New Orleans phone number in mid-April 1963, approximately three weeks *before* Oswald moved to New Orleans.[11] To me, her twenty-one-page narrative strongly suggests that the location of Oswald's apartment was not accidental, and that it had been selected in advance for some reason. Was this reason its close proximity to the U.S. Public Health Service Hospital? Had Lee Harvey Oswald been sent to New Orleans to spy on the secret experiments at the U.S. Public Health Service Hospital?

Now the timing of Sherman's murder comes into focus. With Oswald in the picture, the fact that Mary Sherman's murder happened underneath the noses of the Warren Commission's investigators takes on a whole new light. Had someone sabotaged the linear particle accelerator in order to create a high-profile incident that would blow the cover off the secret laboratory and call attention to its connection to Lee Harvey Oswald? And what would have happened to the "lone nut" theory if the public began to suspect that Lee Harvey Oswald had been spying on a top-secret U. S. Government laboratory? Would it have seemed unusual that the doctor who ran that same secret government laboratory had also arranged the radio debates which discredited the soon-to-be-accused assassin of the President?

In my opinion, if this event was intentional sabotage of this laboratory, whoever planned it was well aware of Oswald's proximity to the lab, Ochsner's involvement with Oswald, the FBI investigation of the U.S. Public Health Service Hospital, and to whom the trail of accountability would lead, once the public discovered that the government was secretly mutating monkey viruses because they had released a polio vaccine contaminated with such cancer-causing viruses.

Sabotage of the linear particle accelerator may have been a hardball tactic in a big-league game of power. In this bold arena, our celebrated concepts of truth and justice give way to more fundamental questions like "Who rules?"

Mary Sherman may have been the incidental victim in a war between political Titans. Luck was not on her side. If Dr. Ochsner had grabbed the circuit breaker, things would have been different, at least for Mary Sherman. If such a plan to expose the secret medical experiments at the Infectious Disease Laboratory of the U.S. Public Health Service Hospital in New Orleans had worked, American history may have turned out differently.

---

1   FOIA stands for Freedom of Information Act, a U.S. law which gives citizens access to government documents. It is used as a verb by researchers to refer to the process of using the law to request documents from the government. Ultimately, the government still decides what gets revealed and what does not. Each agency has a FOIA officer who functions as a censor, deleting words, sentences, and paragraphs for a variety of reasons. To "redact" is to cross out with a black marker so that the requester cannot read the section. A heavily redacted document is one where many things have been blacked out. An unredacted document is one where the requester has protested the redaction and the government has agreed to issue a new version of the document with no redactions. FOIA was originally set up by LBJ in response to the argument that the government did not have the legal right to keep documents secret. The original law was so restrictive, critics called it the Freedom *From* Information Act. There are whole books written about how the process works.

2   While Harvard's name is universally respected, it is seldom mentioned in the popular press in connection to the development of nuclear technology. Instead, the stories recount once-secret, but now familiar, events like the Manhattan Project, which developed the atomic bombs that the U.S. dropped on Japanese cities during World War II. The featured names are usually Einstein, Fermi, and Oppenheimer. The featured locations are

usually Chicago and New Mexico. I did not question this perspective until I found a photograph of a scientist *dismantling* a particle accelerator for use in the Manhattan Project. I had not thought about centers of nuclear research that existed before the project. The caption explained that the accelerator (and the scientists) were about to be shipped to New Mexico for the super-secret Manhattan Project. The accelerator that they were dismantling was at Harvard. The point was so simple and so obvious. It was Boston, not Chicago or New Mexico, that was the actual intellectual headwaters of nuclear research in the United States. Of course, Boston would have been where the first commercial linear particle accelerators were built. At least Mr. Y was from the right place.

3    But he *did* say that Dr. Ochsner was involved.

4    The Children's Hospital used to be named the Crippled Children's Hospital. The name was changed around 1973.

5    The building appears to be two stories from the outside, but the attic was finished, and functioned as the third floor.

6    Jim DiEugenio and Lisa Pease sent me the FBI file on Mary Sherman. The New Orleans Police Department had requested the FBI's help. Asst. Director DeLoach, speaking on behalf of the Director of the FBI, turned them down, saying it was a local murder and that it was not within the FBI's jurisdiction. Agents were ordered not to participate in any manner other than routinely researching published sources. No FBI interrogation was allowed. An FBI agent in New Haven was threatened with a reprimand when he interviewed a doctor about Mary Sherman. Had Mary Sherman's body not been moved from the U.S. Public Health Service Hospital, the case would have automatically been in the FBI's jurisdiction. Did the FBI take this position to preserve the secrecy of this covert government operation?

7    The idea of Ferrie working under Sherman's direction in this lab makes a lot more sense to me than the claim that Sherman worked alongside Ferrie in his lab.

8    11/25/63 was the Monday following the JFK assassination (Friday 11/22/63) and the day after Oswald had been murdered (Sunday 11/24/63).

9    A.J. Hidell was an alias that Lee Harvey Oswald used during his first month in New Orleans.

10   Warren Commission, Volume XIX, Exhibit # 2012, memos from the New Orleans FBI office. Also HSCA, Cadigan 23 & 24.

11   Dr. Edisen said she was given Oswald's phone number by Jose A. Rivera, M.D., Ph.D., a Director of NIH's Institute for Neurological Diseases and Blindness. Subsequent research proved Dr. Rivera to be Colonel Jose A. Rivera of the U.S. Army's biowarfare unit and that he had lived in uptown New Orleans during 1960-61, a fact which he later concealed from the U.S. Civil Service Commission. Rivera may have been involved in the secret experiments at the U.S. Public Health Service Hospital.

Oswald's 4907 Magazine St. apartment was a small flat usually rented by Tulane or Loyola students. The phone number given to Edisen belonged to the building's landlord. Like the other tenants, the Oswalds borrowed their landlord's phone and never had a phone of their own. Dr. Edisen eventually called the phone number and spoke to Oswald himself. She was surprised to hear Oswald say that he did not know Dr. Rivera, and cautioned him: "Well, he sure knows who you are."

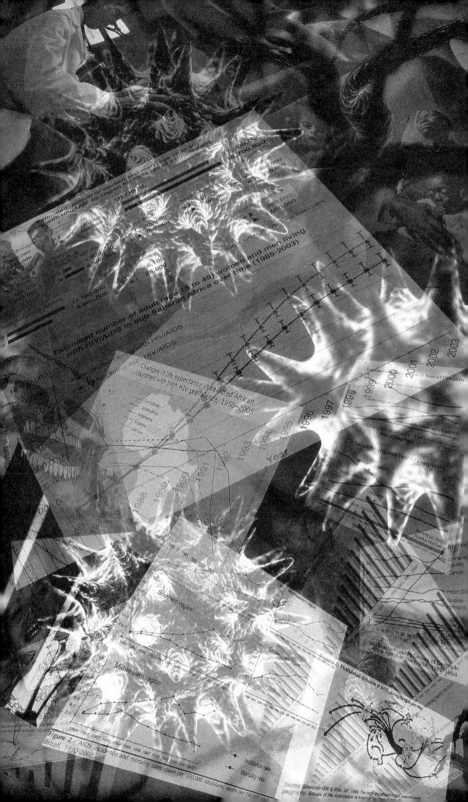

# CHAPTER 12

# That Other Epidemic

A S WE ENDED THE TWENTIETH CENTURY, a new plague stalked our planet. The official projections from the World Health Organization predicted that, by the millennium, 30 million people would be infected with this new virus. Other experts put the number over 100 million.[1] According to the Joint U.N. Program on HIV/AIDS, the actual number was 30.4 million; 18.8 million had by then succumbed to the disease.[2]

The damage would be worst in the Third World, where population and poverty are the highest and where education and sanitation are the lowest. But this plague knows no borders and, in time, will likely infect every city in the world. In the words of a WHO spokesman, this is "the worst public health disaster ever — beyond anything in our comprehension."[3]

Most articles published in the American press about "where AIDS came from" concentrate on the spread of the virus. The theories published in the United States tend to say that AIDS came from either Haiti or Africa. In Haiti, they prefer to say it came from the U.S. or Africa. And in Africa, they'd rather say it came from the U.S. or Haiti. And many people have heard about the homosexual Canadian flight attendant whose promiscuous activities helped spread the virus in the late 1970s and early 1980s.[4] This flight attendant story is an interesting example showing how fast a sexually transmitted disease can travel over great distances and how slow a bureaucracy can be about responding to something that it does not want to see.

When I ask Americans where AIDS came from, most of them say Africa. This is primarily due to publicity about the huge number of HIV-1 cases in Zaire in central Africa, about the relationship between the AIDS virus and an African monkey virus, and about the discovery of HIV-2 in Senegal on the western coast of Africa. But remember, Dr. Robert Biggar of the National Institute for Health said, "There is no conclusive evidence that the AIDS virus originated in Africa, since the epidemic seemed to start at approximately the same time as in America and Europe."[5] It is interesting to note that in 1985, after four years of tracking AIDS globally, there were 9,000 cases in the U.S. but only 2,000 cases in Africa, Europe, Australia, Haiti, and Asia combined.[6]

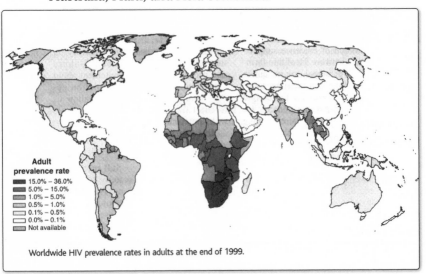

Adult prevalence rate
- 15.0% – 36.0%
- 5.0% – 15.0%
- 1.0% – 5.0%
- 0.5% – 1.0%
- 0.1% – 0.5%
- 0.0% – 0.1%
- Not available

Worldwide HIV prevalence rates in adults at the end of 1999.

*Dr. Mary's Monkey*

Most of the efforts to tie the origin of the AIDS epidemic to Africa are based upon efforts to tie Kaposi's sarcoma to AIDS. While Kaposi's is one of the cancers which frequently accompanies HIV infections, AIDS and Kaposi's are separate diseases. Kaposi's has been recognized as a distinct disease and studied as such since the 1800s.[7] HIV is new. As Robert Biggar titled his article: "Kaposi's sarcoma in Zaire is not associated with HTLV-III [AIDS] infection."[8]

It is interesting to note that in 1983, before Zaire exploded with HIV-1, before the relationship with SIV was discovered, and before HIV-2 was found in Senegal, a researcher named Jane Teas from the Harvard School of Public Health published a theory which suggested that AIDS was caused by a mutation of the African Swine Flu virus to which the Cuban pig population had been intentionally exposed, as an act of political sabotage, and which then spread casually from Cuba to the nearby island of Haiti, where it reached epidemic proportions in the tolerated prostitution environment.[9]

When the monkey virus connection was announced, the pig virus theory evaporated quickly. But because "pig" was wrong does not mean "Cuba-to-Haiti" was wrong. What epidemiological evidence did this researcher from the Harvard School of Public Health have for saying that AIDS spread from Cuba to Haiti? This is an area that needs to be explored further. It is important to note that we have virtually no public health information from Cuba during the 1960s and 1970s. And if we did have it, we probably would not believe it anyway. After all, Communists have always said that AIDS came from an American lab.

But it was a French epidemiologist who suggested that the spread of AIDS between the Caribbean and Africa may have been the result of a Cuban military airlift during the mid-1970s, and from the Caribbean to the U.S. via a Cuban exile boatlift to the US in 1977.[10]

What is known about AIDS in the Caribbean is that HIV-1 cases were reported very early in Haiti. In one particular case, a French engineer received a blood transfusion after he lost an arm in an automobile accident in 1977. Back in France, he developed AIDS and died. This is pretty conclusive evidence that HIV-1 existed in the Haitian blood supply around the mid-1970s. (AIDS was not reported in the U.S. until 1981.)

Further, a highly respected American scientist, Matilda Krim of the American Foundation for AIDS Research, suggested that the sudden and massive outbreak of AIDS among American homosexual males might have been due to infected batches of gamma globulin (an immune system booster commonly given to Third World travelers, and a health fad in the American gay community at the time) which were made from tainted human blood bought in the Caribbean during the 1970s.[11]

IN ORDER TO BE CONSIDERED a possible creator of HIV-1, one would have had to possess both the *capability* of mutating a monkey virus and the *opportunity* to do so within the established *timeframe*.

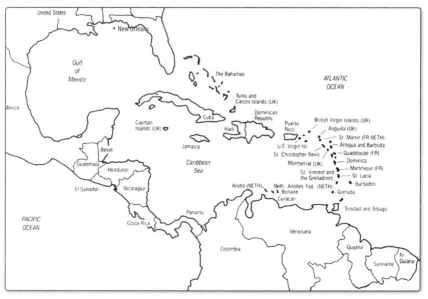

*Dr. Mary's Monkey*

Let's analyze *capability* first. If you were going to mutate a monkey virus, the first thing you would need is *access* to monkey viruses! Where would you get them? Drug stores do not sell monkey viruses. A zoo may have monkeys, but if you asked the zookeeper which one had a given retrovirus, he would not be much help. The obvious answer to "Who would have had access to monkey viruses?" The people who were doing medical research on monkey viruses!

So let's make the question explicit: Who was researching monkey viruses during the late 1950s and early 1960s?

In fact, there was a small group of medical schools,[12] private laboratories,[13] and government research facilities[14] here in the U.S., and a smaller number in Europe and the U.S.S.R. The majority were among those facilities which specialized in either *genetics* or *cancer research*.[15]

Once you had the monkey virus, the next thing you would need is a *means of mutating it* to produce the particular type of genetic change seen between SIV and HIV-1. One possible means of mutation is *ionizing radiation*. Radiation's ability to produce genetic mutations was established as early as 1928 by experiments on fruit flies, and has been confirmed in numerous studies since then. In his book on radiation, Dr. Martin Ecker described the ability of ionizing radiation to cause chemical changes at the atomic and molecular level, thereby causing biological genetic mutations. Acknowledging the reckless nature of such efforts, Ecker likened ionizing radiation to "shooting a gun into a computer." You will change something, but it is difficult to predict what.[16]

Supporting the idea that radiation could trigger such a mutation, we will recall that in 1966 British primatologist Richard Fiennes said,

> There is, therefore, a serious danger that viruses from such closely related groups as simian primates could show an altered pathogenesis in man, of which malignancy could be a feature. The dangers of such happening are enhanced by

man's exposure in crowded cities to oncogenic agents and increased radiation hazards.[17]

Today, there are other more precise techniques for genetic manipulation, techniques (like genetic recombination) which have their roots in the discoveries of the late 1950s and early 1960s. So, minimally, any potential creator of this monkey virus mutation would have needed access to both the monkey viruses and a means of altering genetic chemistry, such as a powerful radiation machine.

Once the virus was mutated, the next step would be to put the mutated virus into living animals to find out how it behaved. One would need a laboratory full of animals to test the various batches of mutated viruses in order to find out which mutations did what. To isolate the most effective mutations, you would need *thousands* of animals, like laboratory mice or hamsters, which are frequently used in blood and cancer research. These animals would need to be kept in cages, so you would need hundreds of cages. Caged animals need food and someone to feed them. The cages need to be cleaned. Records need to be kept. Minimally, it would require a technician and perhaps a maintenance person to handle these tasks.

In order to design the experiments, to handle the viruses safely, to record data accurately, and to recognize significant results, you would need to have a person with a *high level of medical knowledge* on the team, particularly knowledge of techniques used in virus research laboratories, i.e. a medical doctor experienced in virus research.

And labs take money. The animals, the cages, and the food all need to be bought. Space needs to be rented; electricity and water bills need to be paid. So someone on the team has to have money.

Actually, just about every medical school and government research facility could muster the above requirements *if directed to do so*. Therefore, the next ingredient is critical, because it is hard to find in combination with the above resources. You must have an environment which is *tolerant* of "wild card" experiments. So the question is not only who would do such a thing, but also who would allow researchers to play genetic roulette by irradiating monkey viruses in their facility? It would not be surprising if *nobody* wanted it done *in their facility*, due to the enormous risks and possible repercussions.

Thus, if there *was* a reason compelling enough to warrant such risky experiments, it would not be surprising to find the whole effort being conducted in secret, in an "underground" medical laboratory.

Moving on to *opportunity*, any potential creator of HIV would have had to have all of the above capabilities operating within the *timeframe* established by researchers: before 1969, and most likely in the early 1960s.

Finally *motive*. Someone has to have a *compelling reason* to do a project of this scale, to take the time, to spend the money, to organize the resources, and to do it all in secret. What reason could justify such effort and risks? Would a desperate attempt to find a *cure for cancer* explain it, if they were using radical techniques which would not have been accepted in a traditional research environment?

My point: *There was such an underground medical laboratory!*

And between the technician and the doctors involved, they had all the capabilities, opportunities and motives discussed above!

THE FERRIE-SHERMAN UNDERGROUND medical laboratory may have started with the noble and patriotic mission of preventing an epidemic of cancer in America; but once the work started, once the power to move cancer from animal to animal was established, once the ability to change viruses genetically was demonstrated, once the more virulent viral strains were isolated, once the means of transmission was established, once Mary Sherman died, and once Guy Banister died, then *the laboratory, the animals, and the viruses were left in the hands of David Ferrie.* He could have easily perverted the lab's resources into a biological weapon if he wished to do so, picking the most virulent strains and delivering them to a target deep in the heart of the Caribbean.

From David Ferrie's racist perspective, Haiti was a blister in the Caribbean, breeding "niggers," and shedding them and their primitive paganism into the waters off the coast of America. Its neighbor Cuba was worse, the fortified stronghold of godless Communism poised to spring upon weak neighbors with Russian weapons of war and enslave them in brutal captivity. Worse still, Cuba was the lair of the treacherous Fidel Castro, for whom Ferrie held a personal hatred. If there was ever a case of putting *a destructive instrument* into the hands of *a dangerous man*, this was it.

Given his history of violent political activities and his record of mental instability, the question is disturbing: *What would David Ferrie do if he realized he held the power to change history in his hands?*

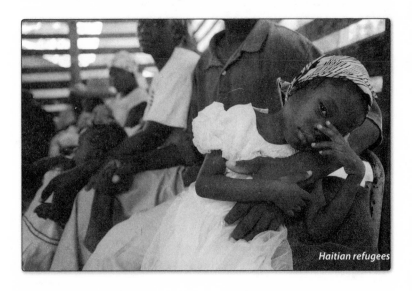

Haitian refugees

*Dr. Mary's Monkey*

1 Christine Gorman, "Invincible," *Time*, August 3, 1992, p. 30.

2 *The World Almanac and Book of Facts 2001*.

3 Hancock and Canin, *AIDS: The Deadly Epidemic*, p. 33. A good factual introduction to the whole subject of AIDS without a lot of political rhetoric..

4 Shilts, Randy. *And the Band Played On: Politics, People and the AIDS epidemic* (New York, 1987).

5 Cowley, "The Future of AIDS," p. 49; also Cantwell, *AIDS: the Mystery & the Solution*, p. 120, also R.J. Biggar, "The AIDS problem in Africa," *Lancet*, 1986, p. 79-83.

6 Hancock and Canin, *AIDS: The Deadly Epidemic*,

7 Kaposi's sarcoma is a deadly cancer, usually of the skin, first reported in medical literature in 1872 by Moriz Kaposi, a dermatologist in Austria; see Cantwell, *AIDS: The Mystery*, p. 20. In the U.S., pre-AIDS appearances of Kaposi's were most frequently seen in elderly people of Mediterranean or African ancestry. Kaposi's was a popular target for radiation therapy in the 1950s and 1960s; see R. Lee Clark, *Tumors of the Bone and Soft Tissue* (Chicago, 1964), p. 10. In Clark's words: "X-ray therapy in the management of soft tissue tumors is almost limited to Kaposi's sarcoma."

8 Biggar, R.J., "Kaposi's sarcoma in Zaire is not associated with HTLV-III infection," *New England Journal of Medicine*, vol. 311, 1984, p. 1051-52.

9 Teas, Jane, "Could AIDS agent be a variant on African Swine Fever Virus?," *Lancet*, 8330, April 23, 1983, p. 923.

10 Leibowitch, Jacques, *A Strange Virus of Unknown Origin*, (New York, 1985), p. 113-114. Quoted by Grmek, *The History of AIDS*, p. 154.

11 Cantwell, *AIDS: The Mystery & the Solution*, p. 188.

12 Between 1962 and 1964 seven federally-funded primate centers were built around the U.S. to provide monkeys for medical research by selected medical schools; see Eyestone 1966.

13 In 1962 the National Cancer Institute awarded a contract to Bionetics Laboratories, one of the U.S. Army's biological warfare suppliers, who inoculated over 2,000 monkeys with various oncogenic and immunosuppressant viruses. See Hatch, "Cancer Warfare," *Covert Action*, p. 17.

14 The National Institutes of Health had operated a major primate lab since the 1940s. The Center for Disease Control also had monkeys, as did the U.S. Army's Biowarfare Center at Ft. Detrick.

15 Virtually the entire science of genetic recombination was developed studying one monkey virus in extreme detail. The virus was Simian Virus #40 (SV-40), which was naturally found in Asian monkeys. In laboratory tests SV-40 caused cancer in a wide variety of mammals, including primates and humans. While SV-40 is a DNA virus, and is not related to SIV or the AIDS virus, cross-infection between African and Asian monkeys was common in American labs. SIV and SV-40 were frequently found together in the blood of laboratory primates.

16 Ecker, Martin D., *Radiation: All You Need to Know to Stop Worrying, or to Start* (New York, 1981).

17 Fiennes, Richard, *Zoonoses of Primates*, p. 144.

# Judy Vary To Continue Research

A summer spent at the Roswell Park Memorial Cancer Research Center in Buffalo, N. Y., has brought 18-year-old Judy Vary closer to the one goal towards which she has dedicated her life—finding a cure for cancer.

Judy arrived home late last night (only six buses late!) to spend a few days with her parents, Mr. and Mrs. D. W. Vary and sister, Linda, at their Gulf to Bay Estates home on Sneads Island. She leaves the latter part of the week for St. Francis College in Fort Wayne, Ind., where she will enter the freshman class under a $1,300 scholarship from the National Science Foundation.

She is one of three students who will continue research under such a grant.

## FIRST FROM FLORIDA

Judy was the first person from Florida to be chosen to spend the summer in research at the Center; it was through the efforts of Mrs. C. R. Watkins, long-time worker in the American Cancer Society, and Col. Phillip Doyle, MHS physics teacher, that Judy was among the 2,000 applicants for the summer work. Only 68 were chosen, from all parts of the world.

Judy was among the five chosen most outstanding among the scientists attending the summer session and her report to the National Foundation was considered the best. Each person chosen for the summer study must be recommended by a doctor at the Center; Judy was selected by Dr. Howard Moore, director of the Center and considered one of the world's outstanding experts on cancer.

Judy is glad to be going to St. Francis College as it is a smaller school and she will have a go-ahead signal to continue research in a new field — that of finding the substances which cause the cancer to become most deadly; Judy herself was a volunteer in one phase of research.

## SMOKED FOR FIRST TIME

Although she had never smoked, she volunteered to smoke after she first gave a half-pint of blood; more blood was taken after she smoked and scientists were elated to find a good many differences in the blood. Judy hopes to pursue this testing this year.

Judy bubbles over with enthusiasm when she speaks of the many people here who have made possible her venture into cancer research; she is particularly proud that Florida is being recognized for the unusual amount of interest in science locally.

## ALSO AN ARTIST

This young girl is not all scientist; she is an artist of note, writes short stories, loves to create poetry. This fall she will have a one-man art show in Buffalo, hopes to sell quite a few canvases for one half of the proceeds will be donated to Research, Inc., which helps young scientists financially.

Judy can't say enough about the people she met in Buffalo this summer; all are such dedicated, stimulating, fine persons. Most all of Judy's findings were verified at the Center: her theory is that anti-radioactive agents plus non-toxic stearates can be injected beneath the cancers to retard the movement of the cancer to other parts of the body.

According to Mrs. Vary, Judy's favorite expression is "when this moment is gone it will never come back." She expects to spend her every waking minute in her fight against cancer; she hates the disease, had seen members of her family die with it; nothing will stop her dedication to finding a cure.

She will meet with several local doctors Thursday to tell them of her findings this summer.

## Senior Attends National Meet With Scientists

With two Nobel Prize winners, and leaders in cancer research, Judy Vary, Manatee High School senior, recently attended the National American Cancer Society Seminar for 1961 in St. Petersburg.

Dr. Howard Moore, head of the Rosewell Park Memorial Institute for Cancer Research in Buffalo, New York, was so impressed by Judy and her cancer project that he offered her transportation to and from the Institute, room and board, plus $150 a month, to continue her research this summer in Buffalo.

### She's Going

Judy is going; she's delighted! Of her work, she explains, "It's never been done before, and that's the reason these people are so interested." And "It's so encouraging," she adds, meaning the definite and positive results of her experiments. What Judy is trying to do is to protect normal tissue from the adverse efefcts of irradiation while this radioactive bombardment destroys cancerous tissue, and to retard the movement of the cancer to other parts of the body. She has tried her theories with white mice, keeping exact records and precise charts of all treatments and results.

### 1st High School Student

Judy was one of three Floridians at the Seminar, and the first high school student ever invited. Just 68 people were invited, Judy explained, and all except herself had doctor's degrees or better. During the five days, March 18-22, they discussed the most recent advances in cancer research, and released much information to the public.

### Bring Home Awards

Arriving home from the State Science Fair last week-end, Judy brought with her six cash awards given to her for her outstanding research work. She was awarded a special scholarship from the American Cancer Society . . . $250 to the college of her choice. The American Medical Association also presented her with a special $25 award.

as she asked for understanding in her work.

The pink mice will develop cancer and will undergo irradiation treatments and the yellow mice will be cast in the most important role — that of testing Judy's theory.

Judy found it difficult to explain her project in simple words, since tongue-twisting scientific terms are such an integral part of her everyday vocabulary.

She managed to explain it this way though.

"Cancer is often treated with irradiation, Beta and Gamma rays. This treatment will kill the cancerous growth, but sometimes has an adverse effect on surrounding normal cells, causing them to become cancerous," Judy explained.

"My theory, which I feel in my heart has worth, is that anti-radioactive agents combined with be extremely happy if she could get additional tranquilizers.

"I also need very badly the use of an X-ray machine. The one at the hospital is too large for mice, so I need to find a laboratory that also experiments with mice," Judy said.

Judy is a young woman very hard to explain with mere words. You must watch her and talk with her to understand the depth with which she experiences life. Very sincerely she related a little of what she likes and believes in.

"I love to count things . . . I love statistics . . . I love fact . . . these things are all so substantial . . . they are solid . . . they are real."

Judy is a girl that never walks, but is always running. Why? "I run because there is so much left to be done, so much to be found,

# CHAPTER 13

# The Witness

I N 1995, ON THE EVE OF PUBLICATION of *Mary, Ferrie &
the Monkey Virus*, a fellow writer cautioned me: "You
have everything except a witness."

Five years later, the phone rang. It was *60 Minutes*, the
CBS News TV show. CBS News was investigating a woman
who said that she had been in the laboratory I had written
about in my book. In the laboratory in David Ferrie's apartment. Did I want to talk to them about what I knew?

Frankly, it was not a good time to ask me that question. In
2000 I was extremely busy doing other things in my profes-
sion, and I was not anxious to get drawn back into the story
that had dominated so many years of my life.

On the other hand, I respected the power of the *60M*
microphone. Whatever they said, whether right or wrong,
critical or favorable, would be heard by millions of people
and would shape the public's understanding of events which
I cared about. I reluctantly decided to participate enough to
keep an eye on the situation. We agreed to meet for an off-
camera interview. They sent me background materials to review, and one of their investigators came to see me — a lawyer. Ironically, it was *60M* that brought me the witness that I
had been missing.[1]

After I had reviewed the materials which they sent me (which did not include any of the photos of the woman nor the other evidence that I will be showing you shortly), they asked me to comment. My opening remark: "Well, she needs to be written up. Either in the history books or the medical books. At the moment, I am not sure which one." Neither were they.

*60M*'s interest in this woman was fueled by the sensational aspects of her story—that she had met Lee Harvey Oswald in New Orleans in the summer of 1963, that they had fallen in love and had an affair, despite the fact that both were married at the time. Any TV executive could see the blockbuster potential for a sizzling story built around the vortex of love, sex, politics and the accused assassin of JFK set in America's most exotic city. They eagerly flew their investigators to New Orleans and interviewed Oswald's girlfriend for hours.

*60M* asked Oswald's girlfriend all the logical questions: "Where are you from? Why were you in New Orleans? Where did you work? Where did you live? How did you meet Lee? What did you do together? Did you ever hear the subject of killing JFK discussed?" And Oswald's girlfriend kept answering them. Before long *60M* realized that their sizzling little romance between a beautiful young woman and a soon-to-be-accused assassin had morphed into an 800-pound gorilla with "serious politics" written all over it.

The adulteress sitting in front of them stated that she and Lee Harvey Oswald stood side by side in an underground medical laboratory located in David Ferrie's apartment on Louisiana Avenue Parkway in New Orleans, and that she was the laboratory technician that handled the cancer-causing monkey viruses which were being used to develop a biological weapon for the purpose of killing Fidel Castro. To put the icing on the cake, the entire project was secretly directed by the famous Dr. Alton Ochsner (former President of the American Cancer Society) and supervised by a prestigious

*Dr. Mary's Monkey*

cancer researcher named Dr. Mary Sherman, who worked for Dr. Ochsner at his hospital.

Further, she said, after successfully killing numerous monkeys with their new biological weapon, this group had tested it on a human subject in a mental hospital, killing the human. Lethal human experiments! Leaders of American medicine and the accused assassin of the American President involved together in developing a biological weapon! Can you hear *60M*'s signature sound-effect ticking in the background?

As the dimensions of the story grew, so did *60M*'s demands for hard evidence. *60M* was not about to risk its credibility over an unsupported story involving a homemade biological weapon and the accused assassin of the President without hard evidence. This is when they contacted me, because I had already written a book that sounded on-point.

Yes, they had my book, but no, they had not read it yet. I insisted that the *60M* investigator read it, every word cover-to-cover, which she later said that she did on her flight back to New York.

No, I did not have the hard evidence about this woman that they were looking for. But I never said that I did. From my perspective, I was particularly concerned that *60M* could easily discredit *her* story as a means of discrediting *my* story. Such were my initial thoughts.

The next problem came when I read the name in the documents they had sent: Judyth Vary Baker. The problem was that I already thought I knew someone named Judyth Vary Baker. And she had said that she had been a close friend of Lee Harvey Oswald!

A woman had been introduced to me (and my girlfriend Barbara) as "Judyth Vary Baker" at a party near Tulane's campus in uptown New Orleans in October 1972. The exact location was on Pitt St. near the corner of Dufossat St., behind the Ladder Library on St. Charles Avenue. It is important to point out that our invitation to this party was the result of an argument that I had had several days earlier concerning David Ferrie's underground medical laboratory, and whether viruses could actually cause cancer in humans. My opponent was the Latin American graduate student, mentioned in Chapter 4, who had previously made comments to Barbara about Dr. Ochsner's connections to Nazi scientists in South America.

At Barbara's suggestion, we had gone as a group to a cafeteria on Tulane's campus for coffee. Several other graduate students joined us there. What began as a polite discussion about local lore and Jim Garrison's investigation into the JFK assassination descended into an argument about the scientific accuracy of my comments about cancer-causing viruses. A particularly volatile point was the fact that I said that this fellow's hero, Dr. Ochsner, had said that "sex could cause cancer." Several days later Barbara complained to me that since that conversation in the cafeteria, none of her fellow graduate students had spoken to her: "You have to make up your mind whether you are going to be the recognized expert on the Garrison investigation, or whether you want to be my boyfriend."

I assured her that I was more interested in being with her than in discussing the JFK assassination, and agreed not to discuss it around her friends. Several days after that watershed conversation, Barbara announced that my "performance in the cafeteria" had gotten us invited to a party. Barbara was anxious to attend the party in hopes of regaining her social standing among her graduate school colleagues. She invited me to accompany her to the party, on the condition that I could "control myself." Therefore, when the hostess of this party told Barbara that she had been a friend of Lee Harvey Oswald when he lived in New Orleans and invited me to discuss the Garrison investigation with her, I asked Barbara if we could leave. Barbara agreed, and we immediately left the party.

Two weeks later, this "Judyth Vary Baker" contacted Barbara, and invited us (as a couple) to dinner at her home (without any other guests). I reminded Barbara that this woman had said that she had been a friend of Lee Harvey Oswald, and I said that I did *not* want to go to any dinner with her. Barbara declined the invitation.

When *60M* said they were investigating "Judy Vary Baker," I thought this was the same person. She was not. Was I being set up to discredit the real Judy Vary Baker should she ever emerge from hiding? Or was I given her name so that I would recognize it when she did? I don't know. For a more detailed account of this incident, see my video interview by Jim Marrs posted on www.DrMarysMonkey.com.

When it became clear that the woman introduced to me by *60M* was not the same person I had met in 1972, I realized that I now had two separate women claiming to be "Judyth Vary Baker," who both claimed to have known "Lee Oswald." Simply stated, one had to be an impostor. With the information available to me at that time, I could not tell *60M* which one was the impostor. I hoped that they would be able to tell me.

At that point, *60M* pulled the plug on the Judyth Vary Baker story. The rank-and-file CBS producers and investigators had worked hard on the story. They were extremely disappointed by the decision of their bosses to terminate it. One insider forwarded me an email written by a senior *60M* executive, in which he stated that *60M* had spend more time and money investigating Judyth's story than they had on any story in their 20-year history. To refuse to air the story after making that kind of investment was a difficult decision for them. It makes one wonder: Who really made *60M*'s decision to abort? And: Why?

After the *60M* debacle, I contacted Judyth Vary Baker directly. I was curious about this unusual woman, and wanted to learn more about her. If she could show me that she was the real Judyth Vary Baker, then it meant the other Judyth

Vary Baker whom I had met in 1972 was the impostor. This raised some very interesting questions: Why would someone have gone to the trouble to impersonate Baker back in 1972? How did she know who Baker was? How did she know about Baker's connection to Oswald? Why was I invited to the party?

Yes, the 1972 incident did cause confusion and distrust among the *60M* team. Their only evidence was my word and my memory. But that was their perspective. I, on the other hand, was the one who was there. I knew what I saw. I knew what I heard. And I remembered the names clearly.[2] The fact that *60M* had a real live person who said that her name was Judyth Vary Baker, and that she had known Lee Oswald, made the 1972 "Judyth Vary Baker" incident even more interesting to me. I decided to learn more about this new "Judyth Vary Baker" to try to sort out the facts.

In 2001, I happened to live in Bradenton, the small town on the west coast of Florida where Judyth was raised. When Judyth said that she would be visiting Bradenton soon to see her aging mother, we agreed to meet.

I took the day off from work so I would not be distracted by business matters. We met in the lobby of the central library and drove to a local restaurant where we could talk. Judyth picked a restaurant where she knew the owner. When we got there, she introduced me to the owner, who remembered her fondly, and we were shown a table in the back where we could talk. For the next several hours, Judyth displayed binders of documents she had collected and neatly organized over the years, and told me her story, page by page. It was only then that I really began to understand the dimensions of what she was saying.

Finally, I looked at her carefully, studying her pensive blue eyes and her coke-bottle-thick glasses, and said, "You are telling me that you personally stood in David Ferrie's apartment with Lee Oswald at your side, day after day, and worked with cancer-causing monkey viruses so that you could develop a biological weapon to kill Fidel Castro?"

"Yes," she said.

I felt that Judyth's story was an important development. So I called the writer who had said that I had "everything except a witness," and told him about Judyth. He had written a book about the JFK assassination. He assured me that Judyth was a walking, talking disinformation machine sent by the CIA to cause chaos and confusion among the JFK assassination research community, and that the documents that I had seen were probably forgeries.

"If these documents are fake," I countered, "they are the best forgeries I have ever seen. I'm talking about 30-year-old newspapers and faded ink."

"Langley does great work," he quipped.[3]

"You once told me that my only problem was that I didn't have a witness," I retorted. "Now my problem seems to be that I *do* have a witness."

I begin my discussion of Judyth this way to show how skeptical I was of her. It was clear to me that Judyth's road to acceptance was going to be a difficult one. Was she crazy? Was she an impostor? Had she made up her story after reading my book? Would people think Judyth and I were some sort of tag team, secretly coordinating our stories?

These are fair questions for the person who has heard her story from others, and has not seen her evidence presented properly. If you harbor some of these thoughts, know that I did too. It is reasonable to be suspicious of claims that challenge our understanding of history. But it is unreasonable to ignore evidence because it might change one's mind or challenge the positions that one has taken in public. History shows us that new information is rarely welcome. And Judyth has new information.

It's time to get to the core questions about Judyth Vary Baker. I consider these three most important:

1. Is "this Judyth" the real Judyth Vary Baker from Bradenton, Florida? Or is she an impostor?
2. Did Judyth know Lee Harvey Oswald in New Orleans in 1963? If she has no reasonable proof to support this claim, then there is little point in pondering her story.
3. Was Judyth trained to handle cancer-causing viruses before she went to New Orleans in 1963? If 1 and 2 above are true, then this point would qualify her as a suspect for the "technician" role.

If the answers to all three questions are "yes," then we need to pay attention to what Judyth has to say, even if it conflicts with both the official and the unofficial stories concerning Oswald and his role (whatever it was) in the assassination of JFK. Even if it disagrees with the self-appointed Oswald experts. And even if it disagrees with some of the things I originally concluded in *Mary, Ferrie & the Monkey Virus*. Let's tackle these questions right now — one at a time.

## 1. Is she the real Judyth Vary Baker from Bradenton, Florida?

Judyth showed me that collection of newspaper articles when we met in 2001. Several had photos of her. Most of the articles were published in the *Bradenton Herald*, one of the local newspapers in the Bradenton, Florida area.

A year later, in February 2002, I started working for the *Bradenton Herald*. My role was to handle its market-research materials, but my position gave me access to the news library and microfilm collection. This microfilm collection had been copied about 10 years earlier, and the copy had been given to the Bradenton Public Library. The public could see the microfilm collection at the public library, but the original microfilm was kept in the news department's research library on the upper floor of the *Herald*, which was not open to the public. No one could have anticipated that I would start working there and would have access to the original microfilm collection. If I could find Judyth's newspaper articles there in the off-limits microfilm collection, I could settle the "forgeries" issue once-and-for-all. I got Judyth to send me a list of publication dates for the articles she had.

In the microfilm library I indeed found all of the *Bradenton Herald* newspaper articles that Judyth had shown me. She had also shown me two other newspaper articles, which I will be discussing later in this chapter.

So the answer to our first question: "Yes, she is definitely the real Judyth Vary Baker from Bradenton, Florida." Her maiden name was Judyth Anne Vary, and she was frequently referred to as Judy in the press of the day. She is easy to recognize in the photos. Bradenton was proud of her. "Judy" was going to find the cure for cancer.[4] She presents copious evidence to support all of this in her book.[5]

## 2. Did Judyth know Lee Harvey Oswald in New Orleans in 1963?

It might help the reader to know that there has never been any dispute over the fact that the person that the press has referred to as Lee Harvey Oswald worked at a coffee company in New Orleans in the summer of 1963. This is reported by the Warren Commission and acknowledged throughout the JFK assassination research community. In fact, I have never heard anyone dispute it. Beyond that, I personally heard Boatner Reily, later the president of that same coffee company, state that they (the Wm. B. Reily Coffee Company) had turned over their employment records of Lee Harvey Oswald to the U.S. Government immediately after the assassination. What is less clear to the casual reader is whether Lee Oswald worked for the Standard Coffee Company or for the Wm. B. Reily Coffee Company, since the names differ on various documents. Both companies were owned and operated by William B. Reily and his family. It is odd that a supposed defector sporting an undesirable discharge from the Marines would work for William Reily, one of the most visible members of the ultra-conservative anti-Communist business community in New Orleans. But he did. Lee Oswald worked for Reily. So did Judyth Vary Baker.

Here is her old W-2 tax form, submitted by Wm. B. Reily & Co. to the U.S. Internal Revenue Service, which shows that she did:

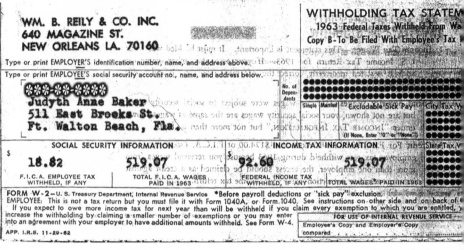

This document was provided to me directly by Judyth Vary Baker, who scanned it from the original. I accept it as authentic.[6] I have blocked out her Social Security number to protect her privacy. I did, however, compare that social security number with a variety of other documents which Judyth provided to me, such as her college transcripts, and I assure the reader that the numbers match.

The name on the document is Judyth Anne Baker. The person we now know as Judyth Vary Baker was known as Judyth Anne Vary until she married Robert Baker, becoming Judyth Anne Baker in 1963. Back then it was not common for women to incorporate their maiden names into their married names.

W-2 forms are mailed out in January of the following year — in this case, in January 1964 for the 1963 tax year. The address on the form shows where the form was mailed, not where the person lived while employed. Judyth left New

Orleans in September 1963, after her employment with Reily ended, and returned to Florida. The Ft. Walton address on Judyth's W-2 form was her husband's family's residence, which he used as his official address while attending the University of Florida in Gainesville.

The amount of money shown on the W-2 form is consistent with Judyth's pay stubs from Reily, of which I also have copies. It should be emphasized that Judyth was referred to Reily by the same employment agency that referred Lee Oswald, and that she started work on the same day. Judyth worked directly for Reily's Vice President William I. Monaghan, an ex-FBI agent who later testified to the Warren Commission about Oswald. But Monaghan did not mention Judyth to the Warren Commission, nor did he mention that another person was hired on the same day that Oswald was hired.

A simple gumshoe investigation of a murder suspect would have started with friends and associates, particularly at the place of employment. A gumshoe investigation of Oswald would have checked out Reily Coffee, found Judyth, and realized that she was close to Oswald. They started on the same day and arrived at Reily together each morning, though they frequently clocked in at different times due to Lee's other activities in the neighborhood. We even find Judyth's initials written on Lee's timecards. Figuring out the connection would not have been difficult.

Consider these obvious points: Neither Lee nor Judyth owned a car. Reily Coffee was located on Magazine Street. Both Judyth and Lee lived along the Magazine Street bus route and rode the bus to work. Day after day, Lee would get on the bus at the 4900 block of Magazine. Several blocks later Judyth would get on at the corner of Marengo Street, and sit next to Lee. Bus drivers recognize their regular customers. The bus driver could have easily confirmed that Judyth and Lee sat together every morning, read the newspaper, and talked — and that they got off the bus together near the Reily

Coffee Company. This would not have been difficult for an investigator to sort out.[7]

Who was this young woman who talked to the accused assassin of the President on a daily basis? What did she know about him? What did she know about the assassination? Did she have prior knowledge? These are good questions, and a competent investigator would have asked them. So why were they not asked?

Did the Warren Commission send in a gumshoe to investigate Oswald at Reily? No, they asked the ex-FBI agent that hired Oswald about him.[8] And that ex-FBI agent did not mention that his own secretary, whom he had also hired, had started on the same day and arrived at his front door with Oswald every morning. How convenient! This raises the question: Did Monaghan intentionally withhold information from the Warren Commission? If he did, was he instructed to do so? And by whom? Was Judyth being shielded in order to protect the bio-weapon project and the people behind it?

Several years after the Warren Commission "investigation," the investigators working for New Orleans District Attorney Jim Garrison tracked down another young woman, Anna Lewis, a waitress who worked at Thompson's Restaurant —a favorite gathering spot for the anti-Castro crowd around Lafayette Square in downtown New Orleans. At the time, Anna was married to David Lewis, who had worked for another ex-FBI agent: Guy Banister.

Today we have video testimony from Anna Lewis recorded in 2003, and made available on the Internet by Dutch JFK researcher Wim Dankbaar. In this interview, Anna clearly states that she knew Lee Oswald and that Oswald was a regular customer at Thompson's in 1963. Further, she states that she and her husband socialized with Lee and Judyth together on a number of occasions. More importantly, Anna Lewis admits that she lied to District Attorney Garrison and his investigators when they asked her about Oswald.

Had Anna Lewis told Garrison the truth, Garrison could have easily tracked down Judyth. Garrison was already suspicious of Ochsner and his role in the media depiction of Oswald. If Garrison had had access to Judyth, and if Judyth told Garrison what she now tells us — that she and Lee were working on a biological weapon project under the direction of Dr. Alton Ochsner, Garrison's investigation (and his whole life) might have turned out very differently. But she didn't. Anna Lewis lied to Garrison because she was afraid. Meanwhile, Judyth hid silently because *she* was afraid.

Two critical pieces of evidence were unavailable to the American people, and their elected representatives (like Garrison), at the time they were pondering who had killed their President. Now that we know differently, is it time to reconsider our history?

### 3. Was Judyth trained to handle cancer viruses before going to New Orleans?

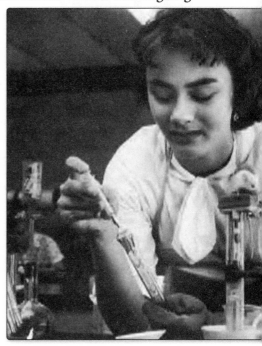

The short answer is "yes," and the evidence to support this is abundant. The photo to the right, taken by the *Herald-Tribune* (a newspaper in the Bradenton area), shows Judyth in her cancer lab with her mice during high school. The numerous newspaper articles published in the *Bradenton Herald* tell a similar tale. Judyth was a star science student who wanted to find a cure for cancer. Everyone wanted her to succeed. After creating lung cancer in her mice faster than anyone known to

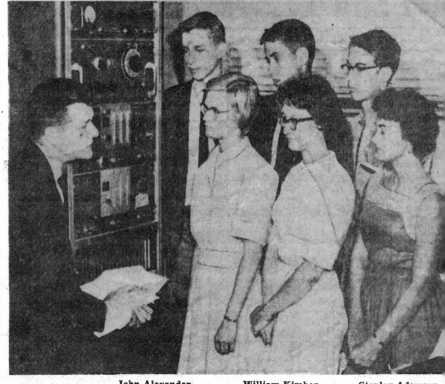

John Alexander     William Kimber     Stanley Adamson

Dr. M. A. Bender     Helsa Servis     Moira Burke     Judith Vary

... *Roswell scientist discusses radioactive isotopes with student*

# Students Start Roswell Park Work

**By PAUL WIELAND**

Scientific research with a high school beat began its eighth summer yesterday, brightening the ever-busy Roswell Park Memorial Institute with young people who want to be "in the know."

A group of 66 high school students and June graduates from five states and Canada started work at the cancer research institute under grants mainly supplied by the State of New York and the National Science Foundation.

**But their work isn't on the high school level. Far from it.**

Working closely with the institute's scientists, the students have plunged into the maze of highly - complicated research techniques being developed to fight cancer.

Officially titled the "Summer Research Participation Program," by its originator, Dr. Edwin A. Mirand, the summer study period provides outstanding science students with opportunities for original and sometimes rewarding research.

### National Recognition

"Last summer we had a young lady studying here whose work in the sex determination of chickens was not only outstanding, but earned her national recognition," said Dr. Mirand, director of the program. "These young people are brilliant," he said, "and we try to give them the opportunity to display that brilliance usefully."

The teen-agers began their eight weeks yesterday with a battery of tests to determine their scientific "I-Q's," tests which will be repeated at the end of the program to ascertain the progress they have made.

**Following tests, the youngsters were taken on a tour of the institute. The tour was punctuated by calculated once-overs of strange and complicated-looking pieces scientific apparatus.**

The conversation of the dents was a strange mixture the usual teen talk and an ab dance of scientific words little or no meaning to the man.

Blond Helsa Servis, an year-old June graduate f Silver City, N.M., said she study neurosurgery technic during her stay here. She'l tend San Jose State in San J Calif., this fall.

### To Study Radio Biology

Dark-haired Judith Vary, from Palmetto, Fla., bub with the serious-sounding servation that the insti would "certainly be intelle ally stimulating." She study radio biology.

Dr. Mirand said "whate they would study, they wo study well," as he strode the corridor to begin discus of radioactive isotopes wit student.

medical science, Judyth was given introductions, financing, opportunities, chemicals, tuition, and training. Her training was world-class.

I know a man in Bradenton who remembers Judyth from high school. He was in an independent-study science class with Judyth, and saw her on a regular basis during their senior year in high school. His comments to me are worth noting: "If you're telling me that Judyth wound up in some secret lab doing some heavy-duty experiments, it wouldn't surprise me in the least. She was always very intense and took herself very seriously."

In upstate New York, the *Buffalo Courier-Express* reported on the cancer-research training program that Judyth attended at the Roswell Park Cancer Center.

This article not only proves that Judyth was trained in cancer research techniques at one of the most prestigious cancer institutes in the country, but it also identifies Dr. Edwin Mirand as running the program. Dr. Mirand was half of the "Grace and Mirand" medical research team that wrote "Human Susceptibility to a Simian Tumor Virus," an article published in the *Annals of the New York Academy of Science* in 1963.

This article has been referenced in everything I have published on this subject since 1995. Since we have proof that Judyth personally knew and studied under these national experts in cancer-causing monkey viruses in 1961, 34 years before I published anything on the subject, this contradicts claims that Judyth read my book and then refashioned herself as a character in it. She did not. All the evidence indicates that she was trained to handle cancer-causing viruses, lived in New Orleans, and knew Lee Oswald decades earlier.

This may be intoxicating news for those concerned about Judyth's credibility and what she can tell us about Lee Oswald, but it is sobering to those of us worried about the fate of the biological weapon. This means that Judyth Vary Baker really did have the technical skills to handle the cancer-causing monkey viruses that might be used to create a biologi-

cal weapon. Yes, Judyth Vary Baker had the technical quali-
fications to be the technician that did the bench work in the
Ferrie-Sherman medical laboratory. Hearing Judyth admit
that as a 19-year-old she assisted Lee Harvey Oswald, David
Ferrie, Dr. Mary Sherman, and Dr. Alton Ochsner in their efforts to develop a biological weapon is … literally mind-boggling. Yes, I have my witness.

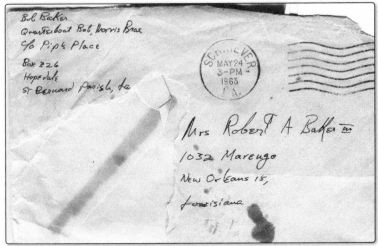

Letter envelope postmarked May 24, 1963 from Robert Baker in Hopedale, St. Bernard Parish, Louisiana, to
Mrs. Robert A. Baker (Judyth Vary), 1032 Marengo, New Orleans (her apartment near Oswald's).

HAVING CONFIRMED THE IDENTITY OF today's Judyth Vary
Baker, our next step is to ask what else she said?

Here is a brief summary of the parts of Judyth's story that
are relevant to our inquiry. A more in-depth account is given
in the Appendix entitled "Judyth's Story":

Judyth went to New Orleans in 1963 at the invitation of
Dr. Alton Ochsner. Ochsner had known Judyth for several
years, and had previously arranged for her to be trained at
the famous cancer research center discussed above.

Ochsner promised Judyth early-admission to Tulane
Medical School in return for her services in Dr. Mary
Sherman's cancer lab at Ochsner Clinic. Ochsner also pro-
vided her with cancer research papers on state-of-the-art

*Dr. Mary's Monkey*

discoveries such as cancer-causing viruses. Judyth wound up working under Sherman's direction in the underground medical laboratory in David Ferrie's apartment instead of in Dr. Mary's cancer lab at the Ochsner clinic.

Judyth met Lee Oswald at the Post Office in what she thought was a chance encounter. In hindsight, she realized that this had to have been intentional, since Lee was already working with David Ferrie, Dr. Mary Sherman and Dr. Alton Ochsner on the bio-weapon at the time. Lee introduced her to "Dr. David Ferrie" the following day, and helped Judyth find an apartment.

When Judyth went to meet Dr. Ochsner in a room within the bowels of Charity Hospital, Lee Oswald accompanied her to the appointment, and went in first to meet with Dr. Ochsner alone.

Lee was working with ex-FBI agent Guy Banister at the time, as has been reported by many sources. Lee took Judyth to meet Banister in his office to satisfy her concerns that the bio-weapons project was really a secret government operation. Banister confirmed that Lee was working with them on a "get-Castro" project.[9]

When Judyth went to Dr. Sherman's apartment for a private dinner, David Ferrie was the only other guest. Sherman and Ferrie discussed the nature of their project with Judyth. They deemed the idea of using cancer-causing viruses to kill Castro as ethical, since it might prevent World War III. Lee phoned Judyth that same night at Sherman's apartment. Dr. Mary Sherman was the operational director of "the project." Ferrie and Oswald were participants.

Lee escorted and transported Judyth all over town, including to Dr. Sherman's apartment, where Judyth routinely dropped off "the product," and provided reports for Sherman's review. Lee was "the runner."

Judyth and Lee were given cover-jobs at Reily Coffee Company, where they were allowed to slip out several afternoons a week to work in the underground medical laboratory in David Ferrie's apartment. [10]

LEE OSWALD'S CONNECTIONS TO THE MAFIA in New Orleans were much stronger than have ever been reported publicly. [11] Judyth and Lee ate gratis at restaurants owned by Carlos Marcello, and went to his headquarters (500 Club and Town & Country Motel).

Lee's role in the kill-Castro portion of the project was to transport the bio-weapon into Cuba. The radio debates and film clips of Oswald's leafleting were arranged by Ochsner (at Oswald's request) to make Oswald appear to be an authentic defector, so he could get into Cuba more easily.

Judyth heard the subject of assassinating JFK discussed at various times by various people, including Ferrie, Sherman and Oswald. Part of the logic that was explained to Judyth was that they had to hurry up and kill Castro with their bio-weapon before Ochsner's friends ran out of patience, and decided to kill Kennedy instead.

After testing their bio-weapon on dozens of monkeys, they arranged to test it on a human "volunteer," a convict brought from Angola State Penitentiary to the Jackson State Mental Hospital in rural Louisiana for that purpose. The weapon was successful. The man died, after 28 days.

Judyth wrote a letter to Dr. Ochsner protesting the use of an unwitting human in their bio-weapon test, and delivered it to his secretary. [12] Upon seeing the letter, Ochsner exploded in anger, and threatened both Judyth and Lee. Everything fell apart for Judyth as a result. Ochsner reneged on his offer to place Judyth in Tulane Medical School. Lee was ordered to Dallas. Judyth went back to Florida with her husband.

For the next few months, Judyth and Lee stayed in contact by telephone, thanks to access to the Mafia's "secret" Miami-to-Las Vegas sports-betting lines, courtesy of David Ferrie. While the phone company and the U.S. Government might not have been able to listen to their conversations, the Mafia could.

On Wednesday, November 20, 1963, Lee told Judyth that there would be a real attempt to kill President Kennedy when he visited Dallas on Friday. That is the last time they talked.

HOWEVER, WE ARE NOT HERE to figure out who killed JFK. We are trying to understand who was using radiation to mutate monkey viruses, and why. Judyth's testimony is an important piece of the puzzle for us to have. Judyth's account means that a witness who participated in "the project" (as they called it) has confessed that both she and Lee Oswald were operational members of the Ferrie-Sherman underground medical laboratory, and that they knew that they were developing a biological weapon. This is a major point.

Think about how difficult it would have been to investigate and prosecute Lee Oswald in a court of law for killing Kennedy without exposing that laboratory, its sponsors, the cancer-causing viruses that had contaminated the polio vaccine, and all of the ethical and medical questions arising from their irradiation of a flotilla of dangerous monkey viruses. Can you imagine the publicity? The political fallout? With one side of Lee's life connected to anti-Communists like Ochsner, Reily, and Banister (and perhaps the FBI and the CIA), and the other side connected to Carlos Marcello and almost everyone around him, Oswald's trial would have exposed everything. Whether Oswald had anything to do with killing Kennedy or not, the exposure of a trial would have created obvious problems for the sponsors of the lab.

Like the cover-up which dumped Mary Sherman's burned and mangled corpse at her apartment, Lee's murder was deemed a "necessity" to protect the underground medical laboratory and its sponsors. Thus was silenced the man who could have explained what really happened (or perhaps what did not happen) in Dallas on November 22, 1963.[13] This may have been part of their plan all along.

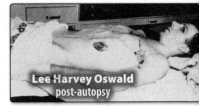

Lee Harvey Oswald
post-autopsy

TODAY, JUDYTH'S GOAL IS TO EXONERATE LEE OSWALD. She will never stop her crusade to clear his name. I consider the bulk of what she has said to be as accurate as she can

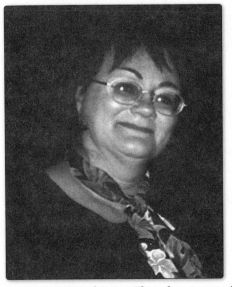

be held accountable for. She is explaining what happened in her life to the best of her ability. I have seen people whom I knew to be in the same room at the same time disagree over what had happened there. Disagreement is not the acid-test of truth. Events are always colored by perception.

Judyth remembers what she heard and knows what she believes, much of which is what she was led to believe by others. Yes, Judyth loved Lee. Judyth believed Lee. Judyth trusted Lee. She also trusted Dr. Alton Ochsner, Dr. Mary Sherman and David Ferrie. She was really there with Lee Oswald in New Orleans. She was young, impressionable, naive and gullible. Somewhere along the line, both she and Lee were betrayed.

But there is a limit to what she knows. Judyth was not in Dallas on November 22, 1963.[14] We all need to distinguish between what she personally saw or heard and what she understands or believes to be the case. Both her critics and her supporters need to make these distinctions. So does she. So do I.

NEXT WE LOOK AT WHAT JUDYTH HAS SAID that disagrees with things I wrote in *Mary, Ferrie, & the Monkey Virus*.

First, I remind the reader that I did not feel that I had strong enough evidence in hand to endorse the claimed connection between Mary Sherman and David Ferrie without reservation, and that I challenged any researcher to come

*Dr. Mary's Monkey*

forward with real evidence or testimony that they were associated.[15]

Judyth clearly states that Mary Sherman knew David Ferrie well. In fact, Judyth had dinner with Sherman and Ferrie at Sherman's apartment. Judyth is adamant that Mary Sherman was definitely part of the cancer-virus research project that was going on at David Ferrie's apartment. In fact, part of Judyth's daily operational cycle was to bring "the extracts" of her cancer-causing virus research from Ferrie's apartment to Mary Sherman's apartment.

She also clearly states that Dr. Alton Ochsner was ultimately in charge of the Ferrie-Sherman lab. And that both she and Lee Oswald were part of the effort to use the cancer-causing monkey viruses to develop a biological weapon. No, David Ferrie had not run off with the mice after the Big Lab was shut down, as I had suggested. Routinely the mice had been delivered to his apartment several times per week for processing in 1963. This has always been what I called the "worst-case scenario" — the confirmed existence of the secret cooperation between talented scientists, dangerous radioactive equipment, monkey viruses and political extremists in an underground medical laboratory.

BUT DID THEY USE RADIATION to mutate monkey viruses?

I wrote to Judyth and said that I needed to know specifically if she had been told that the viruses she was working with at David Ferrie's apartment had been exposed to radiation at another location to change them genetically? I told her I wanted to make sure that no one could find any ambiguity in her statement, or otherwise be able to misconstrue it, so I was going to put a magnifying glass on it. I needed clarification. I needed her to confirm or deny it based on what she knew?

My exact words: "My question is about your time in New Orleans in the summer of 1963.... Do I understand that you are saying that you were told that the extracts that you prepared at David Ferrie's apartment and delivered to Mary Sherman's apartment were being subjected to radiation and then recycled into more mice? Do I have this right?"

Judyth's response was clear: *Exactly ... we all knew it ... Also, into monkeys. Many were killed, but they ordered thousands of pounds of new monkeys ...*

I continued, "By your term 'we all knew it' who are you referring to? Could I ask you to answer 'Yes' or 'No' to each person on this list separately. The question is, Did you personally discuss exposing your tumor extracts to radiation with this person:"

Dr. Sherman — *She was the one in charge of doing this.*

Lee Oswald — *Yes. He once took one batch over to Crippled Children's Hospital and met her there because she didn't have time to get them from her apartment...*

Dr. Ochsner — *He was in charge of the project. Dr. Sherman was afraid he was being exploited and didn't realize the full significance, that others could get their hands on this material. But he kept himself white as snow, though he wasn't. Dr. Mary didn't trust him.*

David Ferrie — *Yes*

Bill Monaghan — *No, he didn't know anything except they needed me for lab work on company time and he had to do work I was supposed to do, which irritated him.*

**SIV** is the Simian Immunodeficiency Virus, one of several monkey viruses known to have contaminated the polio vaccine. The more carcinogenic SV-40 has received most of the press.

SIV, a single-strand RNA retrovirus, is considerably smaller than SV-40 (a double-strand DNA virus). The technology of the 1950s was not able to filter SIV from the viral extracts. Further, researchers of the day did not consider retroviruses to be dangerous, so they basically ignored them. AIDS has taught us how dangerous retroviruses can be.

If "the project" in New Orleans was intentionally exposing SV-40 to radiation, they may have exposed SIV to radiation at the same time. Simply stated, HIV-1 is a mutated form of SIV.

Did the mutation which changed SIV into HIV-1 occur when SV-40 was exposed to radiation? Was this the moment of conception of AIDS? Could this artificially-induced mutation explain why HIV-1 is mutating so rapidly? Why it is behaving so "unnaturally"? If you are a scientist involved in AIDS research, these are the questions I would like you to consider.

*Dr. Mary's Monkey*

Was Judyth the technician in David Ferrie's underground medical laboratory? She admits that she was, despite the obvious legal, ethical and security consequences of doing so. Were they irradiating cancer-causing viruses to develop a biological weapon? Judyth participated in that operation, and has said that their use of radiation was both deliberate and central to the design of the project. Was the operation in David Ferrie's apartment connected to an operation at the U.S. Public Health Service Hospital? Judyth says it was.

The consequences of these statements are terrifying!

Frankly, I would have preferred to have been wrong. It appears that I was not. These were very dark deeds indeed. They may have been dark deeds whose price the population of the planet still pays today. Yet I doubt this connection will ever be proved to the satisfaction of the critics.

But they do not control us, nor do they control the truth!

At least I can finally understand why my father was so upset, when he learned what was going down at the U.S. Public Health Service Hospital.

> **Q**UESTIONS that neither Judyth Vary Baker nor I can answer:
> - Which monkey viruses did the project's radiation genetically alter? Was SIV one of them?[16]
> - What happened to their collection of mutated monkey viruses after Judyth left?
> - Did any of these mutated monkey viruses "escape" into the human population?
> - Will Judyth's price for attempting to clear Lee Oswald's name be the sacrifice of her own?
>
> Fortunately we can still ask questions like these. One has to wonder what will happen if we ever stop.

---

1   CBS's legendary anchorman Dan Rather was part of the *60M* management team at the time. Rather was a staunch supporter of the Oswald-did-it-alone theory, and is infamous for his comment about the Zapruder film, stating that it showed that President Kennedy's head had been thrown violently "forward" by the fatal head shot from the rear. Since the public had not yet been allowed to see the film, there was no one to dispute the accuracy of Rather's comment. Now that the film has been viewed by millions, everyone knows Kennedy's head was thrown "backwards." How could Rather have been so wrong? Was *60M* the best place to take Judyth's story?

2   I should add that until I saw the *60M* documents, that I did not know that her middle named was spelled "Vary." But with my Jesuit education, I remembered wondering, (wrongly) when I first heard her name back in 1972, if her middle name was "Veri" (like

*veritas*, meaning truth) or "Vari" (as in various or variable, indicating multiple or changing).

3    Langley is the small town in Virginia where the headquarters of the U.S. Central Intelligence Agency is located.

4    Judyth's knowledge of and personal involvement with the subject of cancer research is remarkable to this day. Upon seeing a 2006 news article about a breakthrough in cancer research involving a mouse whose immune system was extremely good at resisting cancer, Judyth sent me an email which included the following: "We could have cured cancer … decades ago … and here you see that macrophages in mice do it --- and yes, just as I have claimed they could.... This can be turned into an efficient and cheap way to combat cancer. Oh, if only I could have convinced somebody to just give me a chance to direct a lab!… And also because they are still just using murine [mouse] macrophages, a first step that I knew would work way back in 1961. Oh, I feel as if my whole life has been wasted! Have to admit I just sat down after reading this and wept tears of anger and frustration for the millions who have suffered and died from cancer, especially children, and I knew the key, but my mouth had been stopped up with clay. I cannot stop weeping... This is awful, to feel such anger and helplessness. Yet happy that at last they should be able to see what to do…"

5    Baker, Judyth Vary. *Lee Harvey Oswald: The True Story of the Accused Assassin of President John F. Kennedy by his Lover*, Trafford, Victoria, BC, Canada, 2006.

6    The same document was shown on the History Channel in 2003, *The Men Who Killed Kennedy*, "The Love Affair," November 1963, produced by Nigel Turner in association with British Independent Television.

7    On their return trips from Reily, Judyth and Lee exhibited more caution. Though they rode the same bus, they did not sit together. They would ride the bus past their apartments, past the U.S. Public Health Service Hospital, and get off at Audubon Park, where they could speak and socialize freely. Then they would ride the Magazine bus back in the opposite direction to their respective apartments. In an interesting aside, Judyth mentioned to me that she and Lee even rolled down "Monkey Hill" during one of their visits to Audubon Park. Monkey Hill is a 25-foot pile of dirt which is covered with grass. Rolling down Monkey Hill was a great tradition for kids in New Orleans; I did it many times as a child while playing a game called "King on the Mountain." New Orleans is so flat that the City built this artificial hill in Audubon Park so that the local children would know what a hill was. The sight of dozens of school-age children rolling down the hill provided the name: Monkey Hill, because we all looked like a bunch of monkeys.

8    Technically Oswald's employment interview was conducted by a Mr. Prechter, who was head of Personnel. However, as Reily's Vice President in charge of Finance and Security, it was Monaghan (the ex-FBI agent) that had to made the final decision on whom to hire. Monaghan apparently did not think that hiring "a defector" who had lived in Russia and held an "undesirable discharge" from the Marines would be a security problem for the virulently anti-Communist company.

9    While meeting Banister satisfied Judyth, it does not convince me of official sanction for "the project," since Banister was also working with Mafia-boss Marcello. The larger question: "Was Marcello working with the government?" And the ultimate question: "Who *is* the government?"

10   I emphasize that I do not know of any document, testimony or evidence which suggests that William Reily personally (nor his company as an entity) knew about Ochsner's secret medical project nor that his employees were being used to develop a biological weapon while on the company clock. Nothing herein should be interpreted as implying such. What is known is that Reily was fiercely anti-Communist, a member of INCA, and that he provided financial support to some of Ochsner's political activities,

but this can easily be explained by the financial interest of the local business community and the political events of the day. William Reily should be considered as innocent as Oswald, since neither have had a day in court.

11 Lee Oswald's family had been Mafia-connected since he was a child. Lee attended parties at Marcello's house, and was remembered from those days by people that Judyth met. Lee also worked as an errand boy, running between Marcello's clubs and restaurants. Lee personally met with Mafia boss Carlos Marcello on several occasions in 1963. Judyth saw Lee collect fists full of cash from the manager of Marcello's Town & Country Motel and deliver it to his uncle, who was involved in Marcello's gambling operations.

12 The secretary was a temp. Ochsner's regular secretary (a nurse) was on vacation at the time.

13 Jack Ruby visited David Ferrie's apartment one day when Judyth and Lee were there. Ferrie introduced him to Judyth as Sparky Rubenstein. Judyth was surprised that Ferrie briefed Ruby on their bio-weapon project. (Why not? They all worked for Marcello.) Ruby recognized Lee, and said that he used to see him at parties when he was a boy. This means that Jack Ruby knew about Oswald's connection to the underground medical laboratory when he shot him, and he knew about the cancer cocktail that could be used to silence him as he awaited trial for Oswald's murder. It is no wonder he wanted to get out of Dallas. And it is no wonder that the Warren Commission did not accept his offer to talk in exchange for safer accommodations. Jack Ruby told Al Maddox (his Dallas Police guard) that he had been injected with cancer cells. Maddox has said that the doctor that gave Ruby injections came from Chicago. Maddox was present at Parkland Hospital when Ruby died of an embolism caused by galloping lung cancer.

14 Publicly, I have always taken the position that Oswald's guilt or innocence is ultimately irrelevant to whether an underground medical laboratory in New Orleans was using mutated monkey viruses to develop a biological weapon, and whether that project is responsible for epidemics we see today. My neutrality on Oswald is a position that has become increasingly difficult for me to maintain. To my eyes, Lee was the perfect patsy —one that could not be investigated without getting into his connections to the Mafia, to the CIA, to Ochsner, to the particle accelerator, to the biological weapon and (most importantly) to his ultimate sponsor. Who was the person who had helped the "defector" return to the United States from the Soviet Union with his wife and child at the height of the Cold War? Who was Oswald's ultimate sponsor? Is the need to hide this key piece of information the reason why Lee Harvey Oswald's tax returns have never been made public? Was it Marcello using his influence on the Louisiana politicians that he was so famous for bribing? Or was it Bobby Kennedy himself —who was U.S. Attorney General at the time Oswald returned and had the power to declare that he was still a citizen and allow him to return. Either of these sponsors could have arranged for the State Department to lend him the money to pay for his family's transportation back to the U.S. These are the type of penetrating questions that the "lone nut" theory was constructed to suppress. They are the questions we still need to ask today.

15 Credit Dr. Howard Platzman for taking Judyth Vary Baker to *60 Minutes* and later to me.

~~~~~~~~~~

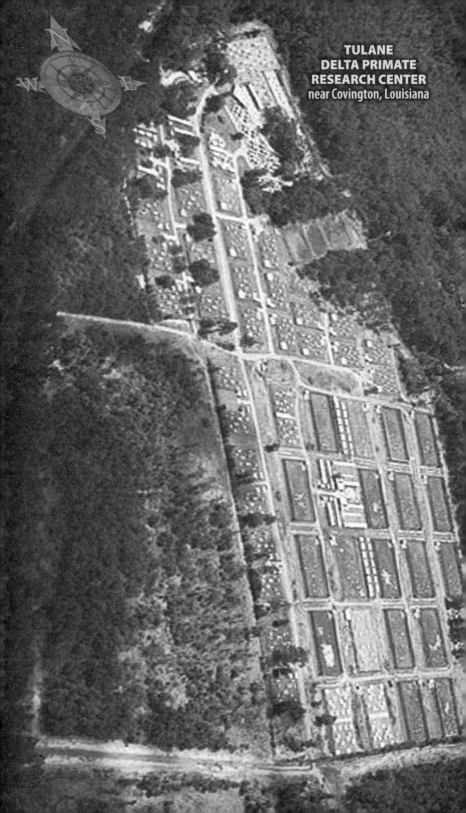

TULANE
DELTA PRIMATE
RESEARCH CENTER
near Covington, Louisiana

# CHAPTER 14

# The Teacher

W E HAVE LOOKED AT WHAT IS KNOWN (and unknown) about Dr. Mary Sherman and her murder,
as well as at David Ferrie and the cancer treatise
which was found at his apartment. In the process, we stumbled onto some very disturbing information indicating that
the polio vaccine was contaminated with monkey viruses
which might be responsible for America's unprecedented
epidemic of soft tissue cancers.[1] It also appears that powerful
forces have shaped our understanding of these events to protect themselves and that there are mysterious relationships
between medicine and politics which raise significant questions about the health care decisions we face as a nation.

We have also looked at what the mainstream scientists
have said about the origin of AIDS, and compared that to
what we know of these secret experiments and the people
around them. Along the way, we pondered the dangers of irradiating cancer-causing viruses with nuclear devices capable of mangling their genetic structure.

But since that evidence is incomplete, I will not draw any
conclusions concerning a direct relationship between this
underground medical laboratory and the origin of the AIDS

epidemic. We may never know. And if we did know, what could we change? In the meantime, we are still free to ask the obvious question: Was this bizarre new epidemic caused by a mutated monkey virus engendered during the more than forty years of intensive scientific research, medical experimentation, and genetic manipulation of simian viruses?

BEFORE WE CONCLUDE, I do want to answer one final question. It was the first question ever asked me in a public presentation of this matter, and over time it has been the most frequently asked question: "How did you originally learn about this subject?"

When I first heard this question, all I could say was that I have known about the generality of these things most of my life. But the more I thought about it, the more I realized that most of my understanding of the dangers we faced from monkey viruses came from a particular incident. But it was not from my father; it was from another source whose words are worth recalling.

About a year after the pirate incident dashed my hopes for a pet monkey, a remarkable elderly woman entered my life. Her name was Mrs. Ellis,[2] and she taught history and English to my class at New Orleans Academy. Her grandmotherly appearance and out-of-date clothes could not conceal her unique spirit. Her specialty was sculpting rowdy teenage boys into disciplined young men, and she did so with uncommon precision. During her forty-year career, she had nearly a thousand students to her credit.

She worked us hard, and rewarded us with her recognition. Demanding and loving, she offered her students a respect which we returned. When combined with the high expectations she placed upon us, it was hard for us not to feel like her grandchildren.

Philosophically, however, Mrs. Ellis was a Darwinian who loved all forms of competition — the rougher the better. She even watched our playground fights with relish, because she saw them as demonstrations of character.

In her own family, she raised three sons, and put each through college and then law school. Then she shepherded their entrance into Louisiana politics. All three of them became elected judges in Covington, Louisiana, across the lake from New Orleans. Very little went on in Covington that "Mama Judge" did not know about.

Mrs. Ellis was very systematic about her teaching, but she always reserved time to talk to us about the important things that were on her mind. Most of these had to do with activities across the lake, where she spent her summers and weekends.

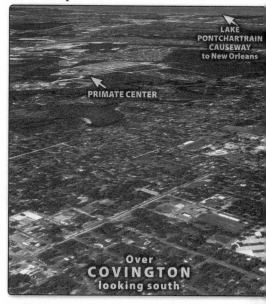

One day, in 1963 or 1964, she concluded her lesson and turned our attention to the new monkey laboratory that the U.S. government was building near Covington. As you can imagine, my ears perked up. She talked about the research that Tulane and LSU medical schools were doing at "the Yerkes lab." She cautioned us that it was "not the famous Yerkes lab," but it was "like the Yerkes lab."

As she praised these new efforts to make the monkey research safer and more humane, I was busy thinking about the African monkey viruses that my father feared more than rabies. Then she started talking about polio. At first I did not get the connection. Then she told us that the polio vaccine had been contaminated with monkey viruses. The medical experts admitted that they did not know what effect these monkey viruses in the human blood supply would have, and they acknowledged that a new generation of diseases might result — diseases which the world had never seen.

And she told us about the response of prominent doctors like Alton Ochsner who had supported the mass inoculation of the polio vaccine. Ochsner's position, she explained, was that it was better to get rid of a known disease today and deal with the possibility of a new disease tomorrow, than to do nothing. Further, Ochsner believed that if these monkey viruses did produce new diseases, then medical science would be able to meet the challenge, as it had with so many other diseases. I remember hoping that he was right.

When class was over, I had to stay late and finish some work before going home. Another boy had to stay late, too. We both finished our work at the same time, and handed her

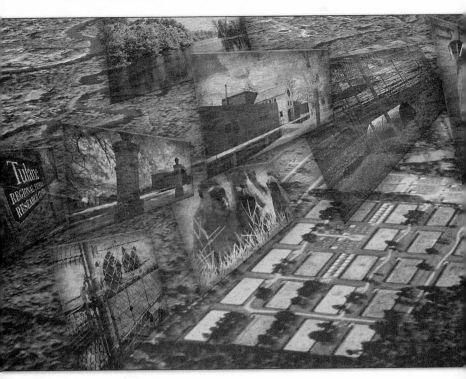

*Dr. Mary's Monkey*

our papers. As we were leaving, I turned to Mrs. Ellis and thanked her for telling us about the monkey laboratory. I realized she had told us information that we would not hear through normal channels. She accepted my comment and added a few of her own, expressing her personal bewilderment over the people calling the shots. Her frustrations were not hard to see.

Then the other student said solemnly, "This is pretty serious stuff you're talking about ... the government, contaminated vaccines and the possibility of epidemics in the future. Don't you think *it's dangerous* to be talking about this?"

"Oh, they can't hurt me," she chuckled at him.

"Well, that's not exactly what I meant," the other boy said apologetically. "Do you think you should be *telling us* about these things?"

"Why shouldn't I?" she said in a snap. Then lowering her head to study both of us over the rim of her glasses, she concluded:

"This is going to be your country soon, and you are the ones that are going to have to deal with these problems. You have the right to know what they did."

---

1  When the debate quietly raged over the contamination of the polio vaccine with monkey viruses, it focused on one virus, SV-40, a DNA virus that produced pathogenic results fairly quickly. NCI eventually claimed that SV-40 was not a significant threat to humans, and declared the debate over. But the reason that SV-40 was named "SV-40" was to remind us that there were 39 other monkey viruses already identified.

What about all the other monkey viruses in the polio vaccine, especially the slow acting retroviruses which can take decades to produce disease. These retroviruses baffled the scientists of the 1960s, but today we understand how they breed by inserting themselves into the genetic material of other cells. In 1994 Dr. Michael McGrath, a medical researcher from San Francisco, demonstrated that retroviruses can cause cancer *directly*, by invading a cell's genetic material and triggering the cancer process, rather than only causing cancer indirectly through the suppression of the immune system, as previously believed; Associated Press, "AIDS virus can cause cancer," *St. Petersburg Times*, April 8, 1994, p. 8A. Look at the cancer statistics presented in Chapter 9 and decide for yourself if there might have been a problem, even if honest scientists are not yet able to explain it.

2  I never knew her first name. When we wanted to be familiar, we called her "Mrs. E."

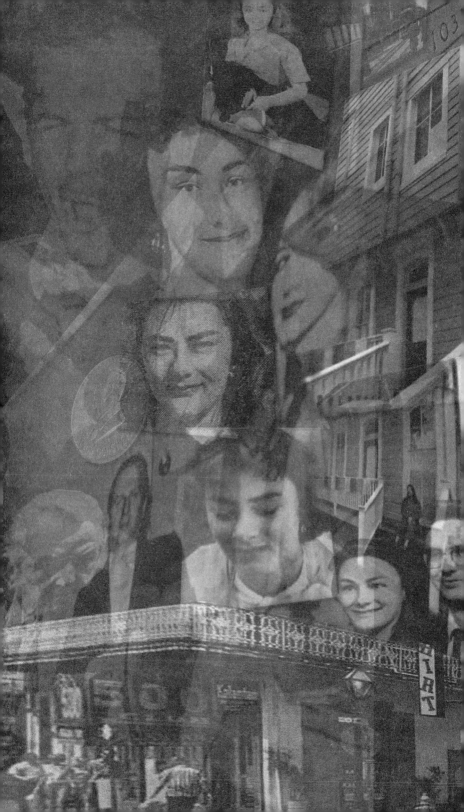

# Appendix

# Judyth's Story

I N THE CHAPTER ENTITLED "The Witness," I explain how I came to know Judyth Vary Baker, present key evidence about her, and give a top-line summary of her story — which was admittedly focused on points that related to my interests: Mary Sherman, the underground medical laboratory at David Ferrie's apartment, the contamination of the polio vaccine, Dr. Alton Ochsner, and irradiating cancer-causing monkey viruses. As important as these points are, I want to enable the reader to see a broader overview of the rest of her story.[1]

Judyth's story helps us understand what happened in New Orleans in that very important summer of 1963, both with the Ferrie-Sherman underground medical laboratory and with the broader activities of Lee Harvey Oswald in the months prior to Kennedy's assassination. Judyth's narrative provides an important, if not essential, perspective on these matters. In what follows you will read what I consider to be the salient points. The text font will vary so that you may distinguish between when I am relating her story to you, and when I am adding my commentary.

Judyth has been kind enough to corroborate (and correct) my version of her account:

Judyth's story begins in Bradenton, Florida during her high school years, which ended in 1961.[2] Due to her success as an award-winning science student, she attracted the attention of teachers and press. Doors were opened, and Judyth was given access to support that a high school student would not normally have. This early success led to introductions to important contacts in the medical community, including Dr. Alton Ochsner, a famous physician from New Orleans, and his friend Dr. Harold Diehl, Vice President for Research Projects at the American Cancer Society. Ochsner helped Judyth by arranging a summer position for her assisting his friend Dr. George Moore in his laboratory at the prestigious Roswell Park Cancer Institute in upstate New York.

After a false-start at a Catholic college,[3] and a year at the University of Florida, Judyth was invited by Ochsner to New Orleans to work in a cancer lab at his hospital for the summer, and to be part of a project which she understood to be of national-security importance. For her services, Judyth was promised advanced admission to Tulane Medical School, a stipend as compensation for her involvement, as well as the opportunity to work under the direction of a distinguished cancer researcher named Dr. Mary Sherman. Due to a fluke in her college schedule and problems at home in Bradenton, Judyth headed to New Orleans several weeks ahead of Ochsner's schedule.[4]

Upon her arrival she got a room at the YWCA, which she shared with several female roommates. One of these roommates was a stripper at the 500 Club. The stripper explained to Judyth that New Orleans was run by organized crime, particularly by her boss Carlos Marcello. The club had just been raided that night by the police, but that was understood to be Marcello's way of persuading Jada, the headline act, to relocate to Dallas to work for his friend Jack Ruby. A few evenings later, the stripper invited Judyth to the 500 Club to help her with her makeup. Eager to broaden her horizons, Judyth went to the 500 Club.

*Dr. Mary's Monkey*

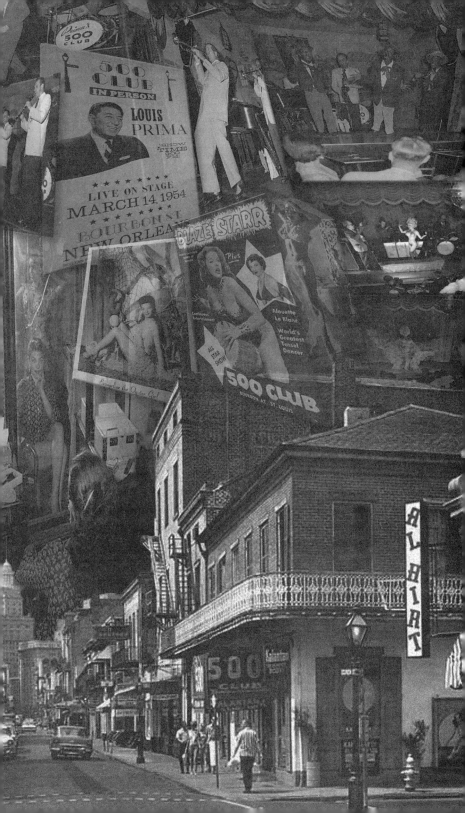

Another roommate encouraged Judyth to get a job with "more of a future to it," like the one she had — learning to work as a bunny at the Playboy Club. But Judyth declined this offer as well, and followed the advice of yet another roommate, who convinced her to work at a hamburger joint called the Royal Castle out by the airport. This Royal Castle was next to the Town & Country Motel, headquarters of Carlos Marcello, the infamous Mafia boss.[5]

Lonely and scared in this strange city and anxiously expecting a letter from her fiancé, Judyth headed to the Post Office to pick up her letter, But fate sent her a protector — Lee Harvey Oswald.[6]

At the Post Office Judyth gets in line, and a clean cut young man gets in line behind her. He is close enough to read what she is carrying under her arm and to hear what she is saying to the clerk. Then Judyth drops her newspaper, and Lee picks it up. They meet.

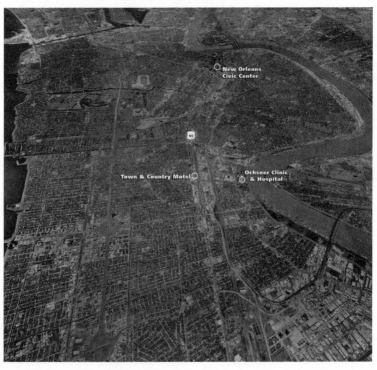

*Dr. Mary's Monkey*

Lee befriends her and offers to walk her home. She accepts. Judyth tells Lee that she has come to town at Dr. Ochsner's request and will be working in Dr. Mary Sherman's cancer laboratory. What a coincidence! Lee was just talking about Dr. Sherman the night before with a good friend who was also interested in cancer research — Captain David Ferrie. Lee tells her that Captain Ferrie also works with Carlos Marcello as a pilot, ever since he had a problem with his job at Eastern Airlines.

The next morning Lee visits Judyth at her new job at the Royal Castle outside of Marcello's headquarters, and waits for her to finish her work. Lee then borrows a car from his uncle. The uncle used to be "an enforcer" for Carlos Marcello on the docks, but got promoted to bookmaking and collecting gambling debts.[7] Lee is concerned that Judyth has to live at the YWCA with the strippers and offers to help. Judyth is expecting her fiancé, who obviously can't stay with the women at the YWCA, so Lee helps Judyth find a nicer place — a boarding house on St. Charles Ave. where she can be with her new husband. Lee pays part of her rent and helps her move in.

The fiancé arrives, he stays for a day, marries Judyth, and then he leaves to go work offshore in the Gulf of Mexico, working on a boat for most of the summer. As soon as her husband is gone, her new residence is raided by the police as a house of prostitution. Luckily the negligee-clad Judyth has her marriage license handy, and is not arrested. Meanwhile, Lee Oswald keeps showing up at both Judyth's apartment and the Royal Castle. A day or so later, Lee is asked to run an errand for the uncle whose car he borrowed. He has to pick up something for his uncle at the Town & Country Motel.

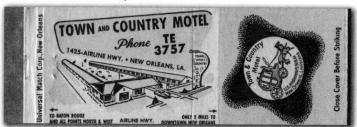

Lee brings Judyth with him to Carlos Marcello's headquarters, but Lee warns Judyth that the hotel does offer the services of prostitutes to its patrons.[8] Judyth sees the manager pass a fistful of rolled-up bills to Lee under the table for him to courier back to his uncle. Once the wad of cash was delivered, the grateful uncle gave Lee $200 (1963 dollars) for his trouble.

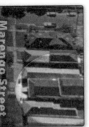

Supposedly embarrassed by the police raid on her last residence, Lee comes to Judyth's rescue again, by helping her find a small quiet apartment on Marengo Street in uptown New Orleans, near Magazine Street. The house is owned by Susie Hanover, a woman Lee has known since he was a child. Susie's husband also worked for Carlos Marcello, and she remembered Lee fondly from parties at Marcello's house during his childhood.

**Have you noticed a pattern here? Lee was surrounded by New Orleans Mafia.**

Lee then takes Judyth to lunch with his friend David Ferrie, who invites them to his apartment to see his cancer laboratory. She accepts and the trio goes to Ferrie's apartment. There they talk cancer research for hours. Judyth is very impressed with Ferrie's knowledge of cancer research. It is there in Ferrie's kitchen that he explains that he and Dr. Mary Sherman are cooking up a cancer cocktail to kill Cuban President Fidel Castro.

Ferrie is hoping that Judyth will agree to work with them in their patriotic venture. They really need the help, and they are behind schedule. Ferrie invites Lee and Judyth to a party at his house the next night, promising that Mary Sherman will be there. Ferrie is right, Mary Sherman does come to the party, but she totally ignores Judyth, preferring to practice her fluent Spanish on Ferrie's Cuban friends. Sherman does not stay long, but before she leaves, Judyth sees her remove a jar of tumors from Ferrie's refrigerator. As the night progresses, Judyth hears Ferrie talk to the Cubans about how President Kennedy could be killed. The police finally shut the party down at 2:00 A.M.

At this point, Judyth is getting concerned that she might be falling in with the wrong crowd, and asks Lee if Ferrie's

*Dr. Mary's Monkey*

secret get-Castro project is really a U.S. government project. Lee offers to prove that it is by introducing Judyth to Mr. Guy Banister, the former head of the FBI's Chicago office, who is now a private investigator in New Orleans. Banister assures Judyth that Lee is OK because he is working with them to get rid of Castro. Impressed by Banister's credentials hanging on the wall, and the large gun under his arm, Judyth concludes that things are on the level.

Lee then takes Judyth upstairs, and shows her some of the military equipment that he will be using to help make a training film for the Cuban exiles. Lee mentions that Banister also happens to work with Carlos Marcello and his attorney, handling "private investigations." Oswald explains that Banister used to work for the New Orleans Police Department, until they fired him. Now he gets back at them by blackmailing cops for Marcello.

But what about Ferrie's talk about killing Kennedy? Oh, that. Judyth is told that Ferrie was just saying that stuff about Kennedy so that the Cubans would trust him. He doesn't really mean it.

A few days after her lunch with David Ferrie, Lee takes Judyth to Charity Hospital for a meeting with Dr. Alton Ochsner. The date is May 7, 1963. Lee goes in first and meets with Ochsner alone for 45 minutes. When he comes out, Judyth goes in and meets with Ochsner alone.

This is a profound point. If Oswald met with Ochsner in the same room privately before Judyth entered the room to meet with Ochsner, it implies that Ochsner already knew (or knew of) Oswald prior to Judyth's arrival. As her story unfolds, we learn that Oswald is already operationally involved in Ochsner's kill-Castro project, running the supplies between a string of secret laboratories stretched across New Orleans. This is a remarkable development because of Ochsner's public position that Oswald was a Communist and the lone assassin who killed Kennedy.

Publicly they were enemies. Privately they were evidently working together. If Oswald was secretly working with

Ochsner, this certainly discredits the idea of Lee Oswald being a "lone nut." And it makes us ponder the "Sensitive Position" for the U.S. Government that Ochsner held! So much for the "accidental meeting" of Judyth and Lee at the Post Office.

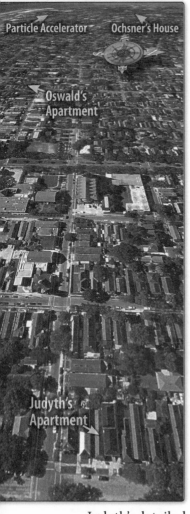

Shortly after her meeting with Ochsner, Judyth is introduced to Dr. Mary Sherman herself. This time, Judyth is invited to dinner at Sherman's apartment. When Judyth arrives, she finds David Ferrie waiting for her inside Mary Sherman's apartment. Now Mary is gracious and attentive. The conversation is a smorgasbord of cancer talk, of why we need to kill Castro before he nukes us, and, more importantly, of why we need to do it soon, before Ochsner's Texas friends run out of patience and decide to kill Kennedy instead.

Judyth's confusion over the politics subsides when Mary shows her a collection of microscope slides of a "galloping cancer" that Mary had developed by exposing the cancer-causing monkey viruses to radiation. Judyth knows enough about cancer to realize that she is holding the world's most aggressive cancer cells in her hands. She's hooked.

Before the night is over, Lee Oswald calls Mary Sherman's apartment just to check in. Judyth is given a key to Sherman's apartment so that she can drop off "the product" of their experiments when Mary is not there.[9] Judyth is instructed to address Sherman as "Dr. Mary." The trio joke about their names: "Mary, Ferrie and Vary."

Judyth's detailed description of the bio-weapons work she was doing at Ferrie's apartment places Dr. Mary Sherman at the operational center of the project, not on the edge as I had

*Dr. Mary's Monkey*

originally suspected. The ensuing chapters of Judyth's book detail their two- or three-day-per-week routine at David Ferrie's apartment.

The basic routine at the Ferrie-Sherman lab was that Judyth and Lee were given cover jobs at the Reily Coffee Company.[10] Judyth would conceal Lee's various comings-and-goings at the building (for him to work with Banister and do other things) by punching his time card for him when he was not there. Lee was given a key to Adrian Alba's garage, next door to the Reily Coffee Company.[11] Then, three days per week, in the afternoons, Judyth and Lee would meet at David Ferrie's apartment for their cancer-virus work. There was obviously a large supply of mice somewhere nearby, because cardboard trays of 50 mice would be brought to the apartment by some Cubans for processing.

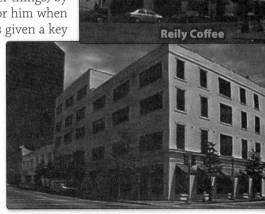

Reily Coffee

Judyth's job was to look for the mice with the most aggressive tumor growth. Judyth terminated the mice, dissected them, removed their tumors, ground the tumors in a blender to make "the product," and then cleaned up Ferrie's kitchen to laboratory standards.[12] The Cubans who always seemed to be nearby then disposed of the mice carcasses.

Judyth identifies the two Cubans that brought the cardboard trays of mice to Ferrie's as Carlos and Miguel. Is this the Miguel of Chapter 4 whom I met in 1972 when he lived in the apartment above Barbara? Were these two Cubans inoculating "the product" back into the mice after its return from being irradiated at the U.S. Public Health Service Hospital?

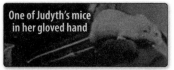
One of Judyth's mice in her gloved hand

Were they the people responsible for raising the sick mice in the Little Lab on Louisiana Avenue Parkway until the tumors were ready to be harvested?

Judyth was grinding up tumors in Ferrie's apartment when she was supposed to be working at Reily's. Her supervisor at Reily (William I. Monaghan) covered for her by picking up her workload, and punching her time clock when she was not there. "The product" (tumor extracts) was then delivered to Dr. Mary Sherman's apartment, for analysis later the same day. (Mary Sherman lived near the corner of Louisiana Ave. and St. Charles Ave., a short bus ride down Louisiana Ave. from David Ferrie's apartment.) Sherman had a microscope and a device for holding test tubes that she jokingly called "Ferrie's wheel."

Next, the extracts were "enhanced" by exposing them to more radiation at the U.S. Public Health Service Hospital. The roasted viruses were then re-injected into other mice (and monkeys) to see which viruses were "best" at producing deadly tumors. On occasions when Dr. Mary Sherman did not have time to return home to pick them up, Lee Oswald was asked to take the products of Judyth's experiments from Ferrie's apartment directly to her at the Children's Hospital. The Children's Hospital was next door to the U.S. Public Health Service Hospital, home to the linear particle accelerator and guarded by U.S. Marines.

I want to emphasize that Judyth was led into this bio-weapon project with patriotic zeal. We have heard over and over that these experiments were to develop a cancer-causing virus to kill Fidel Castro — or so Judyth was told. Judyth was hoping to develop the knockout punch to rid the world of a Communist dictator who had threatened the United States with nuclear missiles. She believed what she was told. She was not told that the project was run by maniacs who may actually have wanted to rid the world of its promiscuous, impoverished and unproductive underclass by perfecting a sexually-transmitted disease. Nor was she told that the project might give the Mafia and others a covert means to silence

*Dr. Mary's Monkey*

inconvenient witnesses as they awaited trial. Personally, I doubt Judyth would have cooperated under these latter circumstances. She has a conscience. Eventually it got her into trouble with Ochsner, and destroyed her promising future.

But Judyth *does* say that Mary Sherman expressed concerns over the safety of the project to her, and that she also thought Alton Ochsner was overconfident in his belief that he could control who got their hands on his biological weapon. Given that the genetically-altered monkey viruses were being couriered around New Orleans by people (like Lee Oswald and David Ferrie) with conspicuously close contacts to the Mafia (and who knows who else?), I think Mary's concerns about the safety and control issues were well founded.

The Sherman-Ferrie-Vary experiments successfully created aggressive cancers in mice and (at Judyth's suggestion) these new cancers were tested on monkeys. They worked, killing the monkeys quickly. But there was a missing link — they needed to know if their cancer cocktail would actually kill a human. It was decided to test their concoction on a prisoner from Louisiana's Angola State Penitentiary who had "volunteered" for the experiment. They brought him to the Jackson State Mental Hospital (near Clinton, Louisiana) where he was injected with their new bio-weapon, and died.

Upon discovering that the "volunteer" had no idea what he had signed up for, the outraged Judyth wrote a letter protesting the use of their product on an unwitting human patient, and delivered it to Dr. Ochsner's secretary.[13] In doing so, she violated the security rules that Ochsner had mandated (Don't write anything down!), jeopardized his reputation, and forever crossed-swords with one of the most powerful men in American medicine.

It was a serious tactical error on her part, but Judyth has always been very strong-willed and uncompromising on certain issues. Dr. Ochsner was equally strong-willed and uncompromising in his response, before slamming the telephone down: "You and Lee are expendable!"

From there, the situation fell apart rapidly. Lee and Judyth were released from their cover-jobs at Reily. The game-plan had been that Judyth would enter Tulane Medical School, and Lee would go to Mexico to work as a CIA informant. But Lee was ordered to return to Dallas, and Ochsner reneged on his offer to place Judyth in Tulane Medical School. Judyth watched Lee read a newspaper as she drove off with her husband back to Florida.

Judyth fell deeply in love with Lee Oswald that summer and recounts numerous trysts that they had, ranging from the back of a Volkswagen van parked in the Orleans Garage to a suite at the Royal Orleans Hotel provided by their friend Clay Shaw.

Roof-top Swimming Pool

ROYAL ORLEANS HOTEL

*Dr. Mary's Monkey*

David Ferrie had also grown found of Judyth, and arranged a job for her back in Gainesville, Florida doing laboratory work. Ferrie also arranged for Judyth to stay in contact with Lee by phone calls which used the Mafia's sports-betting phone lines, which were supposedly untraceable.[14] Judyth's phone conversations with Lee Oswald continued until Wednesday, Nov. 20, 1963.

During the final emotional phone call, Lee made it clear to Judyth that there would be a real attempt to kill President Kennedy on Friday at one of three locations in Dallas. Lee told Judyth that he believed a man named David Atlee Phillips was organizing it.[15] He told Judyth to remember the name.

However he got there, Lee was now inside the assassination plot trying to kill President Kennedy, and considered it his duty to stay in position and undercover until it was over, telling Judyth, "If I stay, there will be one less bullet fired at Kennedy." Lee did not know if he would make it out alive, but if he did, he was prepared to elope with Judyth. They would go to Merida (a city in Mexico's Yucatan peninsula), where they could both get quickie Mexican divorces from their respective spouses, and then Lee would marry Judyth. If he didn't make it out alive, he encouraged her to go on with her life and have babies.

It is a fact of history that both Jack Kennedy and Lee Oswald were murdered within the week. Judyth remained with her husband Robert, and had her babies — five of them.

After the assassination, David Ferrie spoke to Judyth for the last time. In that phone call, he told her in blunt language that if she opened her mouth, she too would be killed — as Lee had been.

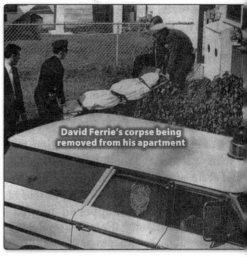

David Ferrie's corpse being removed from his apartment

Judyth took Ferrie's warning seriously, and maintained her silence for decades.

This is the basic outline of Judyth's story. She tells it differently, and in much more detail. Her book is 700 pages long. Having known her now for six years, it is clear to me that Judyth loved Lee, and that she suffered the horror of seeing the man she loved murdered on national television. She is very angry about all of this. Who wouldn't be?

She has chosen to come out of hiding after more than 35 years, at considerable risk to herself. Personal risk and legal risk. She admits that she was party to the murder of the patient in the Jackson mental hospital. She admits to developing a biological weapon intended to murder Fidel Castro. She has placed herself at the center of a heated, and often angry, debate over the murder of the President, on the side of the accused assassin. She has been treated disgracefully in Internet newsgroups, and subjected to vicious insults from people hoping to humiliate her back into silence. She begrudgingly accepts all this as the price that she has to pay to tell the world about the Lee Oswald she knew — about his wit, his intellect, his sensitivity, his liberal political leanings, his admiration of President Kennedy, his courage, his innocence in JFK's murder, and especially the personal risk he took (and price he paid) in hopes of preventing President Kennedy's assassination. Her take: Lee infiltrated the plot to kill President Kennedy, was set up as the patsy, and was then murdered to protect the real assassins by silencing him.

I EMPATHIZE WITH JUDYTH as a person. She has paid a terrible price both for what she did in the 1960s, and for what she says today. I hope you will read her story for yourself, if you are able to obtain it, and make your own decisions about her story.[16] I hope *60 Minutes* will complete their story about Judyth. I hope the History Channel will re-instate "The Love Affair" episode in *The Men Who Killed Kennedy* series for a wider audience to see. The public has the right to hear what

Judyth Vary Baker has to say, and the right to make up its own mind about the government's highly contested claims that Lee Oswald killed President Kennedy — whether alone (1964) or as part of a conspiracy (1972).

In 2006 Judyth sent me an email saying there was something else she wanted to discuss and asking me to call her. I did. In the middle of the hour-long conversation, Judyth started talking about a letter from Guy Banister that she had seen lying on a desk in Congressman Willis' office in New Orleans, one that she thought might be important. With her typical love of detail and analysis, she began explaining about a note that was handwritten in the margins of the letter, and took off on a tangent that I did not follow.

"Judyth! Time Out!" I interrupted. "What were you doing in Willis' office?"

"Oh, Monaghan used to send me over there to deliver messages ... a couple of times a week. They were always in sealed envelopes so I didn't know what the content was. I think it was INCA-related information.[17] Willis was hardly ever there, but the staff all knew who I was. Monaghan took me over to introduce me to the staff so they would know who I was when I showed up with an envelope. It was on Lafayette Square, right by Reily's." In the summer of 1963, Congressman Willis was Chairman of the House Committee on Un-American Activities (HUAC).[18]

Now, let me see if I am following this:

In the morning, the young cancer-researcher rides the bus to work with the "defector" who is about to be accused of assassinating the President. In the afternoon, she goes to the underground medical laboratory run by a known Mafia-asset to develop a biological weapon. In between the two, she works at a cover-job under the supervision of an ex-FBI agent, who sends her on errands to deliver "envelopes" to the office of the Congressman who chairs the House Committee on Un-American Activities.[19]

What was in all those envelopes from the coffee company? Coffee? Would violating the Neutrality Act by conspiring to murder Fidel Castro be considered an Un-American Activity? Would developing a biological weapon be considered an Un-American Activity? Would someone be willing to bribe the local Congressman (or his staff) to make sure that it was not? You have to wonder if Congressman Willis even

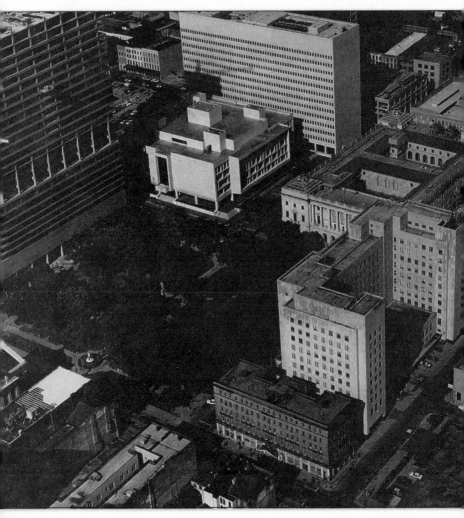

*Dr. Mary's Monkey*

knew his office was being used in this manner? Or whether he was a key player who organized the others? Or whether he was just Marcello's tool?

Whatever the answers may be, they lie in the buildings around Lafayette Square — within a stone's throw of where the Warren Commission held its hearings in New Orleans.[20] Next to the Federal court house. Under the noses of the most powerful Congressmen in the land. With the cooperation of former members of the FBI. With the knowledge of the CIA. With the participation of the press. With the cooperation of leaders of American medicine.

In hospitals guarded by Marines. With the help of organized crime. And in the name of freedom. With flag-waving allegiance to colors and slogans that mask a contempt for law. With smoldering hatred and flaring impatience. With the cynical belief that you really can't tell the people what you need to do, because they might not let you do it. That you can't trust democracy to produce the right answers or the right leaders. That it as patriotic to intervene illegally in the politics of our own country as it is for us to intervene illegally in the politics other countries. These are the lessons of our Labyrinth. And we have Judyth Vary Baker to thank for bringing them to our attention.

---

1   Frankly, I would prefer that Judyth present it herself. I have watched her for five years. She has tried and tried to get her story out. In fact, in 2003 the History Channel presented an excellent documentary which featured Judyth Vary Baker as part of their legendary series entitled *The Men Who Killed Kennedy*. This well-produced narrative presented Judyth and her story clearly and powerfully, but it was bundled with two other episodes which erupted into lawsuits. Though I never saw news of any legal complaint involving Judyth's story, it was withdrawn along with the other two episodes. This was not because it was not popular. Over 50,000 copies of the DVD were sold in the first week. A week later all three were withdrawn. If that DVD were still available, I would not feel the need to provide such a detailed review of her story; but right now it is not.

2   Judyth's father was an electrical engineer who invented various TV components. After the family moved to Florida, the money from selling his patents ran out.

3   Judyth was considering becoming a nun. Her family strongly objected. Her father drove to the college and essentially kidnapped her in the middle of the night, bringing her home to Florida.

4  Tulane University was on a traditional semester schedule. Judyth's university in Florida switched to a new trimester schedule in 1963. The result was that Judyth's campus shut down (cafeterias, etc.) three weeks earlier that normal. Due to Judyth's problems at home, she headed to New Orleans early.

5  Lee Oswald advised Judyth that this Royal Castle was a favorite dead-drop spot for Bobby Kennedy's agents who were spying on Carlos Marcello, who was not only the local Mafia boss, but one of its national leaders.

6  Complicating Judyth's story (and her life) was the impending arrival of Robert Baker, her fiancé. She explains this part of her story in detail in her book, but it is extraneous to our discussion here, and. I therefore ignore it.

7  Also, Lee's mother dated Sam Termine when Lee was a teenager. Termine had been Carlos Marcello's chauffeur.

8  Imagine how easy it would have been to discredit a whistleblower if she had first been rounded up in a brothel and then photographed at the Mafia boss' motel. Who would believe such a person? Was all this a safety precaution?

9  Remember Elmener Peterson, Mary's maid? Judyth was given her work schedule, so that she could arrange her visits when Elmener was not there. I wish I had known about Judyth when I spoke to Alvin Alcorn.

10  We have no way of knowing if the Reily management knew about the events going on in their building. Until we do, I will assume that they did not. But professional investigators might want to explore this question.

11  Was Lee able to borrow cars from Alba's garage to carry out his activities? Imagine how difficult it would be to track his activities in different cars belonging to different people each time he went somewhere!

12  The question of whether there were actually mice in David Ferrie's apartment in the summer of 1963 has been the subject of debate in the news groups and on the Internet. One JFK researcher, who has interviewed a lot of Ferrie's "young male friends" about this, points out that none of them recall seeing mice at Ferrie's apartment on Louisiana Avenue Parkway in the summer of 1963. Even Perry Russo, a witness that I interviewed who had seen Ferrie's mice at a previous apartment, said that he did not see any in Ferrie's apartment when he attended a party there in the summer of 1963. So I asked Judyth whether David Ferrie kept mice in his apartment. Judyth said that she did see a small collection of live mice in Ferrie's apartment the first time she went there (April 27, 1963), but he removed them when he cleaned up his apartment for the party (April 28, 1963). After that, she did not see any mice living in cages in Ferrie's apartment on a regular basis. I think the answer is simply that once they cranked up the secret lab work, he realized that having a bunch of people seeing mice at his apartment was not good security, so he moved the few mice he had in his apartment to the apartment across the street. Judyth told me that the mice she used for her research sessions in Ferrie's apartment were brought there in cardboard boxes from another location somewhere nearby. Each box contained about 50 mice. They were all killed and disposed of the same day.

13  The secretary involved was a temporary covering for Dr. Ochsner's regular secretary (a nurse) who was on vacation. Involving an outside person in the communication between Judyth and Ochsner was a risky move, to which Ochsner strongly objected. He told Judyth that she should have communicated her concerns to him directly.

14  These untraceable phone calls between Lee and Judyth were arranged by David Ferrie using the Mafia's secret sports-gambling telephone network, which deliberately did not keep records of the phone calls. This Mafia connection seemed reasonable to Judyth because she and Lee had gone together to the 500 Club (a famous strip-club and bar in

the French Quarter), where they had spoken to Carlos Marcello himself.

**15** David Atlee Phillips is a well-known name in the JFK assassination research circles. He was a CIA officer stationed primarily in Mexico City at the time. He has long been suspected of being the organizer behind the JFK assassination by those who believe that it was the CIA that murdered Jack Kennedy. We now have a real, live witness, who can prove that she worked with Lee Harvey Oswald, state that Oswald (the man accused of the JFK assassination by former-CIA Director Allen Dulles, FBI Director J. Edgar Hoover and the others on the Warren Commission) personally told her two days before the JFK assassination that Kennedy would be killed on Friday, and that a CIA officer name David Atlee Phillips was organizing the hit. This is a serious charge which should not be ignored. And it raises serious questions about the composition of the Warren Commission.

**16** Judyth's book entitled *Lee Harvey Oswald* was released in June of 2006. It was published by Trafford press and could be ordered on their Web site. After about two weeks, it was suddenly withdrawn without explanation. I do not know why and will leave that for others to explain and to discuss. I was given my copy directly by Judyth Vary Baker. Used copies may be available from time to time: Check the Internet.

**17** It was INCA's Executive Director Ed Butler who said that the newspaper clipping about Oswald's defection to the Soviet Union used in the WDSU radio debate from Congressman Willis' office.

**18** Edwin Edward Willis (1904-1972) had been a U.S. Congressman representing the Cajun parishes of Louisiana since 1949. A senior liberal Democrat, Willis was a loyal LBJ ally in building the "Great Society." From 1963 to 1968 Willis chaired HUAC, once the anti-Communist bludgeon of Senator Joe McCarthy.

**19** Judyth assured me that Willis knew about Lee, and knew that his defection to the USSR was not a real one — which is why he was allowed to work for Reily: the ex-FBI agent at Reily's would have never hired a defector with an undesirable discharge to work for one of the city's most prominent anti-Communists.

**20** On July 21, 1964 (the day Mary Sherman's murder was discovered), LBJ suddenly headed from the White House to the Pentagon for an unscheduled visit. After that meeting, he stopped at Arlington National Cemetery, and stood alone at JFK's grave for the first time since the assassination. One has to wonder if this was LBJ's epiphany? Was this the day LBJ finally understood the dimensions of the forces that Kennedy had faced? Was this the day LBJ was told about Mary Sherman's murder and the bio-weapon that she had been developing with Lee Harvey Oswald? The timing does make one wonder.

~~~~~~~~~~~~~~

DALLAS

ATLANTA

NEW ORLEANS

•MIA

•NO-NAME

•HOUSTON

HAVANNA

NEW ORLEANS LA
112 723

DALLAS
POLICE
54018
11 23 63

HYCTOTL
MRZYM CALLED 4 JLEST WEDN 74
FOR THE COAST. MEET AT A.O. IS WINDA
OSWALD IS OUT OF THE WAY. WE LOOK US
INJECTED WITH 24C 4 WITH NO MONEY ELSE
LEFT INTACT GOOD WILL THE FIGHT IS ON

HANDS
OFF
CUBA!
Join the Fair Play for
Cuba Committee
NEW ORLEANS CHAPTER
MEMBER BRANCH
Free Literature Lectures
LOCATION

# The Perfect Patsy

## *Rethinking Lee Harvey Oswald*

I TRIED TO STAY OUT OF THE ENTANGLED DEBATE surrounding the JFK assassination. I really did. Simply said, my book is not about the Kennedy Assassination. My public position about Oswald's role in the JFK Assassination had always been one of shoulder-shrugging neutrality. Whatever Oswald's role was (or wasn't) in the JFK assassination, it did not affect the basic facts of Mary Sherman's murder, the cancer-causing monkey viruses in the polio vaccine, or whether Ferrie and Sherman irradiated cancer-causing monkey viruses to develop a biological weapon.

But once I realized the connection between Dr. Alton Ochsner (the former President of the American Cancer Society, who was working on a secret project for the U.S. Government) and Lee Harvey Oswald (the accused assassin of President Kennedy), my aloof position became more difficult to maintain. Connecting Ochsner to Oswald not only rules out "lone nut" as a realistic description of Oswald, it helps us understand how convenient "lone nut" was for protecting Ochsner (and others) from inconvenient questions about both the bio-weapon project and the JFK assassination. Using "lone nut" to cut off further discussion about

Oswald protected Ochsner, his circle of powerful contacts, the CIA, the FBI, the Mafia, and Oswald's hidden sponsor — the person who brought him back from Russia. It was a great political compromise worthy of the skillful politicians on the Warren Commission. But it simply was not true.

It is not difficult to demonstrate that Dr. Alton Ochsner had some connection to Lee Harvey Oswald in the summer of 1963. After all, Ochsner had INCA produce and distribute an audio recording featuring Lee Harvey Oswald.[1]

The fact that Dr. Alton Ochsner financed, produced and distributed this record is itself a connection to Oswald. The Oswald radio appearance was aired on WDSU radio, and the TV footage of Oswald passing out pro-Castro leaflets was filmed by WDSU-TV camera crews. Both stations were owned by a close Ochsner associate named Edgar Stern.[2] It has long been suspected that it was Ochsner who asked Stern to provide the media coverage of Oswald. This suspicion was so strong that at one point the New Orleans District Attorney spoke of arresting Ochsner for conspiracy in the Kennedy assassination. Garrison's staff talked him out of it.

Further connecting Ochsner to Oswald, I reported that I personally saw Guy Banister's files in the offices of Ochsner's political organization INCA. It was INCA's Executive Director Ed Butler himself who told me that they had been Banister's files.[3] Banister was widely regarded as "Oswald's handler" in New Orleans during 1963, and was considered to be the operational leader of the paramilitary training camp outside of New Orleans that Bobby Kennedy shut down later that sum-

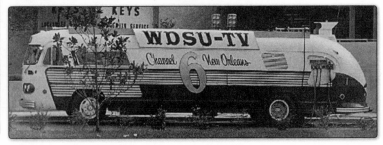

*Dr. Mary's Monkey*

mer.[4] Banister and Ferrie were training Cubans and mobsters as a strike force to enter Cuba and assassinate Fidel Castro.

Additionally, it has been said for many years that Oswald was helping make training films to teach Cubans how to use certain military weapons in support of this kill-Castro project.[5] So the connection between Ochsner and Banister is also a connection between Ochsner and Oswald.

The *extent* of Ochsner's connections to Oswald, and his motives for setting up the media coverage, have always been less clear to me. Unlike Garrison, who thought that the media coverage was part of the "sheep dipping" of Oswald to make him a convincing patsy for the JFK assassination, it is hard for me to imagine that Dr. Ochsner knew that he was setting up Lee Harvey Oswald as part of an effort to kill the President of the United States. Ochsner's role was too high-profile, and, frankly, his reputation was too valuable for him to risk in such a manner. In the same breath, one might ask why would a wealthy and prestigious doctor bother at all with Lee Harvey Oswald? Perhaps there was another reason behind their association, and a different reason for arranging the media coverage.[6]

Judyth Vary Baker has told us that there was. Judyth reports that Lee Oswald secretly worked as a team member on Ochsner's bio-weapon project, that Oswald met with Ochsner personally, and that it was actually Lee Oswald who requested that Dr. Ochsner set up his media coverage to help position him as a pro-Cuban activist, so that he could get into Cuba more easily and deliver their bio-weapon to sympathetic doctors, who would use it to kill Castro.

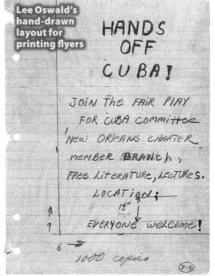

Lee Oswald's hand-drawn layout for printing flyers

Before we move on, I want to focus on a detail of the dialog between Lee Oswald and INCA's Ed Butler during the radio program. The debate was evidently Lee's idea in the first place, to portray himself as a pro-Cuban activist who would seem more "acceptable" to Cuban authorities who could grant him a visa to visit Cuba. But Butler (Ochsner's front-man at INCA and a staunch anti-Communist himself) was not privy to that part of the story. Butler had another objective.

He thought his role was to discredit Oswald as being a Communist. In the middle of their debate, Butler pulled out two 1959 newspaper articles from the Washington *Evening-Star* and the *Washington Post,* and read quotes that accused Oswald of "defecting" to the Soviet Union. Now there is a *big* difference between being a sympathetic pro-Cuban activist who might be welcome in Cuba and being an American military defector. Oswald was surprised by Butler's unexpected comment, and was obviously annoyed by the accusation. In a tense exchange, he defended himself against the defector accusation: *"The obvious answer to that is that I am back in the United States."*

This is a really good point. Take some time to think this one through. It has been glossed over for years. In my opinion, the pivotal issue for understanding Lee Harvey Oswald is the fact that Lee managed to return to the United States with his Russian wife and infant daughter at the height of the Cold War, and after leading American newspapers had claimed that he had defected and renounced his citizenship. Following up on Oswald's remark may tell us for whom he really worked after his return.

My take is that in 1959 Lee was sent to Russia on an undercover assignment for an American intelligence effort, and became marooned there when he lost his sponsors, either in the Eisenhower-to-Kennedy changeover or after the Bay of Pigs debacle, both in 1961. As part of his cover assignment, he had walked into the American Embassy in Moscow and

*Dr. Mary's Monkey*

announced his intention to renounce his American citizenship (but was careful not to sign anything). Later he married Marina, and she became pregnant. It is then that he realized that, unless he returned to the United States, his child would be trapped in the Soviet Union. His problem was that the people who had sent him (and who know about his real mission as an agent and not a defector) were no longer around to vouch for him.

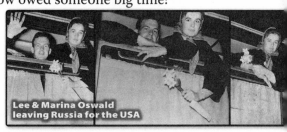

The new people thought that he was really a defector and were unwilling to help him return. Lee wrote to his mother and asked her to help. Lee's mother called and wrote everyone she could (in both New Orleans and Washington) trying to get her son and his family into the United States. Someone finally came through, but to this day we do not know who it was.

The U.S. State Department lent Lee the money to travel, and gave him the proper documentation for his family to enter the United States. Whoever authorized this, there are two things we now know. First, this person had a lot of power and influence with the United States government (enough to overrule staff opposition and to tell the State Department what to do), and, secondly, Lee now owed someone big time!

Did Lee cut a deal to get back into the U.S.? If so, with whom? Who has the power to say if you are (or are not) "an America citizen"? Who has the power to say that you are (or are not) really "a defector"? Who has the power to pick up the telephone and tell the State Department to loan you money to buy your tickets to go home? The right answers to these questions would reveal the person who shaped the rest of Lee Oswald's life.

Lee & Marina Oswald leaving Russia for the USA

TENS OF THOUSANDS OF PAGES have already been written about Lee Harvey Oswald. The debate over his role in the JFK assassination is polarized, opinionated, and often angry. It will not end here. Many people on both sides of the issue have so much personal equity invested in their positions that there is no amount of evidence, nothing that could sway them to change their positions publicly. But these pundits are not the ones I am addressing my comments to.

I laugh at the loyalists who insist that Lee brought a rifle with him to work, but rushed back to his apartment upon hearing about the assassination to get his pistol. I roll my eyes at the "experts" who quote evidence prepared under the direction of J. Edgar Hoover, whom we now know was being blackmailed by Mafia-boss Meyer Lansky.[7] And I shake my head at the Garrison-bashers who insist that that everything the New Orleans District Attorney ever said was wrong, as if all of the rapists, murderers, and robbers that he put in prison during his twelve years as the chief public prosecutor should be freed because of his over-statements.

Instead, I write to you, the thoughtful reader, because (now that we know how close Lee Oswald was to the Mafia in New Orleans and about his involvement in the bio-weapon project) there is plenty of room for new ideas about Oswald and his role in history, and you have the right to hear them. Yes, I have more questions than answers. My goal is to expand the discussion, not to narrow it. Here I offer you what should be fresh information on Lee Oswald, should you wish to consider it.

I am going to present several different scenarios which might explain how Lee Oswald got back into the United States. If I were conducting an investigation in 1963 to determine who Lee Harvey Oswald ultimately worked for, I would have been investigating these possibilities. When you see who the players were, and how unwelcome such an investigation would have been to them, you will understand why it was not done.

Scenario A — The Attorney General. Officially, the officer of the U.S. Government who has the final word on whether you have lost or renounced your citizenship is the Attorney General. In 1961, the U.S. Attorney General was Bobby Kennedy. The normal administrative request to re-solve a question of whether one had renounced one's citizenship would have come to his desk. At that time, Bobby had his own set of problems. He was busy fight-ing a war against the Mafia (particularly Carlos Marcello) and was trying to figure out what the CIA was really doing with the millions of dollars missing from its budgets. Bobby was particular-ly concerned about renegade CIA paramilitary operations involving the Mafia, since they de-fied the authority of the White House. Bobby needed one or

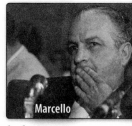

Marcello

more competent undercover agents to get inside these operations and report back to him (through intermediaries, of course). Lee was a trained spy who had done under-cover work in the Soviet Union. Normally, the AG would rely on the FBI for this type of counter-intelligence help, but the FBI Director was his sworn enemy, was black-mailing his brother the President, and had connections to the Mafia himself. So Bobby needed his own off-the-books agents to do this work. Bobby Kennedy arranged for Lee and his family to return to the U.S. The price: You work undercover for me, and use your family contacts to spy on Carlos Marcello and the Mafia in New Orleans.

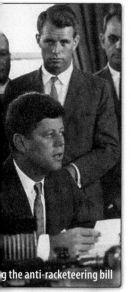

g the anti-racketeering bill

Scenario B — The Mafia Boss. Lee's mother, Marguarite Clavier Oswald, had been a personal friend of Carlos Marcello for decades. She went to the Mafia boss and asked him to use his influence (which was enormous) on the Louisiana poli-

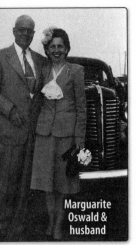

Marguarite Oswald & husband

ticians (which were among the most powerful in Washington) to pressure the right people to let her son and his family back into the U.S. Marcello had considerable influence with virtually all the Louisiana politicians, but he had a special relationship with one in particular — Congressman Edwin E. Willis, Chairman of the House Committee on Un-American Activities.[8] As such, he had the de facto power to decide who was a defector and who was not, and cleared Oswald's reentry in good standing to this country. The price: You now work for Carlos Marcello, and you owe him a very big favor.

SCENARIO C — THE DOUBLE WHAMMY. Bobby Kennedy was at war with the Mafia and was prosecuting organized crime figures in record numbers. His primary target was Carlos Marcello. Kennedy openly said that he would use underworld tactics to fight the underworld. He had Marcello kidnapped and dropped him in Guatemala without a U.S. passport. Marcello was so powerful that he was able to get back into the United States without a passport, and despite the pressure against him by the U.S. Attorney General.[9] Needless to say, Bobby Kennedy was watching every move Marcello made. His attention was attracted when politicians that he knew to be Marcello-connected started pressuring the organs of the U.S. government to let someone believed to be a defector back in from the U.S.S.R. Kennedy had his people quietly deliver a message to Oswald: "We know you want to bring your family home, and we know that Carlos Marcello is pressuring people to make it happen. We have the power to stop it, leaving you and your family in the Soviet Union. But we are willing to let you in, if ..." The price: You work for us and use your family contacts (with Marcello) to spy on the Mafia and get inside their CIA-related projects, but Marcello still thinks you owe him the favor.[10]

*Dr. Mary's Monkey*

In my opinion, these are all plausible, and have a real-world feel to them. Any one could easily explain his jobs at the map company in Dallas, at Reily in New Orleans, and at the Dallas Book Depository.[11] But none are compatible with the "lone nut" theory.

COULD OSWALD HAVE BEEN WORKING FOR the CIA, the Mafia, *and* the Attorney General? The CIA would have known that he was Mafia, because they were already working with the Mafia to kill Castro. Oswald was part of that project. And, of course, the Mafia would have known that Lee was working with the CIA, because they set it up. Was it Lee Oswald who identified the location of Banister's secret paramilitary training camp near New Orleans, which Bobby Kennedy's men raided? Did Lee infiltrate the CIA-Mafia bioweapon project and report back to Bobby on it? If the Mafia and/or the CIA figured out that Oswald was really spying on their operations for their archenemy Bobby Kennedy,[12] then Lee's days would have been numbered from that moment on. Is this why he was ordered back to Dallas?[13] Were they putting him in position to be the patsy in the JFK assassination?

FINALLY, LET'S LOOK AT THE JFK ASSASSINATION from the perspective of the plotters. Yes, they needed a patsy, but why would they choose Lee Harvey Oswald to be that patsy? Was it merely because he had lived in Russia, or did he bring something else to the party? Here is how I explain it:

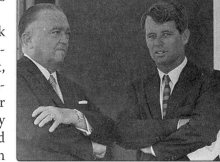

If you're planning to shoot Jack Kennedy in the head with high-powered rifles in broad daylight, you'd better spend some time thinking about his brother. His brother is Bobby Kennedy, the Attorney General, and he has the power and the resources to come after you. In order to get away with killing Jack, you must neutralize Bobby at the critical moment. If you stymie Bobby, you might get away it. If you don't, you could be in really big trouble.

The question: *How do you paralyze Bobby at the critical moment?*

The answer: *By publicly accusing one of his agents of the crime!*

If Bobby says, "But Lee's legitimate; he's with me," then J. Edgar Hoover is able to say, "If Lee's with you, then you have just murdered your own brother, you ambitious little bastard."

DID LEE HARVEY OSWALD SECRETLY WORK for Bobby Kennedy?[14] Was Lee Harvey Oswald chosen as the patsy because accusing him would neutralize Bobby?[15] Is this why Bobby failed to act at the critical moment?[16]

Far from being a "lone nut," Oswald was connected to so many powerful and/or corrupt people that no one wanted him to get into a courtroom and start talking. Not even the Attorney General.

It was brilliant planning. The work of professionals. And they got away with murdering the President.

At least ... that's the way it looks to me today.

---

1   Recall that the first photo on the back cover (see page 164) is of Hale Boggs, who was Congressman from the District where the linear particle accelerator was located. He was later a member of the Warren Commission, and was the father of NPR's political analyst Cokie Roberts.

2   Edgar Stern was a close associate of Dr. Alton Ochsner. Stern was a major financial backer of Ochsner's hospital and a member of INCA, Ochsner's anti-Communist crusade. Edgar Stern and his wife Edith organized press parties to support their friend Clay Shaw when Garrison accused him of conspiring to assassinate Kennedy.

3   Guy Banister is a well-known figure to JFK assassination readers. He was briefly Agent-in-Charge of the FBI's Chicago office and briefly Deputy Chief of the New Orleans Police Department. He founded a small private investigations agency in New Orleans, where he was famous for collecting and distributing anti-Communist intelligence. The fact that he worked with and for Carlos Marcello's attorney is well known.

4   Bobby Kennedy was President Kennedy's brother. At the time he was the U.S. Attorney

General and was responsible for enforcing the Neutrality Act. Training an assassination squad to assassinate a foreign leader was a violation of federal law. So was possession of the explosives found at the training camp.

5  Judyth Vary Baker said that Lee Oswald took her to Banister's office, introduced her to Banister, and showed her military weapons stored on an upper floor there.

6  As we discovered in his FBI file, Dr. Alton Ochsner had been cleared for a "Sensitive Position" for the U.S. government in October 1959. With Oswald's trail at Ochsner's feet, it was virtually impossible for anyone to investigate Ochsner without coming into conflict with the U.S. government over disclosing his sensitive assignment. Conversely, it would be difficult to investigate Ochsner's assignment without dredging up the JFK assassination. What was his "Sensitive Position"?

7  Imagine the Director of the FBI being blackmailed by the organized crime figures whom some say supplied (and paid) the actual shooters in this assassination. How could anyone rely upon Hoover's evidence at this point without questioning his ability to shape the "evidence" to align with his motives? Which may have really been the Mafia's motives!

8  In the 1960s, I heard this Willis-Marcello connection discussed on several occasion by various people, some of which were staff members who worked for other members of Louisiana's Congressional delegation. It appeared to be common knowledge among people inside Louisiana politics at the time.

9  Carlos Marcello was born in Sicily and came to the United States as a child. He never formally acquired citizenship, despite the fact that he lived here for decades. Technically, he was not an American citizen. But when you control the political machine of Louisiana, such technicalities don't really matter very much.

10  Judyth Vary Baker tells us that Lee's favorite TV show was *I Led Three Lives*, based upon the story of an American agent posing as a "card-carrying Communist." If his fantasy was to be a double-agent, this scenario would have given him that opportunity.

11  It should be noted that in both Dallas and New Orleans, Lee Oswald worked virtually next to the Federal Courthouse. Is this a coincidence? Was he there to be close to his handlers? Was he spying on crooked judges for the Attorney General? Was he there to deliver bribes on behalf of the Mafia? Was he working for RFK or Marcello? Or both?

12  The phone log of J. Edgar Hoover shows calls to Banister in the summer of 1963. Did Hoover figure out that Oswald was working for Bobby, and use Banister to alert Marcello?

13  According to Judyth Vary Baker.

14  The idea of Lee Oswald working for Bobby Kennedy was first presented to me by Mrs. Ellis. I did not understand it at the time, but I remembered it. Over the years, I slowly realized that it would explain many things. And I have never heard it discussed publicly.

15  Upon hearing that Lee Harvey Oswald had been arrested, Bobby Kennedy picked up the phone and called CIA Director John McCone, and asked him if the CIA had killed his brother. Bobby and McCone had been working together to track down renegade CIA operations, especially those involved with anti-Castro Cubans.

16  The Attorney General should have sent agents into the Dallas Police Station immediately to make sure that the suspect's safety was assured, and to make sure that everything was handled by-the-books, so that the suspect could be prosecuted successfully in a court of law. Was it to Bobby Kennedy that Lee Oswald was directing his comments when he looked in the camera and requested legal representation?

---

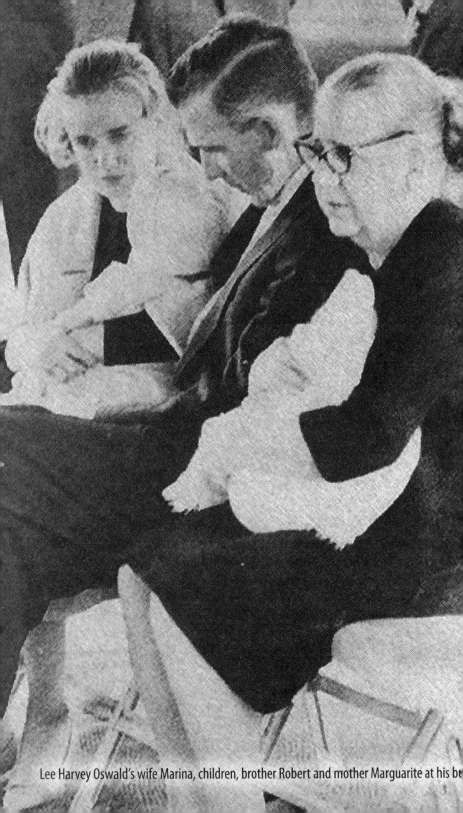

Lee Harvey Oswald's wife Marina, children, brother Robert and mother Marguarite at his bu

# DOCUMENTS

## Document A – The Treatise

REPRODUCED AT THE NATIONAL ARCHIVES

Collection: HSCA (RG 233)

Chief Ed M.

MEMORANDUM FOR:   LEAD FILE

RE:                NOTES MADE BY DAVID FERRIE

-----------------------------------------------------------------

At the bottom of FERRIE'S article on cancer, there is a portion of notes made by him but on another piece of paper. This was apparently picked up in the photostat machine when they made copies of his cancer article and obviously was not intended to be preserved. It appears that a letter or memo which he had made concerning his private activities was accidentally stuck in the photostat machine leaving us the bottom portion of his memorandum.

The portion which was reproduced reads as follows:

". . .round faced - cross-filed file.

". . .man - Bill Dazell (Billie Littlehorse) Some of B's microfilm were sent to Atlanta right-wingers - many of original files are at Guy Johnson's"

JIM GARRISON

347

REPRODUCED AT THE NATIONAL ARCHIVES Collection: HSCA (RG 233)
-25-

maxillae, and on the ears. Finally, the animals were subjected
to small doses of x-ray over a period of three weeks.

## Group I

This group consisted of 20 hamsters; 10 test, 10 control, of
the same strain and family, and more or less the same age. They
were treated with carcinogens as described. Of the 10 test animals
4 developed malignancies. None of the          animals developed
malignancies.

Extracts were made from the malignant tumors which appeared
in animals in the test group. These extracts were then injected
into other animals of the  test group. A variety of malignancies
appeared: Leukemia, chorioepithelioma among them. Extracts of the
malignant tissue heated to 56°C for one hour and then injected
into animals of the control group produced no malignancies. In
some of these latter animals papillomae appeared, however.

One of the cancerous hamsters was isolated for special
treatment including an extract from his own tumors. The method
of Helen King and her group in Philadelphia was followed. The
hamster had been previously treated for cancer regression, a
subject which will be discussed in Chapter Nine. With this
extract in the hamster, to date it seems that this animal will
not produce new malignancies. This is referred to here because
of a discussion, later in the paper, on the use of vaccines in
cancer prevention.

## Group II

This group consisted of 20 R-III pure strain white mice.
Ten were test and ten were control. The animals were all of
the same age. The mice were treated with carcinogens in the
manner previously described. In the test group seven mice
evidenced malignant tumors. None of the control group exhibited
malignancies.

As with the hamsters, extracts made from the malignant
tissue and injected into other animals was able to effect new
malignancies. If the extracts were treated with heat at 56°C
for one hour, and then injected into animals, malignancies failed
to appear.

In both the mice and hamsters to malignancies which appeared
after injections of tissue extract appeared to be the same as the
original malignancies. This would seem a clear indication of the
Koch Postulate had been proved.

It was noted in the tests that the application of carcinogen
does NOT always produce a malignancy. Hence, Cowdry's "final
common path" seems at work. Thus the term "carcinogen" has
reservations. It is to be noted that methylcholanthrene failed
to give a 100% result. Of course it could be argued that there
may have been a conflict since two other items were used in the
carcinogenesis.

Suffice it to say: as with Gregory's work, so here, the
Koch Postulate seems fulfilled. Cancer seems caused by a virus

REPRODUCED AT THE NATIONAL ARCHIVES    Collection:  BSCA (RG 233)

often ma ........ .... ...., performing hypophy-
stomies, adrenalectomies, prostectomies, castrations and the
like. A desperate and not too desirable form of therapy.

## Mercaptopterin

The author has not worked with this drug. However,
there are several encouraging reports circulating which suggest
that it may become a powerful therapy against cancer.

## Aminopterin

This is a successful drug in causing malignant tumor regression,
but its continued use causes death from avitaminosis as aminopterin
prevents formation of folic acid. Tumor growth needs folic acid,
but so do the patients.

## Antivin

Antivin is an antibiotic, developed by a mold. by Dr. John
. Gregory. This author has had the happy opportunity of using
t with small laboratory animals with happy results. Of course
he therapy needs to be controlled. This will be discussed in
he next section. Dr. Gregory has used Antivin on many of his
atients with an altogether satisfactory result. Antivin has
ot as yet been released for general trial, however.

Dr. Gregory is available to come to any part of the country
o demonstrate Antivin. From this writer's experience. to invite
r. Gregory to demonstrate the antibiotic is well worth its while.

Antivin has limitations. rapid tumor regression produces
hosphates which tend to elevate the non-protein nitrogen in the
lood and lower the blood calcium level. However, these items
nd the associated albuminuria can be easily handled by employing
requent laboratory tests, controlling dosage and regulating
iquid and solid intake.

## Magnesium Trecinate

Following Gregory, the author wishes to present an interesting
xperiment which is well worth the time and trouble of the inter-
sted researcher. This is another antibiotic, which Gregory has
ow used on human patients with excellent results. The following
s the process for manufacturing it.

(1) Obtain Bacillus Subtilis, Tracy I and grow over
high protein agar.
(2) Catch up the culture in solution and heat at 55°C
for an hour.
(3) Filter thru a number 11 Berkfeld filter for a
cell-free filtrate.
(4) Combine 100cc of the filtrate with 100cc of
Magnesium Sulphate.
(5) Place in electrophoresis for recovery.
(6) Wash out the magnesium hydroxide.
(7) Catch up the crystals in normal saline. 1500 mg
to 50cc saline.

In treating laboratory mice, begin with 5mgms daily and

REPRODUCED AT THE NATIONAL ARCHIVES   Collection:  HSCA (RG 233)

| Benign | Malignant | Tissue of Origin |
|---|---|---|
| Glomus tumor | | cutaneous glomus |
| | myeloma | bone marrow |
| | leukemia | bone marrow |
| | endothelial sarcoma | bone marrow |
| | endothelioma | lining of body cavity |
| | synovioma | synovia |
| | lymphosarcoma | lymphoid tissue |
| | reticulum cell carcoma | lymphoid tissue |
| | thymoma | lymphoid tissue |
| Leiomyoma | leiomyosarcoma | smooth muscle tissue |
| Rhabdomyoma | rhabdomyosarcoma | striated muscle tiss |

3. Mixed Tumors

| Mixed tumors of salivaries | | salivary glands |
|---|---|---|
| Dermoid cyst | | ovary |
| | mixed kidney | renal anlage |

4. Teratomas

| Teratoma | teratoma | gonads |
|---|---|---|
| Teratoma | teratoma | embryonic rests |

*Dr. Mary's Monkey*

REPRODUCED AT THE NATIONAL ARCHIVES

lection: HSCA (RG 233)

-38-

## BIBLIOGRAPHY

| | |
|---|---|
| Allen, E., | Estrogenic Hormones in genesis of cancer, Endocrinology 30,942-952 |
| Amer. Cancer Soc. Facts & Figures on Cancer, 1949, 1952 | |
| Bittner, J. J. | Further Studies in Active Milk in Breast Cancer Production in Mice. Proc. Soc. Exper. Biol. & Med. 45:805, 1940 Breast Cancer in Mice as Influenced by Nursing, Journ. Natl. Cancer Institute 1:155, 1940 Mammary Cancer in Fostered and Unfostered C₃H Breeding Females and their Hybrids, Cancer Research 2:710, 1942 |
| Borrel, A. | Parasitic Theories of Cancer. Annal Pasteur Institute. 15,49-67 1901 |
| Bostick, W. L. | Status of Search for a Virus in Hodgkins Disease Annals N. Y. Acad. Science. 54, 1162-1176 1952 |
| Claude, A., Porter, K., and Pickels,B. | Electron Microscopy Study of Chicken Tumor Cells, Cancer Research 7:421-430 1947 |
| Coman, D. R. | Decreased Mutual Adhesiveness...in carcinomas Cancer Research. 4,625-629 |
| Conklin, E. G. | Cellular Differentiation in Cowdry's General Cytology U. of Chicago Press |
| Cowdry, E. V. | Cancer Cells. Saunders, Philadelphia, 1955 |
| De Ruyck, R. | Isolation of a Filterable Virus in a Hydatiform Mole transforming into a Choriocpithelioma, Extracts Cancer Bulletin, Paris, 38:52-71, 38:252-256, 1951. |
| Dmochowski, L. and Orr, J. W. | Induction of breast cancer by estrogens and methylcholanthrene in high and low breast cancer strain mice. British Journal Cancer 3,376-384, 1949 |
| Dmochowski, L. and Essey, R. | Attempts at Tumor Virus Isolation, Annals N. Y. Acad. Science 54,1035-1066 1952 |
| Fox, J. D. and Nelson, C. | Virus-like bodies in Human Breast Cancer, Med. Arts & Sciences 3,2 1949 |

... collection: HSCA (RG 233)

REPRODUCED AT THE NATIONAL ARCHIVES

...y, J. and ...... ...... ...... with x-rays Cancer
...... Research 7:241-245, 1947

Gregory, J. E.  Pathogenesis of Cancer. Pasadena, Freemont
Foundation, 1948 Microscope Findings in Malign
Tissue. Amp. Med. & Surg. 5:390-394, 1948 Virus
as a Cause of Human & Animal Malignancy. Sou.
Journ. 43:124-128, 1950
Virus as the Cause of Cancer, Mich. State Med.
Journ. April, 1951

Gross, L.  Is Leukemia Caused by a Transmissible Virus?
Blood, 9,557-573

King, Helen  see Journ. Immunology 517-528, 1948; also
60:517-523 and 61:315-319, 1949

Lisco, E.,  Radiology 49,351-353, 1947
Finkel, M.,
Brus, A.

Molnik, J., et al Annals N. Y. Acad. Sc, 1952, 54 1214-1215
electron microscope studies

Oberling, C.  Riddle of Cancer, Yale Press, New Haven:1952
and Rappaport Shulr

Rous, P.  Transmission of avian neoplasm. Journ. Exper.
Med. 12, 696-705, 1910
Transmission of malignancy thru cell-free
filtrate. JAMA 56,198, 1911
Breast Cause of Cancer C. S. M. A. 122,573-581
1943

Warburg, O.  Metabolism of Tumors, Constable, London, 1930

Warren Shields, Neoplasms in Andersons Pathology, St. Louis,
Mosby 1953

# Document B – Cancer Rates

By Primary Cancer Site and Year of Diagnosis

All Races, Males and Females

Year of Diagnosis

| Site | 1973 | 1974 | 1975 | 1976 | 1977 | 1978 | 1979 | 1980 | 1981 | 1982 | 1983 | 1984 | 1985 | 1986 | 1987 | 1988 |
|---|---|---|---|---|---|---|---|---|---|---|---|---|---|---|---|---|
| Oral & Pharynx | 11.3 | 11.1 | 11.4 | 11.4 | 11.1 | 11.6 | 12.1 | 11.5 | 11.7 | 11.5 | 11.5 | 11.7 | 11.4 | 10.8 | 11.4 | 10.4 |
| Esophagus | 3.4 | 3.6 | 3.5 | 3.7 | 3.5 | 3.6 | 3.7 | 3.7 | 3.5 | 3.7 | 3.7 | 3.6 | 3.5 | 4.0 | 3.9 | 3.6 |
| Stomach | 10.3 | 10.0 | 9.2 | 9.5 | 9.1 | 9.1 | 9.4 | 9.7 | 8.7 | 8.7 | 8.6 | 8.3 | 8.3 | 8.1 | 8.0 | 8.1 |
| Colon/Rectum: | 46.4 | 47.7 | 47.3 | 49.0 | 49.5 | 49.4 | 49.3 | 50.3 | 50.7 | 49.7 | 50.3 | 51.6 | 52.7 | 51.0 | 49.6 | 46.0 |
| Colon | 31.7 | 32.9 | 32.8 | 34.1 | 34.6 | 34.5 | 34.2 | 35.4 | 35.5 | 35.7 | 35.9 | 36.5 | 37.6 | 36.6 | 35.3 | 34.2 |
| Rectum | 14.7 | 14.8 | 14.6 | 15.0 | 14.9 | 14.8 | 15.1 | 14.8 | 15.2 | 14.0 | 14.3 | 15.1 | 15.2 | 14.4 | 14.4 | 13.8 |
| Liver & Intrahep: | 2.3 | 2.2 | 2.2 | 2.2 | 2.2 | 2.3 | 2.2 | 2.4 | 2.4 | 2.4 | 2.4 | 2.4 | 2.7 | 2.7 | 2.8 | 2.8 |
| Liver | 2.1 | 2.1 | 2.1 | 2.1 | 2.1 | 2.1 | 2.1 | 2.0 | 2.3 | 2.3 | 2.3 | 2.2 | 2.5 | 2.5 | 2.5 | 2.5 |
| Pancreas | 10.0 | 9.6 | 9.5 | 9.7 | 9.5 | 9.0 | 9.2 | 9.3 | 9.3 | 9.4 | 9.9 | 9.8 | 9.6 | 9.4 | 9.3 | 9.1 |
| Larynx | 4.5 | 4.5 | 4.5 | 4.7 | 4.4 | 4.7 | 4.8 | 4.7 | 4.6 | 4.7 | 4.6 | 4.6 | 4.6 | 4.5 | 4.7 | 4.6 |
| Lung & Bronchus | 42.5 | 43.9 | 45.4 | 47.9 | 49.0 | 50.2 | 50.9 | 52.3 | 53.6 | 55.0 | 55.0 | 57.0 | 56.2 | 56.6 | 58.2 | 57.7 |
| Melanoma of Skin | 5.7 | 5.9 | 6.6 | 6.8 | 7.5 | 7.5 | 8.0 | 8.6 | 8.3 | 9.2 | 9.2 | 9.1 | 10.5 | 10.6 | 10.8 | 9.7 |
| Breast | 44.6 | 51.3 | 47.6 | 46.5 | 45.6 | 45.6 | 46.7 | 46.6 | 46.5 | 46.7 | 50.9 | 53.0 | 56.7 | 58.1 | 61.6 | 60.1 |
| Cervix Uteri | 7.5 | 6.7 | 6.8 | 6.3 | 5.8 | 5.5 | 5.6 | 5.4 | 4.6 | 4.7 | 4.8 | 4.9 | 4.5 | 4.7 | 4.4 | 4.6 |
| Corp & Uterus, NOS | 15.2 | 16.5 | 17.2 | 16.7 | 15.4 | 14.4 | 13.5 | 13.2 | 13.1 | 13.0 | 12.9 | 12.5 | 12.1 | 11.6 | 11.9 | 11.2 |
| Ovary | 7.6 | 7.9 | 7.6 | 7.4 | 7.3 | 7.1 | 7.1 | 7.2 | 7.2 | 7.3 | 7.5 | 7.6 | 7.8 | 7.0 | 7.5 | 7.9 |
| Prostate Gland | 26.5 | 26.6 | 26.6 | 29.6 | 30.8 | 30.3 | 31.4 | 32.0 | 32.9 | 33.2 | 34.3 | 34.1 | 35.6 | 36.9 | 41.7 | 42.5 |
| Testis | 1.5 | 1.6 | 1.6 | 1.6 | 1.6 | 1.6 | 1.7 | 1.9 | 1.9 | 2.0 | 2.0 | 1.9 | 2.0 | 2.1 | 2.2 | 2.0 |
| Urinary Bladder | 14.6 | 15.7 | 15.5 | 15.8 | 15.2 | 16.0 | 16.1 | 16.4 | 16.6 | 16.1 | 16.2 | 16.6 | 16.6 | 17.0 | 17.4 | 16.7 |
| Kidney & Ren. Pelvis | 6.7 | 6.3 | 6.1 | 6.9 | 6.6 | 6.7 | 6.5 | 6.8 | 7.2 | 7.1 | 7.7 | 7.6 | 7.6 | 8.2 | 8.4 | 8.2 |
| Brain & Nervous Sys. | 5.0 | 5.1 | 5.4 | 5.4 | 5.7 | 5.4 | 5.5 | 5.8 | 5.9 | 5.8 | 5.7 | 5.5 | 6.2 | 6.2 | 6.3 | 6.0 |
| Thyroid Gland | 3.6 | 4.0 | 4.1 | 4.1 | 4.6 | 4.3 | 3.8 | 3.7 | 3.8 | 3.9 | 4.1 | 4.2 | 4.4 | 4.5 | 4.3 | 4.2 |
| Hodgkin's Disease | 3.3 | 3.1 | 2.9 | 2.9 | 2.8 | 2.7 | 2.8 | 2.8 | 2.7 | 2.8 | 2.8 | 2.9 | 2.8 | 2.5 | 2.9 | 2.8 |
| Non-Hodgkin's Lymph. | 8.5 | 8.9 | 9.3 | 9.4 | 9.3 | 9.9 | 10.4 | 10.4 | 11.2 | 11.1 | 11.5 | 12.5 | 12.7 | 12.9 | 13.7 | 13.6 |
| Multiple Myeloma | 3.8 | 3.8 | 4.0 | 4.1 | 4.1 | 3.8 | 3.9 | 3.9 | 4.0 | 4.3 | 4.2 | 4.3 | 4.0 | 4.1 | 4.4 | 3.9 |
| Leukemia: | 10.5 | 10.7 | 10.5 | 11.1 | 10.4 | 10.5 | 10.1 | 10.1 | 10.1 | 10.5 | 10.3 | 10.3 | 10.5 | 9.9 | 9.8 | 9.2 |
| Acute Lymphocytic | 1.1 | 1.4 | 1.0 | 1.2 | 1.2 | 1.2 | 1.2 | 1.2 | 1.4 | 1.4 | 1.4 | 1.5 | 1.4 | 1.5 | 1.4 | 1.5 |
| Chronic Lymph. | 3.3 | 3.4 | 3.4 | 3.5 | 3.2 | 3.3 | 3.0 | 3.3 | 3.1 | 3.1 | 3.1 | 3.0 | 2.9 | 2.9 | 2.8 | 2.4 |
| Acute Myeloid | 2.5 | 2.4 | 2.6 | 2.7 | 2.6 | 2.5 | 2.5 | 2.4 | 2.3 | 2.5 | 2.3 | 2.5 | 2.5 | 2.2 | 2.2 | 2.1 |
| Chronic Myeloid | 1.5 | 1.5 | 1.6 | 1.6 | 1.3 | 1.4 | 1.5 | 1.4 | 1.3 | 1.3 | 1.3 | 1.3 | 1.5 | 1.3 | 1.3 | 1.3 |
| All Other | 2.0 | 2.1 | 1.9 | 2.2 | 2.1 | 2.1 | 2.0 | 2.2 | 2.0 | 2.2 | 2.2 | 2.1 | 2.1 | 2.1 | 2.1 | 1.9 |
| All Sites | 319.8 | 332.3 | 331.6 | 337.2 | 336.6 | 336.7 | 340.3 | 344.1 | 349.9 | 350.3 | 355.5 | 362.9 | 369.9 | 371.1 | 382.6 | 375.1 |

## AUTOPSY PROTOCOL
### ORLEANS PARISH CORONER'S OFFICE

No. S64-7-288

Name: Dr. Mary Sherman      Age: 51 Color: W Sex

Date & Time of Death: 7-21-64 at 5:25 A.M.

Date & Time of Autopsy: 7-21-64 at 9:15 A.M.

### FINAL DIAGNOSES

1. Stab wound of chest with penetration of heart.
2. Hemopericardium and left hemthorax.
3. Multiple stab wounds of abdomen with incised wound of liver.
4. Multiple stab wounds of left upper extremity and right leg.
5. Laceration of labia minora.
6. Extensive burns of right side of body with complete destruction of right upper extremity and right side of thoax and abdomen.

Classification of Death: Homicide

Lloyd F. LoCascio, M.D.
Asst.     Coroner

OPSY PROTOCOL
Mary Sherman
te Female, 51

ERNAL DESCRIPTION: The body measures 5 ft. 6 in. in height and weighs
lbs. It appears to be that of a white female. Exact age cannot be
quately ascertained from the appearance of the body. It is tagged with
Orleans Police Department Identification Tag No. 246. This tag is
oved by Dr. Lloyd F. LoCascio, Assistant Coroner of Orleans Parish, who
present at the autopsy. External examination of the body shows the hair
r the head to be long and dark brown to black in color. It shows extensive
rring and there is destruction of hair and scalp over the entire right
poral region of the head and extensive burns. There are extensive drying
e burns over the entire face producing marked shrinkage of the skin, with
ormity of the facial features and drying and shrinking of the eyeballs,
aterally. The nasal cavity, the ears and the mouth appear to be essentially
mal. There are extensive charring burns all over the right side of the
e, the right thorax and the right flank. There has been complete destructi
the right upper extremity. The only portion remaining is a charred fragmen
the proximal portion of the humerus. There is extensive destruction of the
ire right hemithorax with exposure of the lung and the pleural cavity. In
ition there is destruction of the soft tissues of the right side of the
omen and right flank with exposure of the abdominal viscera. The charring
ends over to beneath the left breast and over the anterior abdominal wall
also over the posterior portion of the body, however, it is not as marked
this region. There is desquamation of skin over the right thigh and also
r the posterior portion of the left side of the body. The skin of the neck
ws disruption of continuity due to the action of heat. On the medial aspec
the right knee is a 2-1/2 x 1-1/2 cm stab wound. A probe inserted into the
ad extends a depth of 10 cm. On the left forearm there is a 2 x .4 cm
wound. A probe inserted into this wound extends a depth of 7 cm. Sup-
r to this is a 2 x 1 cm slightly gaping wound extending a distance of
roximately 4 cm into the subcutaneous tissues. On the left index finger
he distal joint on its medial aspect is a 1 cm laceration and there is a
m laceration on the lateral aspect of the left thumb. There is a 16 cm
r abdominal well-healed scar. There are multiple stab wounds present over
anterior abdominal wall. There is a 2 x .5 cm wound present in the right
abdomen. There is a gaping 3 x 2 cm wound in the right lower quadrant.
e is a 2 x 1 cm wound in the superior abdomen in the midline. There is a
1 cm wound in the left upper quadrant. On the anterior chest wall there
stab wound present 1 cm to the left of the midline at about the level of
5th rib which measures 2 x 1 cm in size. Further examination of the body
ws no other evidence of penetrating injuries nor are there any other
ernible identifying marks present. On reflecting the muscles from the
rior abdominal wall and the chest they are seen to be markedly coagulated
pale by the action of heat. The body itself shows a marked increase in
erature. Examination of the left chest wall after removal of the.
oralis muscle and the breast shows a stab wound to pass through the 6th
rcostal space immediately adjacent to the sternum on the left side. On
ving the sternal plate the left pleural cavity is seen to contain approxi-
ly 1000 to 1200 cc of fluid and clotted blood. The pericardial cavity
ains approximately 50 cc of partially clotted blood. Examination of the
cardial sac shows a 1.5 cm slit-like wound on the antero-lateral aspect
he pericardial sac on the left side. Examination of the heart in situ show
it-like wound on the anterior aspect of the right ventricle immediately
cent to the interventricular septum. A probe inserted into this wound
nds into the right ventricular cavity. On removing the heart the coronary
ries are seen to be patent. The posterior and right portion of the heart

Dr. Mary Sherman                                                          -2-

shows changes due to the action of heat. The endocardium is smooth and
glistening. The cardiac valves are normal.

RESPIRATORY TRACT: The right lung is markedly contracted and changed by
action of heat. The left lung appears to be essentially normal. Examin
of the major bronchi shows the lumen to be patent. The pulmonary arteri
normal. Examination of the left thoracic cavity after removal of the lu
the blood shows no other penetrating injuries.

ABDOMINAL CAVITY: The entire left side of the abdominal wall is missing
charred as previously described. The right side of the liver is markedl
hardened and leathery and coagulated. Examination of the surface of the
shows a slit-like wound to be present extending a depth of approximately
into the liver and originating in the stab wound in the midline of the u
abdomen. There is no hemorrhage noted around this particular wound. Th
spleen is essentially normal. The left kidney is grossly normal. The l
adrenal appears normal. The pancreas is normal. -

GASTROINTESTINAL TRACT: Examination of the stomach shows a small amount
recognizable food material within the lumen showing partial digestion.
remaining portion of the gastrointestinal tract except for changed due t
action os heat is essentially normal.

GENITALIA: Examination of the external genitalia shows a through and th
tear through the left labia majora measuring approximately 1 cm in lengt
There is a smaller similar tear in the right labium which does not exter
through and through the structure. Further examination of the external
talia shows it to be essentially normal. There are no areas of hemorrha
around the lacerations of the labium. Examination of the internal genit
shows surgical absence of the uterus and right adnexa. The left tube ap
moderately cystic.

HEAD: On reflecting the scalp there is extensive change due to the acti
heat. The calvarium is intact. On removing the calvarium the brain sho
the cerebral hemispheres to be symmetrical. The cerebral substances are
coagulated due to the action of heat but otherwise show no gross lesions
Examination of the base of the skull shows no evidence of fracture.

PROVISIONAL ANATOMIC DIAGNOSIS:
1.  Stab wound of chest with penetration of heart.
2.  Hemopericardium and left hemothorax.
3.  Multiple stab wounds of abdomen with incised wound of liver.
4.  Multiple stab wounds of left upper extremity and right leg.
5.  Laceration of labia minora.
6.  Extensive burns of right side of body with complete destruction of
    right upper extremity and right side of thorax and abdomen.

*Monroe S. Samuels*
Monroe S. Samuels, M.D.
Pathologist
dba

Lloyd F. LoCascio, M.D.
Assistant Coroner, Parish of Orleans

*Dr. Mary's Monkey*

# BIBLIOGRAPHY

Allison, A.C., "Simian Oncogenic Viruses," *Hazards of Handling Simians* (International Association of Microbiological Associations, 1969).

Altman, Lawrence K., "Earliest AIDS Case Is Called Into Doubt," *New York Times*, April 4, 1995, Medical Science section.

*American Men & Women of Science*, 23rd ed. (2007), p.267; Michael Stuart Gottlieb, vol. 3, p.267; Ruth Kirschstein, vol. 4, p. 383; Alan S. Rabson, vol. 6, p. 17.

Associated Press, "AIDS virus can cause cancer," *St. Petersburg Times*, April 8, 1994, p. A8.

Baker, C.G., et al., "The Special Virus Leukemia Program of the National Cancer Institute," *Some Recent Developments in Comparative Medicine*, edited by Fiennes (London: Academic Press, 1966).

Baker, Judyth Vary, *Lee Harvey Oswald: The True Story of the Accused Assassin of President John F. Kennedy by his Lover*, (Victoria: Trafford Publishing, 2006).

Barbour, John, "The JFK Assassination: The Garrison Tapes," a video documentary, Blue Ridge / Film Trust, 1992.

Biggar, R.J., "Kaposi's sarcoma in Zaire is not associated with HLTV-III infection," *New England Journal of Medicine*, vol. 311, p. 1051.

Bookchin, Debbie & Jim Schumacher, *The Virus and the Vaccine: The True Story of a cancer-causing monkey virus, contaminated polio vaccine, and the millions of Americans exposed* (New York: St, Martin's Press, 2004).

*Bulletin of the Tulane Medical School*, Spring 1967.

Butel, Janet S., Amy S. Arrington, Connie Wong, John A. Lednicky, and Milton J. Finegold, "Molecular Evidence of Simian Virus 40 Infections in Children," *Journal of Infectious Diseases*, v. 180 (1999), p. 884-887.

Cantwell, Alan Jr., *AIDS: The Mystery & the Solution* (Los Angeles: Aries Rising Press, 1984).

Cantwell, Alan Jr., *AIDS & the Doctors of Death* (Los Angeles: Aries Rising Press, 1987).

Carbone, Michele, et al., "SV-40 like sequences in human bone tumors," *Oncogene*, August 1, 1996, pp. 527-35.

Carpenter, Arthur E., "Social Origins of Anticommunism: The Information Council of the Americas," *Louisiana History*, Spring 1989, p. 117.

Clark, R. Lee, *Tumors of the Bone and Soft Tissue* (Chicago: Year Book Medical Publishers, 1965).

Cowley, Geoffrey, "The Future of AIDS," *Newsweek*, March 22, 1993, p. 47.

Curtis, Tom, "The Origin of AIDS," *Rolling Stone*, March 19, 1992.

Davis, John H., *Mafia Kingfish: Carlos Marcello and the Assassination of John F. Kennedy* (New York: McGraw-Hill, 1989).

Davy, William, *Through the Glass Darkly: The Mysterious World of Clay Shaw* (Sherman Oaks, California; CTKA / Citizens for Truth about the Kennedy Assassination, 1996)

Day, Lorraine, *AIDS: What the Government isn't Telling You* (Palm Desert, California: Rockford Press, 1991).

DiEugenio, James, *Destiny Betrayed: JFK, Cuba, and the Garrison Case* (New York: Sheridan Square Press, 1992); interview with Anne Benoit, 1993; interview with Allen Campbell, September 1994.

*Dorland's Medical Dictionary*, 28th ed., s.v. lymphadenopathy.

Ecker, Martin D., *Radiation: All You Need to Know to Stop Worrying, or to Start* (New York: Vintage Press, 1981).

*Encyclopedia Americana*, Vol. 29, s.v. "Yerkes, Robert Mearns."

Essex, Max and Phyllis J. Kanki, "The Origins of the AIDS Virus," *The Science of AIDS* (New York: W.H. Freeman and Company, 1989).

Eyestone, Willard H., "Scientific and Administrative Concepts behind the Establishment of the U.S. Primate Centers," *Some Recent Developments in Comparative Medicine* (London: Academic Press, 1966).

Fiennes, Richard, *Man, Nature, and Disease* (London: Weidenfeld and Nicolson, 1964).

Fiennes, Richard, *Zoonoses of Primates: The Epidemiology and Ecology of Simian Diseases in Relation to Man* (Ithaca, New York: Cornell University Press, 1965).

Fiennes, Richard, *Some Recent Developments in Comparative Medicine* (London: Academic Press, 1966).

*Frontline*, "Who was Lee Harvey Oswald?" a television documentary, Public Broadcasting System (Boston, November 1993).

Gallo, Robert C., *Virus Hunting: AIDS, Cancer, and the Human Retrovirus* (New Republic, 1991).

Gallo, Robert C., and Luc Montagnier, "The AIDS Epidemic," *The Science of AIDS* (New York: W.H. Freeman and Company, 1989).

Garrison, Jim, *A Heritage of Stone* (New York: G.P. Putnam's Sons, 1970).

Garrison, Jim, *On the Trail of the Assassins: My investigations and Prosecution of the Murder of President Kennedy* (New York: Sheridan Square Press, 1988).

Garrison, Jim and Eric Norden, "Playboy Interview," *Playboy*, October 1967, p. 59.

Garry, Robert F., et al., "Documentation of an AIDS Virus Infection in the United States in 1968," *Journal of the American Medical Association*, Oct. 14, 1988, Vol. 260, No. 14., p. 2085.

Garry, Robert F., et al., "Early case of AIDS in the USA," *Nature*, October 11, 1990, Vol. 347, p. 509.

Gladwell, Malcolm, "Researchers immunize monkeys against AIDS," *Detroit News*, December 18, 1992, p. A1.

Gorman, Christine, "Invincible," a report on the Eighth International AIDS Conference, *Time*, August 3, 1992, p. 30.

Gottlieb, A. Arthur, Michael S. Ascher, and Charles H. Kirkpatrick, *Transfer Factor: Basic Properties and Clinical Applications* (New York: Academic Press, Inc., 1976).

Grace, J.T. Jr & Mirand, E.A. "Human Susceptibility to a Simian Tumor Virus," *Annals N.Y. Academy of Science*, 1963, 108, 1123.

Graham, Rex, "Scientist: New Strains of AIDS Virus Complicate Research," *Albuquerque Journal*, May 12, 1993, p. A1.

Grmek, Mirko, *History of AIDS: Emergence and Origin of a Modern Pandemic* (Princeton: Princeton University Press, 1990).

Guillermo, Kathy Snow, *Monkey Business* (Washington: National Press Books, 1993).

Hahmias, A.J., et al., "Evidence of HLTV-III/LAV Infection in Central Africa in 1959," *Lancet*, May 31, 1986, p. 1279.

Hancock, Graham and Enver Carim, *AIDS: The Deadly Epidemic.* (Rev. ed, A Gollancz paperback. London: V. Gollancz, 1987)

Haseltine, William, and Flossie Wong-Stall, "The Molecular Biology of the AIDS Virus," *The Science of AIDS* (New York: Freeman, 1989).

Haslam, Edward T., *Mary, Ferrie & the Monkey Virus: The Story of an Underground Medical Laboratory*, (Albuquerque, 1995; Bradenton, 2002).

Hatch, Richard, "Cancer Warfare," *Covert Action*, No. 39, Winter 1991-92, p. 14.

*Hazards of Handling Simians* (International Association of Microbiological Associations, 1969).

Hinckle, Warren, and William Turner, *Deadly Secrets: The CIA-MAFIA War against Castro and the Assassination of J.F.K.*, (New York: Thunder's Mouth, 1992).

Horowitz, Leonard G., *Emerging Viruses: AIDS and Ebola, Nature, Accident, or Intentional?* (Rockport, Massachusetts: Tetrahedron, Inc., 1996).

Immerman, Richard H., *The CIA in Guatemala: The Foreign Policy of Intervention* (Austin: University of Texas, 1982).

Ivon, Lou, "Present & Past Addresses of David Ferrie," Memorandum to File, Orleans Parish District Attorney, 1966.

Keith, Don Lee, "Ochsner: the Surgeon, the Man, the Institution," *Times-Picayune*, June 3, 1973, s. 2, p. 8.

Keith, Don Lee, "A Matter of Motives", *Gambit*, August 3, 1993.

Knight, David C., *Viruses: Life's Smallest Enemies* (New York: William Morrow and Company, 1981).

Lapin, B.A., et al., "Use of Non-Human Primates in Medical Research, Especially in the Study of Cardiovascular Pathology and Oncology," *Some Recent Developments in Comparative Medicine* (London: Academic Press, 1966).

Lednicky, J. A., et al., "Natural Simian Virus 40 strains are present in human choriod plexus and ependymoma tumors," *Virology*, October 1, 1995, p. 710.

Leibowitch, Jacques, *A Strange Virus of Unknown Origin* (New York: Ballatine, 1985).

Lemonick, Michael D., "A Deadly Virus Escapes," *Time*, September 5, 1994, p. 63.

MacPherson, Karen, "America's Atomic Fallout," *Albuquerque Tribune*, September 29, 1994, p. A1.

Mann, Jonathan, et al., "The International Epidemiology of AIDS," *The Science of AIDS* (New York: Freeman, 1989).

Marks, John, *The Search for the Manchurian Candidate* (New York: McGraw-Hill, 1980).

Marshall, Eliot, "Breast Cancer: Stalemate in the War on Cancer," *Science*, December 20, 1991, p. 1719.

Martin, W. John, "Foreword," *Emerging Viruses* by Horowitz.

Martin, W. John, "SV-40 Contamination of Poliovirus Vaccine," Center for Complex Infectious Diseases, www.ccid.org, California, 1997.

McNeill, William Hardy, *Plagues and Peoples*, (Garden City, NY: Anchor Press, 1976).

Miller, Leslie, "Boomers' cancer risk tops grandparents," *USA Today*, April 9, 1994, p. 1.

Morrow, Robert D., *First Hand Knowledge* (New York: Shapolsky, 1992).

Munroe, Spencer, "Viral Oncogenesis in the Rhesus Monkey," *Some Recent Developments in Comparative Medicine*, edited by Fiennes (London: Academic Press, 1966).

Munroe, J.S. & W.F. Windle, "Tumors induced in Primates by a Chicken Sarcoma Virus (1963)," *Science*, Vol. 140, p. 1415.

Myers, Gerald, Genetic Sequence Database, Los Alamos National Laboratory, correspondence with author, May 31, 1993.

New Orleans Police Department, Reports on Murder of Sherman, Mary S., July 21, 1964, Item # G-12994-64, Louisiana Collection, New Orleans Public Library, New Orleans, Louisiana (1964).

*New Orleans Item*, March 25, 1946, reported Dr. Ochsner received a War Department citation for his patriotic service in connection with medical research.

*New Orleans States-Item*, "Dr. Ochsner Outlines Anti-Red Tape Activity," April 16, 1963, p. 33.

*New Orleans States-Item*, various articles on Mary S. Sherman, July 21 to August 15, 1964.

*Newsweek*, "Human Guinea Pigs Injected With Plutonium," December 12, 1993, cover.

Pass, H, R. Kennedy and M. Carbone, "Evidence for and implications of SV40-like sequences in human mesotheliomas," *Important Advances in Oncology: 1996*, edited by DeVita, Hellman, and Rosenberg (Philadelphia, Lippincott-Raven Publishers).

Piel, Jonathan, "Foreword," *The Science of AIDS* (New York: W.H. Freeman and Company, 1989).

Pope, John, "Crusading pioneer Surgeon Alton Ochsner is dead at 85," *Times-Picayune/States-Item*, September 25, 1981, s. 1, p. 1.

Posner, Gerald, *Case Closed* (New York: Random House, 1993)

Posner, Martin, "Study of the... Reaction in the Coulomb Stripping Energy Region", *Phys. Rev.* 158, 1018 - 1026 (1967) [Issue 4 – June 1967], American Physical Society, 1967. See American Scientific Directory, 1990.

Powell, Rosemary, "Scene of Slaying Reveals Interrupted Busy Routine," *New Orleans States-Item*, July 21, 1964, p. 1.

*Probe*, the newsletter of Citizens for the Truth about the Kennedy Assassination, "License & Registration Please," June 1994, p. 5, and July 1994, p. 1.

*Research Centers Directory*, Vol. 1, s.v. "Yerkes Regional Primate Research Center," (1995).

Ries, L.A.G., et al., *Cancer Statistics Review 1973-88*, National Cancer Institute, NIH Pub. No. 91-2789 (1991).

Riopelle, A. and J.F. Molloy, "Infectious Hepatitis at Yerkes Laboratories of Primate Biology," *Laboratory Primate Newsletter*, Vol. 1-4 (1962), p. 12.

Roberts, John, M.D., surgeon and president of the Medical Legal Foundation, interviews with author, October 3, 1994 and November 11, 1994.

Ruch, T.C., *Diseases of Laboratory Primates* (Philadelphia: W.B. Saunders, 1959).

Russell, Dick, *The Man Who Knew Too Much* (New York: Carroll & Graf, 1992).

*The Science of AIDS: A Scientific American Reader* (New York: W.H. Freeman and Company, 1989).

Sherman, Mary S., "Giant Cell Tumor of Bone," *Tumors of Bone and Soft Tissue* (Chicago: Year Book Medical Publishers, 1964); "Histogenesis of Bone Tumors," *Tumors of Bone and Soft Tissue* (Chicago: Year Book Medical Publishers, 1964);

Shilts, Randy, *And the Band Played On: Politics, People, and the AIDS Epidemic* (New York: St. Martin's Press, 1987).

Shorter, Edward, *The Health Century* (New York: Doubleday, 1987).

Sobel, Lester, *Three Assassinations: A Summary of the House Select Committee on Assassinations* (New York: Facts on File, 1978).

Southern Research Company, Inc., "Background Investigation on David William Ferrie," New Orleans, Louisiana, January 31, 1963, March 3, 1963, and August 12, 1963.

State of Louisiana, Orleans Parish Coroner's Office, "Autopsy Protocol on Mary Sherman," July 21, 1964, Louisiana Collection, New Orleans Public Library, New Orleans, Louisiana (1964).

State of Louisiana, Probate Records, Mary S. Sherman, "Receipt for Special Bequest - Medical Records," New Orleans, Louisiana, (1965).

Summers, Anthony and Robbyn, "The Ghosts of November," *Vanity Fair*, December 1994, p. 110.

Tarleton, Kermit, "Clues Lacking in Killing of Dr. Sherman," *New Orleans States-Item*, July 21, 1964, p. 1.

Teas, Jane, "Could AIDS agent be a variant on African Swine Fever Virus?," *Lancet*, 8330, April 23, 1983, p. 923.

Thomas, Evan, "Sins of a Paranoid Age," *Newsweek*, December 12, 1993, p. 20.

Thomas, Lewis, "Epilogue," *The Science of AIDS* (New York: Freeman, 1989).

*Time*, "The New War on Cancer via Virus Research and Chemotherapy," July 27, 1959, cover story.

*Time*, "Jolly Green Giant in Wonderland," August 2, 1968, p. 56.

*Times-Picayune*, various articles on Mary S. Sherman, July 21 to August 15, 1964.

Tulane University Medical Center, Press Release: "Tulane Researchers Discover Second Pathway to AIDS Infection," June 23, 1990.

Tulane University Medical Center, Press Release: "Tulane Scientists Discover New Virus," November 22, 1990.

U.S. Congress, House Select Committee on Assassins, "Ferrie's Cancer Treatise," Collection # RG 233, National Archive, Washington, D.C.

U.S. Congress, Senate Select Committee on Intelligence, "Project MKULTRA, the CIA's Program of Research in Behavior Modification, August 3, 1977," U.S. Government Printing Office, Washington, D.C.

U.S. Federal Bureau of Investigation, "Edward William Alton Ochsner," Freedom of Information Act, FOIPA No. 329,965, September 18,1992. On file at Loyola Library Archives, Loyola University, New Orleans, Louisiana, 70118.

Waldholz, Michael, "Reason for Hope," *Wall Street Journal*, March 16, 1995, p. A1.

Watson, Russell, et al., "America's Nuclear Secrets," *Newsweek*, December 27, 1993, p. 15.

Wechsler, Pat, "Shot in the Dark," *New York Magazine*, November, 1996.

Welsome, Eileen, "The Plutonium Experiments," *Albuquerque Tribune*, November 15, 1993, p. A1.

Wilds, John, and Ira Harkey, *Alton Ochsner: Surgeon of the South* (Baton Rouge, Louisiana: LSU Press, 1990).

*Who Was Who in America*, Vol. III, s.v. Yerkes, Robert Mearns.

Willits, Stacy, "Escapees Swinging Through Trees," *Times-Picayune/ States-Item*, September 4, 1994, Metro News.

Willits, Stacy, "Primate Center Back in Spotlight," *Times-Picayune*, September 8, 1994, p. B-1.

Zupko, Andrew, "The Origin of AIDS," *Health Freedom News*, 1989, p. 23.

# INDEX

Maison Blanche building 150, 161
Manchester, John 57
Manson, Charles 68
Marcello, Carlos x, 45, 92, 104, 105, 113, 300, 301, 306, 307, 316-321, 330-332, 341-345
March of Dimes 202
Mardi Gras 46, 51, 142
Marrs, Jim vi, viii, xi, 287
Martin, Jack 102, 103, 105, 112, 216, 225, 277, 281
*Mary, Ferrie & the Monkey Virus* xi, 6, 244, 266, 283, 290, 370
Matas, Robert 172
Mayo, William J. 170
Maytag, Bud 186
McClelland, Laurella 208
*Men Who Killed Kennedy, The* 7, 306, 328, 331
Middle American Research Institute 81, 82
Miguel 79, 80, 89, 109, 111, 112
*Mind of the Gorilla, The* 28
MKULTRA 31, 37, 190
Monaghan, William I. 293, 294, 306, 324, 329
monkey viruses 1-7, 14, 17, 18, 20, 22, 34, 46-49, 76, 77, 106, 138, 207, 208, 216, 218, 219, 222-225, 241, 264, 270, 277-279, 284, 289, 297, 301, 303-305, 307, 309-313, 315, 322, 325, 335
Moore, George 316
Moran, Sam 121, 129
Morrow, Robert 100, 113
"Mr. Y" 247-253, 256, 266, 271

"Mr. Z" 256-258
Murchison, Clint 180, 181
Murret, Charles "Dutz" x

# N

*Naked and the Dead, The* 61
NASA 37, 180
*Nashville Banner* 188
National Airline 186
National Banks of Florida 186
National Cancer Institute (NCI) 5, 26, 187, 200, 206, 211, 212, 216, 217, 219, 221, 222, 225, 281, 313
National Institutes of Health (NIH) 25, 30, 187, 191, 200, 201, 203, 205-209, 216, 217, 219-221, 224, 225, 263-265, 271, 281
Nazis 54, 78, 79, 178, 286
New Leviathan Oriental Fox Trot Orchestra 71
Newman Building 147, 148, 149
New Mexico Agricultural College 205
New Orleans, LA iv-x, 1, 2, 5, 9, 11, 12, 14, 19, 23, 26, 28, 29, 33-41, 47, 48, 53-56, 60-65, 68, 73-88, 93, 96, 97, 101-108, 112, 113, 118-120, 125, 126, 133-139, 142, 144-148, 154,-161, 166, 167, 172-191, 194, 219-222, 232, 233, 244, 248-253, 256-259, 262, 265-271, 284-286, 290-307, 310, 311, 315, 316, 320, 321, 325, 329-331, 336, 339-345, 361-364, 371

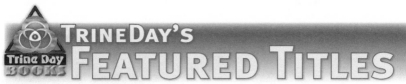

# TrineDay's Featured Titles

## The True Story of the Bilderberg Group
### BY DANIEL ESTULIN

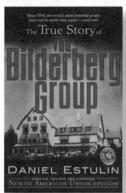

**More than a center of influence, the Bilderberg Group is a shadow world government, hatching plans of domination at annual meetings ... and under a cone of media silence.**

THE TRUE STORY OF THE BILDERBERG GROUP goes inside the secret meetings and sheds light on why a group of politicians, businessmen, bankers and other mighty individuals formed the world's most powerful society. As Benjamin Disraeli, one of England's greatest Prime Ministers, noted, "The world is governed by very different personages from what is imagined by those who are not behind the scenes."

Included are unpublished and never-before-seen photographs and other documentation of meetings, as this riveting account exposes the past, present and future plans of the Bilderberg elite.

Softcover: **$24.95** • ISBN: 9780979988622 • 432 pages • Size: 6 x 9

## THE 9/11 MYSTERY PLANE
### And the Vanishing of America
#### BY MARK GAFFNEY
#### FOREWORD BY DR. DAVID RAY GRIFFIN

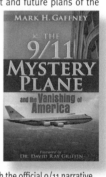

Unlike other accounts of the historic attacks on 9/11, this discussion surveys the role of the world's most advanced military command and control plane, the E-4B, in the day's events and proposes that the horrific incidents were the work of a covert operation staged within elements of the US military and the intelligence community. Presenting hard evidence, the account places the world's most advanced electronics platform circling over the White House at approximately the time of the Pentagon attack. The argument offers an analysis of the new evidence within the context of the events and shows that it is irreconcilable with the official 9/11 narrative.

Mark H. Gaffney is an environmentalist, a peace activist, a researcher, and the author of *Dimona, the Third Temple?*; and *Gnostic Secrets of the Naassenes*. He lives in Oregon.

Softcover • **$19.95** • ISBN 9780979988608 • 336 Pages • Size: 6 x 9

## The Oil Card
### Global Economic Warfare in the 21st Century
#### BY JAMES NORMAN

***Challenging the conventional wisdom surrounding high oil prices, this compelling argument sheds an entirely new light on free-market industry fundamentals.***

By deciphering past, present, and future geopolitical events, it makes the case that oil pricing and availability have a long history of being employed as economic weapons by the United States. Despite ample world supplies and reserves, high prices are now being used to try to rein in China—a reverse of the low-price strategy used in the 1980s to deprive the Soviets of hard currency. Far from conspiracy theory, the debate notes how the US has previously used the oil majors, the Saudis, and market intervention to move markets—and shows how this is happening again.

Softcover **$14.95** • ISBN 0977795390 • 288 PAGES • Size: 5.5 x 8.5

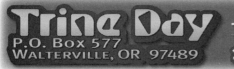

P.O. Box 577
WALTERVILLE, OR 97489

**ORDER BY ONLINE OR BY PHONE:**
**TrineDay.com**
**1-800-556-2012**

## The Franklin Scandal
### A Story of Powerbrokers, Child Abuse & Betrayal
BY NICK BRYANT

*A chilling exposé of corporate corruption and government cover-ups, this account of a nationwide child-trafficking and pedophilia ring tells a sordid tale of corruption in high places.* The scandal originally surfaced during an investigation into Omaha, Nebraska's failed Franklin Federal Credit Union and took the author beyond the Midwest and ultimately to Washington, DC. Implicating businessmen, senators, major media corporations, the CIA, and even the venerable Boys Town organization, this extensively researched report includes firsthand interviews with key witnesses and explores a controversy that has received scant media attention.

*The Franklin Scandal* is the story of a underground ring that pandered children to a cabal of the rich and powerful. The ring's pimps were a pair of Republican powerbrokers who used Boys Town as a pedophiliac reservoir, and had access to the highest levels of our government and connections to the CIA.

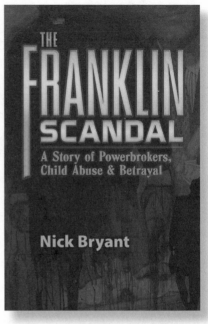

Nick Bryant is a journalist whose work largely focuses on the plight of disadvantaged children in the United States. His mainstream and investigative journalism has been featured in *Gear, Playboy, The Reader,* and on Salon.com. He is the coauthor of *America's Children: Triumph of Tragedy*. He lives in New York City.

Hardcover: **$24.95** • ISBN: 0977795357 • 676 pages • Size: 6x9

**ORDER BY ONLINE OR BY PHONE:**
**TrineDay.com**
**1-800-556-2012**

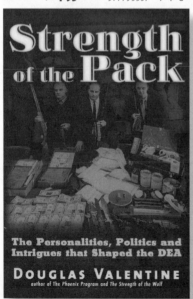

## Strength of the Pack
### The Personalities, Politics and Intrigues that Shaped the DEA
BY DOUG VALENTINE

*Through interviews with former narcotics agents, politicians, and bureaucrats, this exposé documents previously unknown aspects of the history of federal drug law enforcement from the formation of the Bureau of Narcotics and Dangerous Drugs and the creation of the Drug Enforcement Administration (DEA) up until the present day. Written in an easily accessible style, the narrative examines how successive administrations expanded federal drug law enforcement operations at home and abroad; investigates how the CIA comprised the war on drugs; analyzes the Reagan, Bush, and Clinton administrations' failed attempts to alter the DEA's course; and traces the agency's evolution into its final and current stage of "narco-terrorism."*

Douglas Valentine is a former private investigator and consultant and the author of *The Hotel Tacloban, The Phoenix Program, The Strength of the Wolf,* and *TDY*.

Softcover: **$24.95** • ISBN: 9780979988653 • 480 pages • Size: 6 x 9